MANIA

CLINICAL AND RESEARCH PERSPECTIVES

MANIA

CLINICAL AND RESEARCH PERSPECTIVES

Edited by
Paul J. Goodnick, M.D.

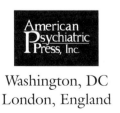

Washington, DC
London, England

Copyright © 1998 American Psychiatric Press, Inc.
ALL RIGHTS RESERVED
Manufactured in the United States of America on acid-free paper
First Edition   01   00   99   98   4   3   2   1
American Psychiatric Press, Inc.
1400 K Street, N.W., Washington, DC   20005
www.appi.org

Library of Congress Cataloging-in-Publication Data
Mania : clinical and research perspectives / edited by Paul J. Goodnick. — 1st ed.
    p.   cm.
    Includes bibliographical references and index.
    ISBN 0-88048-728-3
    1. Mania.   I. Goodnick, Paul J., 1950-
    [DNLM: 1. Manic Disorder.   WM 207 M2774 1997]
    RC516.M34   1998
    616.89'5—dc21
    DNLM/DLC
    for Library of Congress   97-2320
                                                                              CIP

British Library Cataloguing in Publication Data
A CIP record is available from the British Library.

DEDICATION

To my family, teachers, residents, and patients;
With thanks to God, who has given me the
health and strength for completion of this book.

CONTENTS

SECTION 1
DIAGNOSTIC CONSIDERATIONS

SECTION 2
BIOLOGY

SECTION 3
TREATMENT

CONTRIBUTORS

VIRGINIA M. V. BUKI, M.D.
Former Assistant Professor, Department of Psychiatry and
Behavioral Sciences, University of Miami School of Medicine,
Miami, Florida

ANN M. CALLAHAN, M.D.
Assistant Professor of Psychiatry, Mount Sinai School of Medicine,
and Director, Bipolar Research, Bronx Veterans Administration
Medical Center, Bronx, NY

TERESA CARREÑO, M.D.
Assistant Professor, Child and Adolescent Psychiatry, University of
Miami School of Medicine, Miami, Florida

M. BEATRIZ CURRIER, M.D.
Assistant Professor of Psychiatry, and Chief, Psychiatric
Consultation Service, Jackson Memorial Medical Center, Miami,
Florida

LORI L. DAVIS, M.D.
Staff Psychiatrist, Veterans Administration Medical Center, and
Assistant Professor, Department of Psychiatry, University of Texas
Southwestern Medical School, Dallas, Texas

KIRK DENICOFF, M.D.
Clinical Associate, Biological Psychiatry Branch, National Institute
of Mental Health, Bethesda, Maryland

J. RAYMOND DEPAULO JR., M.D.
Professor and Director, Outpatient Psychiatry; Co-Director, Center
for Anxiety and Depression; and Vice-Chairman for Clinical
Services, University of Washington Medical Center, Seattle,
Washington

DAVID L. DUNNER, M.D.
Professor and Director, Outpatient Psychiatry; Co-Director, Center
for Anxiety and Depression; and Vice Chairman for Clinical
Services, Department of Psychiatry, University of Washington
Medical Center, Seattle, Washington

FRANCES R. FRANKENBURG, M.D.
Director, Clozapine Clinic, McLean Hospital, and Associate
Professor of Psychiatry, Harvard Medical School, Belmont,
Massachusetts

MARK S. GEORGE, M.D.
Director, Functional Neuroimaging Division, Psychiatry, and
Associate Professor of Psychiatry, Radiology, and Neurology,
Medical University of South Carolina, Charleston, South Carolina;
and Visiting Scientist, Biological Psychiatry Branch, National
Institute of Mental Health, Bethesda, Maryland

SAMUEL GERSHON, M.D.
Vice President for Research and Associate Vice Chancellor for
Research-Health Sciences, University of Pittsburgh, Pittsburgh,
Pennsylvania

PAUL J. GOODNICK, M.D.
Professor of Psychiatry and Behavioral Sciences and Director, Mood
Disorders Program, Department of Psychiatry and Behavioral
Sciences, University of Miami School of Medicine, Miami, Florida

DAVID S. JANOWSKY, M.D.
Professor of Psychiatry, University of North Carolina School of
Medicine, Chapel Hill, North Carolina

Richard C. Josiassen, Ph.D.
Associate Professor of Psychiatry, Allegheny University of Health
Sciences, and Director, Norristown State Hospital Clinical
Research Center, Philadelphia, Pennsylvania

Paul E. Keck Jr., M.D.
Associate Professor of Psychiatry and Co-Director, Biological
Psychiatry Program, University of Cincinnati, Cincinnati, Ohio

Terence A. Ketter, M.D., F.R.C.P.C.
Associate Professor of Psychiatry and Human Behavior, and Chief,
Bipolar Disorders Clinic, Stanford University School of Medicine,
Stanford, California

Tim A. Kimbrell, M.D.
Senior Staff Fellow, National Institute of Mental Health, Bethesda,
Maryland, and Research Fellow, Medical University of South
Carolina, Charleston, South Carolina

Gerald L. Kramer, B.A.
Research Biologist and Chief, Laboratory Operations, Department
of Psychiatry, Veterans Administration Medical Center, Dallas, Texas

Beny Lafer, M.D.
Neuroscience Fellow, Department of Psychiatry, Massachusetts
General Hospital, Boston, Massachusetts

Alan G. Mallinger, M.D.
Associate Professor of Psychiatry and Pharmacology, University of
Pittsburgh, and Director, Psychopharmacology of Mania and
Depression, Western Psychiatric Institute and Clinics, Pittsburgh,
Pennsylvania

Lauren B. Marangell, M.D.
Assistant Professor of Psychiatry; Director, Mood Disorders
Research; and Director, Adult Psychopharmacology, Baylor College
of Medicine, Houston, Texas

BARBARA J. MASON, PH.D.
Associate Professor and Director, Division of Substance Abuse,
Department of Psychiatry and Behavioral Sciences, University of
Miami, Miami, Florida

CHARLENE A. MCALPIN, R.N.
Former Faculty, Jackson Memorial Hospital School of Nursing,
Miami, Florida, and current Coordinator, Case Management,
University of Miami/Jackson Memorial Medical Center, Coral
Gables, Florida

SUSAN L. MCELROY, M.D.
Associate Professor of Psychiatry and Co-Director, Biological
Psychiatry Program, University of Cincinnati, Cincinnati, Ohio

CHAND NAIR, M.D.
Senior Research Fellow, Allegheny University/Norristown State
Hospital Clinical Research Center, Philadelphia, Pennsylvania

DAVID H. OVERSTREET, PH.D.
Associate Professor of Research Psychiatry, University of North
Carolina School of Medicine, Chapel Hill, North Carolina

RAYMOND L. OWNBY, M.D., PH.D.
Associate Professor of Clinical Psychiatry, University of Miami
School of Medicine, and director, Wien Center for Alzheimer's
Disease and Memory Disorders, Miami, Florida

PEGGY J. PAZZAGLIA, M.D.
Assistant Professor of Psychiatry and Human Behavior, University
of Mississippi Medical Center, Jackson, Mississippi

FREDERICK PETTY, M.D., PH.D.
Medical Director, Mental Health Clinic, Veterans Administration
Medical Center, and Professor of Psychiatry, University of Texas
Southwestern Medical School, Dallas, Texas

ROBERT M. POST, M.D.
Chief, Biological Psychiatry Branch, National Institute of Mental
Health, Bethesda, Maryland

GARY SACHS, M.D.
Assistant Professor and Director, Harvard Bipolar Research
Program, Harvard Medical School, Boston, Massaschusetts

RITA A. SHAUGHNESSY, PH.D., M.D.
Assistant Professor of Psychiatry, Allegheny University of Health
Sciences, Philadelphia, Pennsylvania

SYLVIA G. SIMPSON, M.D.
Associate Professor of Psychiatry, Johns Hopkins School of
Medicine, Baltimore, Maryland

SCOTT A. WEST, M.D.
Co-Director, Psychopharmacology Research Program, Psychiatric
Institutes of Florida, Maitland, Florida

MARY C. ZANARINI, ED.D.
Director, Laboratory for Study of Adult Development, and
Assistant Professor of Psychology in Psychiatry, Harvard Medical
School, McLean Hospital, Belmont, Massachusetts

ACKNOWLEDGMENTS

I would like to thank the administrative staff of the University of Miami School of Medicine, Department of Psychiatry, in general, but particularly Cheryl Clemence, for her assistance in the preparation of this manuscript. The suggestions and cooperation of the APPI staff, especially Pamela Harley, were greatly appreciated.

INTRODUCTION

Paul J. Goodnick, M.D.

A lthough mania as an entity has been well known for centu- ries, Kraepelin's description of "manic depressive insanity" in 1895 (Kraepelin 1895/1921) laid the foundation for the current conceptions of the disorder. Kraepelin separated *mania* from *dementia praecox,* known today as *schizophrenia,* and suggested that the criteria for mania include euphoria, irritability, increased activity, distractibility, and so on. However, because psychosis remained an often associated symptom, psychotic mania and schizophrenia were often confused. In particular, this confusion was evident in the fa- mous United States/United Kingdom study in which the same clini- cal pictures were described as schizophrenia by Americans and manic-depressive by the British. Because of both the emergence of lithium in the 1960s as an effective treatment for mania (Johnson 1984) and the identification of the disorder in noteworthy per- sons, somewhat lessening the associated stigma (Fieve 1975), manic- depression became a better-recognized entity. Clinicians in the United States began to look for means to define the disorder more clearly and to choose appropriate patients for lithium therapy (Feigh- ner et al. 1972; Spitzer et al. 1978).

At that time, because of steadily growing assumptions, Belmaker and van Praag (1980) developed and published their edited text *Ma- nia: An Evolving Concept.* The book, a painstaking review of various germane aspects of diagnosis, genetics, biochemistry, and social as- pects, was a major advance for the time. Of particular importance, it emphasized that: 1) the prognosis of mania was not uniformly "excellent," 2) the chromosomal transfer of manic-depression (bipolar disorder) by X-linkage was not proven, and 3) response to lithium did not prove that a patient was "manic" by circular reasoning. With a review of the existing knowledge about catecholamines, serotonin, and γ-aminobutyric acid (GABA), the text attempted to put the different biochemical theories on etiology into perspective.

From 1980 to 1990, many new research techniques became available, including platelet measures of serotonin uptake and imipramine binding, linkage mapping possibilities, and positron-emission tomography (PET). It also became more obvious that after the initial hope that lithium would "cure" all bipolar illness, many patients did not respond to this agent. Thus, in the ensuing decade, more research results became available on the use of other agents, particularly the anticonvulsants. It was within this period that Goodwin and Jamison published the important *Manic-Depressive Illness* in 1990, which remains the most exhaustive review of knowledge on mania and bipolar and unipolar depression. This five-part reference text—consisting of clinical description and diagnosis, clinical studies, psychological studies, pathophysiology, and treatment—enlightens the reader through the necessary three perspectives of their historical background, the present state of information (as of 1990), and a look at the future. This text even provides the novice with the background required to understand the scientific literature by including a section on scales that are used to assess mania and depression. Many of my current patients, in fact, have read significant sections of this publication.

Even in the relatively short time since Goodwin and Jamison's text, there have been a number of significant advances in the knowledge of and therapy for mania/bipolar disorder. This current text is not intended to be exhaustive (as was the Goodwin and Jamison text); rather, it is designed to point out important, and I hope clinically relevant, additions in the past number of years in a smaller, easy-to-read format. This book has been put together by many of those researchers and clinicians who have played key roles in attaining our current level of understanding.

In the broadest context, this book may be divided into three subareas: diagnostic considerations (Chapters 1–5), biological aspects

(Chapters 6–11), and treatment (Chapters 12–17); these subareas are then followed by a summary (Chapter 18). In Chapter 1, Dr. David L. Dunner begins logically with diagnosis. He focuses on factors that were faced by the American Psychiatric Association Task Force for the discussion of bipolar disorder in DSM-IV (American Psychiatric Association 1994): bipolar II, duration of mania, and rapid cycling. In Chapter 2, Dr. Teresa Carreño and I look at creativity and the currently available literature from a historical perspective, along with the rates of symptoms among "creative" individuals and creativity in patients. We conclude with contemporary paradigms of an association of creativity with mood swing. In Chapter 3, Drs. Gary Sachs and Beny Lafer then look at aspects of appropriate diagnosis and differentiation in children and adolescents. Because alcohol can both induce mood swing and be used as "legal" self-therapy for bipolar disorder, it is important to understand how these two areas relate. In Chapter 4, Drs. Barbara J. Mason and Raymond L. Ownby take on the task of helping the reader differentiate mood swing from bipolar disorder. In the last chapter of diagnostic considerations, Chapter 5, Drs. Sylvia G. Simpson and J. Raymond DePaulo attempt to update knowledge concerning the questions: Did I get this illness from my parents, and will I pass it on to my children? Drs. Simpson and DePaulo provide the reader with an understanding of generational changes and the current information on inheritance and linkage of this disorder by reviewing the current state of knowledge on family, segregation, and linkage studies.

The following six chapters focus on the next area, the state of biological knowledge: four regarding biochemistry and two regarding other biological techniques. In Chapter 6, I attempt to review our current state of knowledge on various measures of serotonin function with a focus on the "permissive hypothesis" of bipolar disorder from older studies on cerebrospinal concentrations and more recent neuroendocrine and postmortem results. Where relevant, the application of this hypothesis to the treatment of mania is presented (i.e., the use of serotonin precursors and lithium). This discussion is followed by an examination of the more complex picture of catecholamines in Chapter 7. Dr. Virginia M. V. Buki and I attempt to look at individual symptoms (e.g., agitation, as a biochemical point of its own) in addition to the diagnosis of mania as a single entity. The possible role of cholinomimetics in the induction of mania is discussed by Drs. David S. Janowsky and David H. Overstreet in Chapter 8. The opposite and antagonistic effects of acetylcholine and catecholamine pathways as well as biological considerations, including sleep studies, round out the chapter. In Chapter 9, Dr. Frederick Petty and associates follow with a focus on GABA as a putative vulnerability factor in mania and bipolar disorder. This topic is discussed in the context of results of plasma GABA in studies of treatment of mania, including results from the latest valproate protocols. In Chapter 10, Dr. Richard C. Josiassen and associates follow with an update on the use of electrophysiology— for example, P300 waves and brain mapping (computerized electro-encephalogram [EEG]) in the diagnosis and therapy of bipolar disorder. Finally, in Chapter 11, Dr. Mark S. George and associates review the current state of imaging techniques (e.g., computed tomography), followed by a discussion of the knowledge of the state and trait of mania. They discuss the strategy of "imaging" mania by inducing manic-like symptoms in control subjects, as well as changes in imaging that have been found as a consequence of treatment for mania.

The final area consists of Chapters 12–17 and focuses on updating information regarding treatment of mania for the clinician. Given that lithium is the most well-established treatment for mania, Dr. Raymond L. Ownby and I begin in Chapter 12 by updating recent findings on relevant points for the use of lithium. These findings include an update on the true risk of lithium in pregnant women and in neonates, on the relationship of lithium level effects produced by mood state and other factors, and more recent data on its mechanism of action as reflected from studies with inositol and G protein. The application of the con-ventional popular treatment alternatives to lithium—the anticonvul-sants carbamazepine and valproate—to bipolar disorder are reviewed, respectively, by Dr. Terence A. Ketter and associates in Chapter 13, and by Dr. Scott A. West and associates in Chapter 14. Each unit carefully presents information on their use in acute mania and prophy-laxis, pharmacology and pharmacokinetics, and drug interactions. Drs. Frances R. Frankenburg and Mary C. Zanarini and I follow in Chapter 15 with a view of antipsychotics, focusing on the newer atypi-cal alternatives not available in 1990: clozapine and risperidone. This original approach to treatment of mania was discontinued (mostly because of the risk of tardive dyskinesia) when lithium first became an established treatment. However, the "atypicals" are now reasonable options because of limited risk of induction of both tardive dyskinesia and extrapyramidal symptoms. In Chapter 16, Dr. M. Beatriz Currier and I focus on results of a group of agents that have been gradually gaining supporting evidence since the early 1980s: the calcium-channel inhibitors or calcium antagonists. Another alternative that appears to have less risk and require less blood monitoring than both lithium and the anticonvulsants, this group of medications (particularly verapamil) may be particularly useful for patients who are unwilling or unable to tolerate the side effects or process of alternative treatments. The most recent evidence points to the possibility that another agent of this class, nimodipine, may become useful for patients with very rapid or ultra-rapid mood cycling. Finally, in Chapter 17, Ms. Charlene A. McAlpin and I present an updated review for the use of psychotherapy with bipolar patients. In this chapter, we focus on both theoretical concepts and results from studies conducted on individual, group, and milieu therapies as well as a consideration of patient compliance to therapy.

In the final summary, Chapter 18, Drs. Alan G. Mallinger and Samuel Gershon provide a brief historical perspective and follow with directions for future research. These authors also look at explanations for lithium's therapeutic benefit, membrane cell studies in bipolar patients, and implications for use of the calcium antagonist therapies.

Thus, the rationale for this text is to set the backdrop for current information with brief considerations of established knowledge in the etiology and therapy of mania. At the same time, the content is intended to bring into focus a look into the future (treatments that were little known at the time of the Goodwin and Jamison 1990 text) of 1) diagnosis, 2) vulnerability information in genetics, 3) biology (in particular, brain imaging), 3) biological theory (e.g., GABA data), and 4) treatment (valproate, atypical antipsychotics, and calcium-channel blockers). It is hoped that this text will complement Goodwin and Jamison's 1990 book by providing for the general clinician as well as the academician an understandable and briefly readable account of the status of basic and applied research in mania with a guiding path toward future research and development.

▶ REFERENCES

American Psychiatric Association: Diagnostic and Statistical Manual of Mental Disorders, 4th Edition. Washington, DC, American Psychiatric Association, 1994

Belmaker RH, van Praag HM: Mania: An Evolving Concept. New York, SP Medical & Scientific Books, 1980

Feighner JP, Robins E, Guze SB, et al: Diagnostic criteria for use in psychiatric research. Arch Gen Psychiatry 26:57–62, 1972

Fieve RR: Moodswing: The Third Revolution in Psychiatry. New York, William Morrow, 1975

Goodwin FK, Jamison KR: Manic-Depressive Illness. New York, Oxford University Press, 1990

Johnson FN: The History of Lithium Therapy. Macmillan, London, 1984

Kraepelin E: Manic-Depressive Insanity and Paranoia (1895). Translated by RM Barclay, edited by Robertson GM. Edinburgh, Scotland, E & S Livingstone, 1921. (Reprinted, New York, Arno Press, 1976)

Spitzer RL, Endicott J, Robins E: Research Diagnostic Criteria. New York, Biometric Research, New York State Psychiatric Institute, 1978

SECTION

1

Diagnostic Considerations

CHAPTER 1

DIAGNOSTIC REVISIONS FOR DSM-IV

David L. Dunner, M.D.

I n this chapter I review the diagnostic revisions proposed for DSM-IV (American Psychiatric Association 1994) in the area of bipolar mood disorders. DSM-III (American Psychiatric Association 1980) was a major advance in developing a diagnostic system for American psychiatrists. DSM-III was a symptom-based diagnostic system that resulted in a narrowing of the diagnosis of schizophrenia and a broadening of the diagnosis of affective disorders, particularly bipolar affective disorders. Furthermore, with DSM-III, the diagnostic interrater reliability among clinicians increased as compared with earlier classifications.

Before DSM-III, studies had shown a higher rate of patients diagnosed as having schizophrenia and a lower rate of patients diagnosed as having affective disorders among American psychiatrists as compared with their British counterparts (Cooper et al. 1972). The development of lithium as a treatment for mania was perhaps instrumental in realigning the American diagnostic system more toward the European system. DSM-III, based largely on the Washington University criteria for psychiatric diagnosis (Feighner et al. 1972), provided the framework for a symptom-based diagnosis. If affective symptoms were present, DSM-III forced a clinician toward a diagnosis of affective disorders.

In DSM-III, the bipolar mood disorders included bipolar disorder, cyclothymic disorder, and atypical bipolar disorder. Bipolar disorder required a week or more of manic symptoms or hospitalization. Atypical bipolar disorder included all bipolar disorders that did not specifically meet diagnostic criteria and particularly included patients who were described as bipolar II (those who had depression and hypomania). Bipolar disorder was meant to reflect bipolar I (patients who had severe mania) (Dunner et al. 1976b).

In DSM-III-R (American Psychiatric Association 1987), the mood disorder definitions were slightly modified. The bipolar mood disorders included bipolar disorder, cyclothymia, and bipolar disorder not otherwise specified (also including bipolar II), and the duration criterion for a manic episode was deleted.

One of the problems that faced the Work Group on Mood Disorders for DSM-IV was reviewing the disorders in DSM-III-R to determine whether there were data to support revisions in the nomenclature, particularly revisions that might correlate with clinical outcome or treatment. Two aspects not included in DSM-III or DSM-III-R were rapid cycling bipolar disorder and bipolar II as a separate disorder. In discussing the inclusion of rapid cycling into DSM-III-R with Dr. Spitzer, who was head of the DSM-III-R Task Force, we noted that some rapid cycling patients had depressions that lasted less than 2 weeks and manic or hypomanic episodes that were of brief duration (Dunner and Fieve 1974). Indeed, 48-hour cycling patients had been reported in the literature (Bunney et al. 1965; Jenner et al. 1967). It was because such patients would not meet criteria for "major depression" that rapid cycling was excluded from DSM-III-R. It is not clear why bipolar II was excluded from DSM-III or DSM-III-R because there was considerable literature regarding bipolar II and the separation of such patients from other types of depression, including both unipolar and bipolar I affective disorders (Dunner 1983; Fieve and Dunner 1975).

The Work Group on Mood Disorders for DSM-IV reviewed available literature and agreed that changes would not be recommended in the absence of data, at least at the Work Group level. This process involved reports from the Work Group to the DSM-IV Task Force and final decisions made at the Task Force level. ICD-10 (World Health Organization 1992) was developed parallel to DSM-IV. Unfortunately, some conditions noted in ICD-10 are based on insufficient data and therefore do not merit inclusion in DSM-IV.

The major areas of concern regarding bipolar disorders resulted in a review of the evidence for inclusion of bipolar II as a separate disorder (Dunner 1993), review of rapid cycling (Bauer and Whybrow 1993), and clarification of rapid cycling. In dropping the duration criteria for mania in DSM-III-R, some confusion existed in the literature between rapid cycling, cyclothymia, and bipolar mixed type.

▶ Bipolar II

The review of bipolar II revealed a considerable body of data from multiple centers supporting the separation of patients with depression and hypomania from patients with mania (bipolar I) and from patients with depression only. These data were summarized and reviewed (Dunner 1993). The data supported the separation of bipolar II using clinical, family history, course and outcome data, and biological factors. The strongest data for the separation for bipolar II were three family studies that indicated that relatives of bipolar II patients had the highest morbid risks for bipolar II as compared with relatives of unipolar or bipolar I patients (Coryell et al. 1985; Fieve et al. 1984; Gershon et al. 1982).

In terms of defining the syndrome, the initial definition proposed by Dunner et al. (1976b) had posited a 3-day or longer duration of hypomania. This definition was based on a study of "normal" women who were being assessed for a premenstrual mood disturbance and who on interview were sometimes found to have 1–2 days of hypomanic symptoms. Because 1–2 days of hypomania could occur in "normal" women, the proposed minimal criteria for the duration of hypomania for bipolar II patients became 3 days or more. There were no data to support the minimal duration criteria for hypomania, and the ICD-10 group had arbitrarily chosen 4 days or more as minimal criteria. The Work Group opted for that definition in order to be consistent.

The other side of the duration question was the duration of depression. In this instance, the duration of depression of 2 weeks or more was adopted (i.e., the minimal duration of major depression). Thus to have a bipolar II condition, one must have at least 4 days of hypomanic symptoms and 2 weeks of depression.

There was a sense from the Task Force that bipolar conditions should not be overdiagnosed in the community; if they are, lithium might be too broadly applied to patients with mood disorders. This is an interesting opinion because there are several studies supporting the use of lithium as a maintenance treatment for recurrent unipolar depression, although not all studies agree (Fieve et al. 1976; Prien et al. 1984; Schou 1979). The criteria for bipolar II were defined in a way that is somewhat restrictive. The period of hypomanic symptoms was required to be noted by others as different from the "normal" self. Furthermore, hypomanic episodes occurring in response to treatment with antidepressant pharmacotherapy would not count toward the diagnosis of bipolar II but would instead be termed *substance-induced hypomania*. Frankly, this latter option makes little sense to me and is inconsistent with the natural course of bipolar disorder. Many patients with bipolar disorder have depression followed by hypomania (Dunner et al. 1976a). The fact that they are treated for depression and become hypomanic does not necessarily mean that the hypomania was induced by the medication at all—it might have happened anyway. In reviewing treatment outcome data for unipolar depression, the package inserts for several of the available antidepressants indicate that treatment-emergent hypomania among patients with major depression (who were presumably screened for bipolar disorder) is about 1%. This low rate likely represents a rate of misdiagnosis of bipolar II in such patients. The point is, it is difficult to induce mania and hypomania in a true unipolar patient; there is a likelihood that patients who develop hypomania in response to treatment are actually bipolar.

Rather than including bipolar disorder as an entity that could be separately coded out for severity of episodes, bipolar II disorder will be coded in such a way that the severity and course criteria are not easily demarcated. For example, for major depression and bipolar I disorder, there are sufficient coding numbers for one to include a reference indicating that the most recent episode was manic or depressed and that the current status is mild, moderate, or severe. The coding of the current mood status will not be easily effected with the proposed coding for bipolar II disorder (296.89). Parenthetical modifiers (with melancholia, with atypical features, with seasonal pattern, with rapid cycling) can be applied to bipolar II.

▌ Duration of Mania

The deletion of duration criteria for mania from DSM-III-R (as compared with DSM-III) was felt to be a problem. Therefore, in DSM-IV, duration criteria for a manic episode were reinstated as 1 week or more or requiring hospitalization.

▌ Rapid Cycling

Once the duration criteria were established for mania and hypomania (and depression), the issue of rapid cycling became relatively easy. The review of rapid cycling conditions indicated that rapid cycling was an important feature of bipolar disorder as a type of course that reflected poor response to maintenance treatment, particularly with lithium carbonate (Bauer and Whybrow 1993). Awareness of rapid cycling would alert the clinician to the difficulty of treating such patients. The Work Group on Mood Disorders decided on a minimal criterion of 4 days for hypomania and 2 weeks for depression, or 18 days for a cycle or no more than 20 cycles per year for a bipolar II rapid cycling pattern. For bipolar I patients with rapid cycling, 7 days or more of manic symptoms and 14 days or more of depressive symptoms were the proposed minimal duration criteria. The cycle frequencies would be in keeping with the early description of rapid cycling, which suggested that the number of patients decreased as the cycle frequency increased (Dunner and Fieve 1974; Dunner et al. 1977).

The minimal cycle frequency of four episodes per year as proposed by Dunner and Fieve (1974) was determined to be a reasonable criterion through a multisite data analysis (Bauer et al. 1994). Gender ratio among bipolar patients was studied in relation to cycle frequency. A higher percentage of rapid cyclers were women as compared with other bipolar patients, and the gender ratio increased toward women when the cycle frequency increased above three cycles per year; these data provided some validation of the minimal criterion of four episodes or more per year (Bauer et al. 1994).

The issue of patients who had briefer cycles or what might be termed *truncated episodes* is complicated, but such patients will be diagnosed as cyclothymic in DSM-IV if they have hypomanic episodes shorter than 4 days or depressive episodes shorter than 2 weeks.

▶ **CONCLUSION**

In summary, the Work Group on Mood Disorders reviewed the major components of bipolar disorders for DSM-IV. The changes made reflect the data regarding the conditions reviewed. The major proposals include establishment of duration criteria for manic episodes of bipolar I disorder, separation of bipolar II from bipolar I and disorders not otherwise specified (NOS), and adding rapid cycling as a parenthetical modifier to bipolar I and bipolar II disorders. Truncated rapid cycling is subsumed in cyclothymic disorder. One area that still requires further research is the definition of bipolar mixed. There is a small but growing database reflecting its differentiation from other more typical manic syndromes (Keller et al. 1986; Post et al. 1989).

▶ **REFERENCES**

American Psychiatric Association: Diagnostic and Statistical Manual of Mental Disorders, 3rd Edition. Washington, DC, American Psychiatric Association, 1980
American Psychiatric Association: Diagnostic and Statistical Manual of Mental Disorders, 3rd Edition, Revised. Washington, DC, American Psychiatric Association, 1987
American Psychiatric Association: Diagnostic and Statistical Manual of Mental Disorders, 4th Edition. Washington, DC, American Psychiatric Association, 1994
Bauer M, Whybrow P: Validity of rapid cycling as a modifier for bipolar disorder in DSM-IV. Depression 1:11–19, 1993
Bauer M, Calabrese J, Dunner DL, et al: Multisite data reanalysis: validity of rapid cycling as a modifier for bipolar disorder in DSM-IV. Am J Psychiatry 151:506–515, 1994
Bunney WE Jr, Hartman EL, Mason JW: Study of a patient with 48-hour manic-depressive cycles. Arch Gen Psychiatry 12:619–625, 1965
Cooper JE, Kendell RE, Gurland BJ, et al: Psychiatric Diagnosis in New York and London: A Comparison Study of Mental Hospital Admissions (Maudsley Monogr No 20). London, England, Oxford University Press, 1972

Coryell W, Endicott J, Andreasen N, et al: Bipolar I, bipolar II, and non-bipolar major depression among the relatives of affectively ill probands. Am J Psychiatry 142:817–821, 1985

Dunner DL: Subtypes of bipolar affective disorder with particular regard to bipolar II. Psychiatric Developments 1:75–86, 1983

Dunner DL: A review of the diagnostic status of "bipolar II" for the DSM-IV Work Group on Mood Disorders. Depression 1:2–10, 1993

Dunner DL, Fieve RR: Clinical factors in lithium carbonate prophylaxis failure. Arch Gen Psychiatry 30:229–233, 1974

Dunner DL, Fleiss JF, Fieve RR: The course of development of mania in patients with recurrent depression. Am J Psychiatry 133:905–908, 1976a

Dunner DL, Gershon ES, Goodwin FK: Heritable factors in the severity of affective illness. Biol Psychiatry 11:31–42, 1976b

Dunner DL, Patrick VJ, Fieve RR: Rapid cycling manic depressive patients. Compr Psychiatry 18:561–566, 1977

Feighner JP, Robins E, Guze SB, et al: Diagnostic criteria for use in psychiatric research. Arch Gen Psychiatry 26:57–63, 1972

Fieve RR, Dunner DL: Unipolar and bipolar affective states, in The Nature and Treatment of Depression. Edited by Flach FF, Draghi SC. New York, Wiley, 1975, pp 145–166

Fieve RR, Dunner DL, Kumbaraci T, et al: Lithium carbonate prophylaxis of depression in three subtypes of primary affective disorder. Pharmako Psychiatri Neuropsychopharmakologie 9:100–107, 1976

Fieve RR, Go R, Dunner DL, et al: Search for biological/genetic markers in a long-term epidemiological and morbid risk study of affective disorders. J Psychiatr Res 18:425–445, 1984

Gershon ES, Hamovit J, Guroff JJ, et al: A family study of schizoaffective, bipolar I, bipolar II, unipolar and normal control probands. Arch Gen Psychiatry 39:1157–1167, 1982

Jenner FA, Gjessing LR, Cox JR, et al: A manic-depressive psychotic with a persistent forty-eight hour cycle. Br J Psychiatry 113:895–910, 1967

Keller MB, Lavori PW, Coryell W, et al: Differential outcome of pure manic, mixed/cycling, and pure depressive episodes in patients with bipolar illness. JAMA 255:3138–3142, 1986

Post RM, Rubinow DR, Uhde TW, et al: Dysphoric mania: clinical and biological correlates. Arch Gen Psychiatry 46:353–358, 1989

Prien RF, Kupfer DJ, Mansky PA, et al: Drug therapy in the prevention of recurrences in unipolar and bipolar affective disorders: report of the NIMH Collaborative Study Group comparing lithium carbonate, imipramine, and a lithium carbonate-imipramine combination. Arch Gen Psychiatry 41:1096–1104, 1984

Schou M: Lithium as a prophylactic agent in unipolar affective illness: comparison with cyclic antidepressants. Arch Gen Psychiatry 36:849–851, 1979

World Health Organization: The ICD-10 Classification of Mental and Behavioural Disorders: Clinical Descriptions and Diagnostic Guidelines. Geneva, World Health Organization, 1992

CHAPTER 2

CREATIVITY AND
MOOD DISORDER

Teresa Carreño, M.D., and
Paul J. Goodnick, M.D.

I am the poet of the Body and I am the poet of the Soul,
The pleasures of heaven are with me and the pains of hell
are with me,
The first I graft and increase upon myself, the latter I trans-
late into a new tongue.

Walt Whitman, *Song of Myself*
(Mack et al. 1979)

To the sufferer, the pain of mood disorder is palpable and
deep. It throbs steadily through history, echoing in the
words of great poets such as Emily Dickinson, George Gordon (Lord Byron), and Victor Hugo; in the words of writers such
as Honoré de Balzac, Leo Tolstoy, Emile Zola, Maxim Gorky, and
Ernest Hemingway; in the music of great composers such as Schumann, Tchaikovsky, Beethoven (Hershman and Lieb 1988), and
Rachmaninoff; and in the art of Vincent van Gogh, Paul Gauguin,
Georgia O'Keeffe, and Michelangelo (Jamison 1993). Great world
leaders such as Alexander the Great, Napoleon Bonaparte, Abraham

Special thanks to Jon Shaw, M.D., for his guidance and to Ruth Richards, M.D.,
Ph.D., for the references by correspondence.

11

Lincoln, Winston Churchill, and Benito Mussolini, among many others, have also shared this pain (Goodwin and Jamison 1990; Jamison 1995).

In a partial list of great writers, artists, and composers with probable cyclothymia, major depression, or manic-depressive illness, Jamison (1993) listed 83 poets, 41 writers, 30 composers and musicians, and 41 artists of stature equivalent to those just mentioned here. She also listed approximately 16 great political, military, and religious leaders with probable mood disorders (Goodwin and Jamison 1990). Is it a coincidence that so many creative contributors to human expression and history share the common thread of mood disorder?

This association was recognized in the time of Aristotle, put aside for centuries, and rediscovered in the Renaissance and the romantic period (Goodwin and Jamison 1990; Hershman and Lieb 1988). The question of mood disorder possibly enhancing the creative state versus a chance association is the focus of renewed interest in this topic, at a time when scientific methodology has opened the doors to a systematic approach to finding the answer. This interest extends beyond the scientific community, having received media attention (Angier 1993; James 1994). In this chapter, the history of the age-old concept of the "mad genius" is revisited. Current studies supporting the association of mood disorders and creativity are reviewed, focusing on sharpened methodologies and research tools. Then, relevant treatment and theoretical issues are addressed. Finally, comments regarding the significance of the balance between the mood-altered state and the creative state in the talented individual with bipolar disorder are presented.

▶ HISTORY

In the time of Aristotle, the association of outstanding creativity in the arts and melancholia was documented (Goodwin and Jamison 1990; Jamison 1993). Plato felt that the poetry of sane men "is beaten all hollow by the poetry of madmen" (Hershman and Lieb 1988, p. 8). Socrates is quoted as saying that the poet has "no invention in him until he has been inspired and is out of his senses" (Hershman and Lieb 1988, p. 8). The Middle Ages closed the door to this association, but it reemerged in the Renaissance. Marsilio Ficino, a Renaissance philosopher, linked Aristotle's melancholic genius with Plato's mad poet, alluding to a manic-depressive genius (Hershman and Lieb 1988). In the Age of Reason, when reserve and moderation were perceived to be akin to genius, Diderot stated, "These reserved and melancholy men owe their extraordinary, almost godlike acuteness of insight to a temporary disturbance of their whole mechanism. One may notice how it brings them now to sublime and now to insane thoughts" (Hershman and Lieb 1988, p. 76). In the romantic period, reference to madness can be found in the works of great poets such as Emily Dickinson:

> Much Madness is divinest Sense—
> To a discerning Eye—
> Much Sense—the starkest Madness—
> 'Tis the Majority
> In this, as All, prevail—
> Assent—and you are sane—
> Demur—you're straightway dangerous—
> And handled with a Chain.—

> Emily Dickinson,
> "Much Madness is divinest Sense"
> (Mack et al. 1979)

This observation has sparked the curiosity of scientists of this modern age.

Review of the more recent scientific literature regarding this association begins with references to the work of Cesare Lombroso, who wrote about genius in 1864 (Andreasen and Canter 1974; Jamison 1993; Juda 1949; Myerson and Boyle 1941). He is reported to have believed that any deviation from the norm was degenerative, genius being at one end of the degenerative spectrum in which mental illness, crime, perversion, and mental retardation followed (Myerson and Boyle 1941).

With the birth of the study of psychiatry and psychology, a new perspective began to emerge. Lombroso's theory of polymorphism faded, and a more objective correlation of mental disease and great ability came under methodical scientific scrutiny (Myerson and Boyle

1941). As diagnostic criteria and research methods have become sharper, the relatively limited amount of research in this area has developed over time. With the introduction of lithium treatment for bipolar disorder by Cade in 1949 (Andreasen and Canter 1974; Benson 1975; Schou 1983) and reports of its possible ill effects on creativity (Kocsis et al. 1993; Marshall 1970; Schou 1979), another stratum of significance has been laid over this interesting question.

▶ RESEARCH

Are mood disorders and creativity associated? If so, might the latter be enhanced by the former? These seemingly simple questions have been difficult to approach from a research perspective. Studies testing the putative association of creativity and mental illness can be grouped into three categories: biographical studies, studies of creative individuals, and studies of the creative abilities of the mentally ill (Goodwin and Jamison 1990; Jamison 1993). A first logical step in conducting such research is to find a consensual definition for *creativity*, a seemingly elusive and ubiquitous human quality.

Biographical Studies

To bypass this requisite, biographical studies have focused on renowned figures such as Virginia Woolf (Bond 1985, 1986; Feinstein 1980), Vincent van Gogh (Destaing 1972; Jamison and Wyatt 1992; Monroe 1991; Ravin 1981), John Ruskin (Joseph 1969), Robert Fergusson (Rooney et al. 1977), Isaac Newton (Hershman and Lieb 1988; Lieb and Hershman 1983), Charles Meryon (Fama and Thompson 1973), Robert Schumann (Fromm-Reichmann 1990), and others whose creativity is undisputed. The biographies of many political leaders who have made contributions to human history, such as Oliver Cromwell (W. D. Henry 1975) and King George III of England (Roth 1967; Salzmann 1970), have also been reviewed for evidence of mood disorder. King George III is believed to have suffered from porphyria as well as manic-depressive illness. Using a retrospective historical design, researchers have attempted to find evidence of mental illness in these individuals and their families. The conclusions that can be drawn from such studies are necessarily limited because, with such a design, it is difficult to seek to disprove the hypothesis of an association. In fact, the researcher must actively work to prove it. What follows is an illustrative point from a biography of Ludwig van Beethoven.

This biographical sketch of the life of Ludwig van Beethoven is summarized from *The Key to Genius* (Hershman and Lieb 1988) as an illustration of the life of a creative individual who is reported to have suffered from bipolar disorder. Figure 2–1 and Figure 2–2 demonstrate his family tree, significant events occurring in his lifetime, and their correlation to possible mood symptoms. He was born in Bonn, Germany, on December 16, 1770, to an alcoholic father who was a violin teacher and a mother who was relatively stable emotionally. Beethoven's father began teaching him the violin at the age of 5 and was a strict disciplinarian. For example, when Beethoven was still a child, his father is reported to have come home at night while drunk and dragged his son out of bed to play the piano until morning, striking him when he made mistakes. During his latency and early adolescence, Beethoven held different jobs playing the piano and organ. His first composition was published at the age of 13. When he was 17 years old and visiting Vienna for the first time, he received news of his mother's death from tuberculosis. This event marks the time of Beethoven's first depressive episode. He remained in Bonn for 5 more years, supporting his father and brothers. At age 18, he began to suffer from auditory loss of high tones and mild tinnitus. In 1790, he moved to Vienna, the "mecca" of the music world at that time, where he remained for the rest of his life.

Beethoven is reported to have shown first evidence of progressive deafness in 1798 at age 28. At age 29, he suffered another bout of depression that lasted 2 years. During this time, his physician first recognized his excessive use of ethanol. In 1801, his mood shifted into a highly energized state. He wrote to a friend: "My physical strength has for some time past been steadily gaining and also my mental powers. . . . At my present rate of composing, I often produce 3 or 4 works at the same time" (Hershman and Lieb 1988, p. 76). It was in 1801 that Beethoven composed his first symphony. His work that year also included a string quartet (Opus 18, No. 6), the final

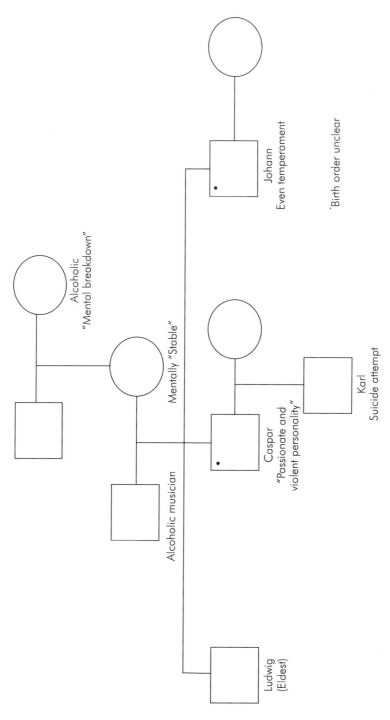

Figure 2–1. Family tree of Ludwig van Beethoven as extrapolated from Hershman and Lieb's 1988 biography. Focus is on mental health.

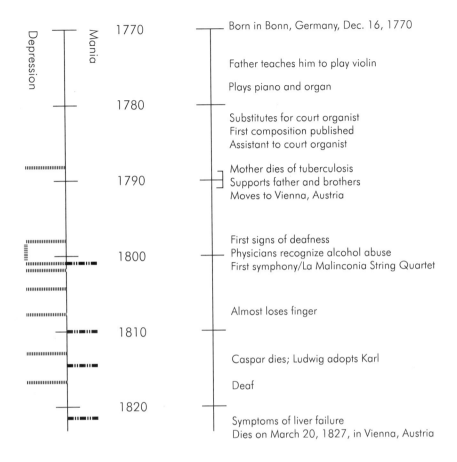

Figure 2–2. Significant events in Ludwig van Beethoven's life superimposed on his presumed manic and depressive episodes.

movement of which has been carefully studied for its fluctuations of mood (Caldwell 1972).

During his lifetime, Beethoven had at least five more depressive episodes (in addition to the two already mentioned). He possibly had one hypomanic episode in 1801, as described, and three episodes of mania. During his episodes of presumed mania, he is reported to have described an elated mood, compared himself to God, worked day and night on his compositions with little sleep, and suffered from paranoid delusions. He described his cyclicity of productivity: "In winter I do but little. I only elaborate and score what I have written during the summer. Yet even that consumes a great deal of time" (Hershman and Lieb 1988, p. 76). Some episodes of reported mood shift occurred at times of psychosocial stress (see Figure 2–2); however, this correlation does not appear to be without exception. Similarly, hypomanic mood states may have affected his comportment with women. Although he never married, it is reported that he was often passionately in love and always with aristocratic women. His social behavior was so inappropriate that it was found at times to be repulsive to his prospective romantic lady friends. His family history is significant for his maternal grandfather suffering from alcoholism and a "nervous breakdown," his alcoholic father, his sibling Caspar with a "passionate and violent personality," and his nephew Karl who attempted suicide.

Individuals like Beethoven who produce such outstanding and valuable creations share, in addition to talent, some strong environmental influences, which engender in them the motivation to create. The most powerful of these forces is found in early family experiences. When the feelings that family members verbally communicate are different from what they actually feel, children develop an ability to read subtle nonverbal cues to understand their environment. Creative individuals typically have at least one parent who is psychologically healthy. Also, in the early family environment of a creative individual, there is almost always one parent who has demonstrated interest but lack of success in a particularly creative field. With regard to Beethoven, his mother was psychologically healthy, but his father was a mediocre musician. He may then have striven "to fulfill a parent's implicit, unrealized yearnings" (Rothenberg 1990).

Individual biographies such as Beethoven's have been compiled in an attempt to answer questions about the relationship between psychopathology and creativity. To date, this relationship remains controversial, as illustrated by three recent studies.

In 1992, Ludwig published the results of an extensive biographical study of 1,005 individuals in an attempt to determine the relationship between creative activity and psychopathology. Each individual was classified according to profession, and Creative Achievement Scale scores and psychopathology ratings based on ICD-9 (World Health Organization 1978) were extrapolated from biographical data. Results indicated significant symptomatology in fiction writers, poets, and theater personnel as contrasted with others. When all "creative arts professions" (art, architecture/design, musical composition, musical performance, theater, expository writing, fiction writing, and poetry) were compared with 10 other professions, significantly higher rates and levels of psychopathology and treatment were noted in the artists. Total lifetime depression and anxiety scores were found to "significantly predict the level of creative achievement (across all professions)" (Ludwig 1992, p. 352), but further study was suggested.

In 1994, Post extracted data from the biographies of 291 world-famous men, searching for lifetime prevalence of various kinds of psychopathology in a variety of outstandingly creative individuals of different fields, using DSM-III-R (American Psychiatric Association 1987) criteria. Six series of subjects were studied posthumously: 48 visual artists, 50 scholars and thinkers, 45 scientists, 46 statesmen and national leaders, and 52 composers. Depressions (major depressive episodes, adjustment disorders, and depressions not otherwise specified [NOS]) were found to occur in 72% of novelists and playwrights. In this study, among mood disorders, only depressive disorders were found to have a higher prevalence than in the population at large. A high prevalence of psychic abnormalities, including character pathology, subjective personality problems, alcoholism, and depressions were found in prominent creative individuals (Post 1994).

In the same year, Schildkraut (1994) reported on the prevalence of psychopathology (focusing on mood disorders) among 15 abstract expressionist artists (12 of whom were deceased) of the New York School, who were considered masters of 20th century art. On evaluation of information collected from published biographies and archival material, a high prevalence of psychopathology based on DSM-III-R was found, with a predominance of depression and depressive spectrum disorders. In response to this publication, it was suggested that perhaps early years of relative failure and marked poverty might have contributed to the increased incidence of psychopathology (Corwin 1995). In contrast, Rothenberg (1995a) questioned the significance of 50% prevalence of affective illness in such a small sample.

Studies of Living Creative Individuals

A type of research design that allows more investigative freedom, still bypassing the requisite for a consensual definition of creativity, is the study of societally acclaimed living creative individuals who are often willing to participate actively in a prospective research design. Such studies date back to Ellis in 1926 (Andreasen and Glick 1988), who studied 1,020 creative and eminent people from different fields selected from the *British Dictionary of National Biography.* Ellis looked for prevalence of mental illness by the diagnostic criteria of his time, which limits the applicability of his work today.

Myerson and Boyle (1941) studied the incidence of manic-depressive psychosis that tended to occur in 20 socially important families as an argument against sterilization of psychotic manic-depressive individuals, which was apparently seriously debated in the World War II era. Juda (1949), from a prospective investigation of 19,000 persons (5,000 of whom were interviewed personally), found 294 individuals (113 artists, 181 scientists) to be highly gifted and creative; however, there was no criterion given for *creativity.* An increased rate of suicides was found among the artists, whereas an increased rate of major depressive illness occurred among the scientists.

The next three studies focused on families. Might creativity have an inherited component? Does it covary with mood disorders?

In 1971, McNeil studied the prevalence of mental illness in adoptees who either were nationally recognized for creativity or pursued creative occupations, their biological parents, and their adoptive parents. He found psychiatric illness present in 30% of the probands, 28% of the biological parents, and 5% of the adoptive parents. He found that approximately half of the illness was "reactive psychosis," which was later seen as affective disorder (Andreasen and Glick 1988).

Another study focused on women writers, looking at both familial basis and predictability of creativity and psychopathology. Ludwig (1994) administered a questionnaire based on DSM-III-R criteria to 59 writers and 59 control subjects matched for age, educational level, and father's occupational status. Results indicated that writers displayed higher rates of mental disorders, including depression (56% versus 14%, $P < .0000$), mania (19% versus 3%, $P < .01$), and panic attacks (22% versus 5%, $P < .01$). Rates of multiple disorders were higher in female writers (51%) than in the comparison group (14%). Parents of the writers were more likely to suffer from mental illness (20% versus 10%). A higher percentage of female writers reported sexual (24% versus 5%, $P < .004$) or physical (25% versus 7%, $P < .01$) abuse before age 13 than members of the comparison group.

In 1970, Karlsson reported on results that indicated that as compared with control subjects, the relatives of psychotic individuals were listed with more frequency in *Who's Who* in Iceland for "creative endeavors." His reference sources, aside from *Who's Who*, were three books on genealogy (individuals born from 1881 to 1910, totaling 3,793 persons) that generated three kindreds, and records of the Kleppur Mental Hospital. The proportion of his general population that were listed in *Who's Who* overall was 181/1,959 or 9.2% and "creative persons" was 13/1,959 or 0.7%. For manic-depressive persons, the rates were, respectively, 29/124 or 23.4% overall and 6/124 or 4.8% for "creative persons," a much higher rate. Thus, Karlsson focused on an association between giftedness and schizophrenia. It has since been observed that the data reveal an even stronger association between giftedness and mood disorder (Andreasen 1988; Andreasen and Canter 1974; George et al. 1988).

This observation followed the work of Andreasen and colleagues, who published three hallmark studies that focused on living creative writers at the University of Iowa Writer's Workshop (UIWW), an elite and nationally recognized creative writing program (Andreasen 1987; Andreasen and Canter 1974; Andreasen and Powers 1975). Fifteen writers from the UIWW and 15 control subjects matched for age, education, and sex were given structured diagnostic interviews pertaining to themselves and their family history. Results revealed a strong family history of psychiatric disorder: 21% in writer's relatives versus 4.4% in relatives of control subjects ($P < .01$). In particular, a significant increase was found in the prevalence of mood disorders in writers' relatives and in writers themselves: 67% in writers versus 13% in control subjects ($P < .02$).

The second study focused on specific cognitive aspects of creative individuals in comparison with bipolar and schizophrenic individuals (Andreasen and Powers 1975). Sixteen manic persons, 15 schizophrenic persons, and 15 writers from the UIWW were compared in terms of behavioral and conceptual overinclusion, idiosyncratic thinking, richness of thought, and underinclusiveness. They found that the writers as a group tended to resemble the manic persons in terms of behavioral and conceptual overinclusion. However, the manic subjects showed more idiosyncratic thought (bizarre associations), whereas the writers showed more richness of thought (imaginative recognition). Interestingly, of the 15 writers, 2 had suffered from manic episodes in the past, and 9 had described symptoms consistent with cyclothymia.

By 1987, Andreasen had expanded her group of writers to 30 and tested them for patterns of creativity, history of mental illness, and prevalence of these traits in first-degree relatives by structured interview. The criteria used for creativity were not listed. Intelligence was determined by the Wechsler Adult Intelligence Scale (Wechsler 1981) on 15 writers and 15 control subjects. Findings revealed a significantly increased incidence of mental illness, particularly bipolar disorder, in the writers and in their relatives when compared with control subjects and their relatives (writers versus control subjects with bipolar disorder: 43% versus 10%, $P < .01$; relatives of writers versus those of control subjects with any affective disorder: 18% versus 2%, $P < .001$). According to the structured interview, relatives of writers were significantly more creative than relatives of control subjects (53% versus 27%, $P < .01$). Intelligence quotients of writers and control subjects were comparable; hence, intelligence did not explain the difference in creativity between the two groups.

In 1989, Jamison published another landmark study of the association of creativity and affective disorder. Results showed that among 47 honored British writers and artists, 38% had been treated for affective illness. Further, during periods of intense creative activity, high rates (percentages are approximate) of elevated energy (75%), elevated speed of mental associations (70%), euphoria (70%), rapid thinking (60%), and decreased need for sleep (50%) were reported. She found overlapping cognitive and mood changes when comparing hypomania and intense creative states. She also found a seasonal summer peak in moods, with elevated mood and productivity correlating more closely in the untreated group as compared with the treated group. The conclusions have been questioned because of possible bias and small sample size (Rothenberg 1990, 1995b).

Although a similar critique might be applied, more recent results appear consistent with evidence that within the entertainment industry, a high proportion of individuals reveal data often associated with bipolarity. Although paid very little for their efforts, professional cheerleaders for the National Football League clubs put in long hours as a second job in practice for performing in front of thousands of fans every weekend during the season. Perhaps not surprisingly, their lifetime measures of total cyclothymia and dysthymia on the General Behavior Inventory (9.5 ± 8.2) were much greater than for control subjects without a psychiatric diagnosis (2.8 ± 5.9) and similar to those for bipolar patients in remission (11.5 ± 13.0, $F = 4.94$, $P < .01$) (J. H. Henry and Goodnick 1991). In particular, high incidence rates on the General Behavior Inventory were found for elevated energy (55.3%), physical restlessness (32.9%), insomnia secondary to elevated energy (32.9%), and elevated self-image (31.6%).

One final study of creativity in living individuals is significant because it examines the link between creativity and psychopathology in adolescents, rather than in adults, to evaluate the relationship between creativity, depression, attributional style, and gender in this group (DeMoss et al. 1993). In this study, 71 male and 57 female eighth and ninth graders who were invited to apply to a magnet school that focused on math and science were administered the Torrance Test of Creative Thinking, the Children's Depression Inventory, and the Children's Attributional Style Questionnaire. A negative attributional style in which negative events are ascribed to internal, stable, and global causes has been associated with concurrent and subsequent depression in children and adults (DeMoss et al. 1993). In this study, there were significant correlations between a negative attributional style and depression (females, $r = .24$, $P < .05$; males, $r = .21$, $P < .01$). A significant relationship was found between figural creativity and a "depressogenic attributional style" among both genders (females, $r = .20$, $P < .10$; males, $r = .21$, $P < .05$). Interestingly, only in females was verbal creativity associated with a positive attributional style ($r = .37$, $P < .01$) and low levels of depression ($r = .28$, $P < .05$). The authors concluded that the link between creativity and affective illness may exist among high-achieving adolescents, and that, among females, verbal creativity may serve as a protective factor.

Creative Abilities of Mentally Ill Persons

Another parameter for the study of an association between mood disorders and creativity is the search for creative abilities in patients with mood disorders. The Lifetime Creativity Scale (Richards et al. 1988a) was developed in an attempt to define creativity and then measure it. It is directed at the "maximum level of original and meaningful accomplishment" achieved by an individual during adulthood (peak creativity) and the "relative degree of emphasis on creative vs. other activity over the adult lifetime" (p. 478) (extent of involvement in creative activity). Each of these areas is rated on a 0- to 5-point scale from "not significant" to "exceptional" or by definition from "routine or prescribed endeavors with negligible innovative aspects" to "radical departures from the commonplace; these may require conceptual reorganization to be assimilated." Examples given for "avocational history" are: 0 = None, "Spends most evenings with the new family television . . . does much needlepoint following specified patterns"; 2 = Some, "Active church member who has ushered . . . sung . . . has been volunteering on a committee"; and 4 = High, "Amateur archaeologist who for years has spent summers and other free time seeking new sites . . . researching artifacts . . . collaborating on articles" (p. 481).

In contrasting peak creativity, Richards et al. (1988b) reported mean levels in control subjects, patients, and relatives as follows: 11 first-degree relatives without mood disorders of bipolar subjects (2.8), 16 cyclothymic subjects (2.7), 33 control subjects (2.4), bipolar subjects (2.3), and control subjects with diagnosis (2.2). These findings were hypothesized to be consistent with a trait rather than state phenomenon in which subclinical factors related to risk of bipolarity—rather than mood symptoms themselves—increase creativity. Yet, a follow-up study indicated that of 34 bipolar patients, 20 (59%) believed that their "most creative" mood state was a "mildly elevated" mood state, rather than a very elevated (20.5%) or normal (20.5%) mood state (Richards and Kinney 1990).

❱ Lithium and Creativity

The evidence is strong that mood disorders and creativity are associated. Evidence is mounting to support the idea that mood disorders might confer an advantage on the gifted artist in terms of facilitating the expression of mood states in his or her work at the great cost of the individual's emotional stability. In fact, many a gifted artist has succumbed to depression by his or her own hand by suicide. In fact, if left untreated, the mortality of bipolar disorder by suicidal act is 20% (Jamison 1993). Fortunately, with the advent of effective pharmacotherapy, bipolar individuals can be spared the ravages of extreme mood states. However, for the gifted artist who depends on his or her ability to transduce feelings into form, the question as to whether mood stabilizing agents might interfere with this process is a crucial one.

There is a limited literature addressing this important question, which was raised as early as 1970 in a review of the literature pertaining to the benefits of mental illness (Marshall et al. 1970). The article cites uncontrolled observations made of six nationally recognized artists and businessmen on lithium therapy suggesting that lithium might enhance their creative potential. Five of the six patients on lithium for a mean of 2 years were reported to have experienced more uniform productivity of sounder quality while on lithium. The sixth opted to discontinue lithium after the resolution of mild hypomania.

In 1975, Benson published a case series of 31 manic patients, meeting Feighner's criteria (Feighner et al. 1972), to look at causes for noncompliance with lithium and the impact of additional psychotherapy. Of 12 who had opted to discontinue lithium, 4 based their decision on a perception that their creativity had been adversely affected. Because these patients had had fewer contacts with Benson, he concluded that psychotherapy should focus on the patients' interpretation of impact of medication. In 1979, Judd found, using the Meier Art Tests and the four Christensen-Guilford Verbal Fluency tests, that lithium was equal to placebo in its effect on psychometric assessment of creative functions in subjects without a psychiatric diagnosis. Schou (1979) published a series of 24 case reports of bipolar artists who primarily create (e.g., composers rather than instrumentalists) from a variety of sources. In summary, lithium prophylaxis attenuated or pre-vented recurrences of illness in all 24 artists. When questioned about their creative abilities during treatment, 12 reported increased produc-tivity, 6 unaltered productivity, and 6 lowered productivity. The author indicated that the severity of the illness, individual sensitivity, and in-dividual work habits may influence the effect of lithium prophylaxis on creative output.

In 1986, Shaw et al. systematically examined whether lithium im-pacted on associational productivity in an "A-B-A" half single-blind and half double-blind study of 22 euthymic bipolar patients, twice off lithium and twice on when lithium was restarted. Results indicated that lithium discontinuation was related to a significant increase in number of associations and percentage of idiosyncratic associations. Interestingly, Richards and Kinney (1989) published a letter noting that among Andreasen's (1987) eminent writers, bipolar II disorder occurred more than twice as frequently as bipolar I disorder and that similar results were obtained by Akiskal and Akiskal (1988). They speculate that treatment for bipolar disorder may enhance creative potential by softening extremes of mood states.

In 1993, Kocsis et al. published a second systematic study of the effects of blind lithium discontinuation on "creativity" in 46 patients with bipolar disorder who were taking long-term lithium therapy. The group found that scores on memory measures, tapping speed, and associative productivity tests improved significantly while on lithium but only modestly while off lithium. As expected, patients who had higher pre-discontinuation plasma lithium levels displayed greater im-provement in motor performance and associational productivity.

As is evidenced by this historical review of the literature pertaining to the effects of lithium on creative productivity, more work is to be done to better estimate and minimize any ill effect that this treatment may have on the creative process. There is a notable paucity of literature related to the effects of valproic acid and carbamazepine on creativity.

As more is learned about bipolar disorder and its different sub-types, and as more specific data are gathered pertaining to the effects of mood-stabilizing agents on the creative process, treatment can be better tailored to suit the needs of the gifted individual whose creative productivity is essential to his or her livelihood and quality of life.

Perhaps maintaining a minimal plasma lithium level will provide adequate prophylaxis without significantly interfering with the creative stream of thought. Or, as an alternative, perhaps carbamazepine or valproic acid will be found to be preferable prophylactic agents for some creative individuals with bipolar illness.

▶ **Contemporary Theoretical Paradigms Addressing Cognitive Complexity and Motivation**

The historical development of an age-old mystery was presented at the beginning of this chapter. Questions related to the wellspring of creativity have puzzled humanity for time untold. References to an association between mental illness and creativity appear in recorded history since before 500 B.C., and research attempting to identify and delineate the association systematically is still in progress. However, a central question remains unanswered: What is the mechanism of human creativity, a characteristic that has fueled the innovations and progress of humankind since its inception? If manic-depressive illness and creativity are indeed associated, what are the mechanisms of the association? In this section, we present a number of contemporary theoretical paradigms addressing mechanisms of creativity and their possible link to mood disorders.

As previously described, creative individuals share certain attributes, among which are more complex, richly interconnected thought patterns and motivation. It is believed that mood disorders, particularly bipolar disorder, enhance the complexity of thought patterns. Cognitive complexity has been conceptualized in different forms, three of which are described: 1) Janusian and homospatial cognitive processes (Rothenberg 1990), 2) functional hyperconnectivity of right and left hemispheres (Miller 1988), and 3) open-systems thermodynamic model (Sabelli et al. 1990). The concept of motivation is then addressed. Is motivation biologically enhanced by the mood disordered state or is it of an unrelated psychodynamic origin?

Janusian and Homospatial Processes

Creativity being "the production of something that is both new and truly valuable" (Rothenberg 1990, p. 5), the first concept to be described is in answer to the question: Is there any cognitive pattern common to all types of creativity? Rothenberg's research is based on data derived from extensive interviews of thousands of creative individuals (such as Pulitzer Prize winners) and control subjects paid to create. Each individual has been interviewed with a focus on the psychological roots of creativity both at the inception of the project and during its progression. Rothenberg, as a consequence, suggested the presence of two thinking processes that underlie all types of creativity and are common to art, science, and other productive fields: the Janusian process and the homospatial process. The Janusian process is a mental process by which "multiple opposites or antitheses are conceived simultaneously, either as existing side by side or as equally operative, valid or true" (p. 15). This thinking is not delusional; rather, the individual always remains aware that the concepts are opposites. It is the very necessity of explaining seeming opposites that generates the originality of thought that is then less evident in the final product. The homospatial process is one that operates later in the process of creativity as "conceiving two or more discrete entities occupying the same space, a conception leading to the articulation of new identities" (p. 25). This process is seen as a fleeting one because the mind is not able to experience two concepts simultaneously for long. Rothenberg quoted Beethoven's description of his experience of this process: "the underlying idea [of a musical work] . . . rises . . . grows, I hear and see the image in front of me from every angle, as if it had been cast" (p. 28). These cognitive phenomena are not viewed as psychotic but rather as requiring a clear foothold on reality that produce mental and emotional strain, thus requiring creative resolution.

Two alternative paradigms have been elaborated to attempt to explain creativity: functional hyperconnectivity (Miller 1988) and open-systems thermodynamics (Sabelli et al. 1990).

The first, presented in a review (Miller 1988), is a neuropsychodynamic approach attempting to explain creativity in terms of personality, psychopathology, and cognitive style. This theory postulates that the creative individual has increased right and left brain communication and is based on Hartmann's concept of ego autonomy as the relative freedom of the self from blind obedience to instinct. This psychodynamic principle is then related to the fact that prefrontal regions are essential for organizing intellectual and affective activity as a whole. However, autonomous self-direction also requires a "self-referential conceptual classification system that can imbue the frontal guidance and evaluation mechanism with a framework of personal goals and values, that is, an identity. And this may be the task of the interhemispheric system" (Miller 1988, p. 385). The left hemisphere is specialized for logical descriptive analysis, for example, whereas the functions of the right hemisphere include spatial processing, intuition, and inference. Galin regarded right hemisphere functioning as congruent with primary process thinking or the unconscious. Furthermore, functional hyperconnectivity may result in a cognitive and emotional imbalance such as that of bipolar disorder, as well as allowing the translation of overly accessible right hemispheric processes (primary process) by left hemispheric processes (secondary process), resulting in creative expressions. To support this theory, Miller (1988) presented results of a study of timed word associations of 12 Nobel laureates (NL) (creative scientists), 18 hospitalized patients (HP), and 113 Yale University undergraduate students divided into high creative (HC) and low creative (LC) groups (Rothenberg 1983). The creative group (NL and HC) showed significantly more ability to provide opposite word associations requiring shift of focus (60% and 50%, respectively) than the noncreative groups (HP and LC) (40% and 38%, respectively), with lower latencies of response (NL: 1.1 and HC: 1.3 versus HP: 1.5 and LC: 1.6).

Sabelli et al. (1990) proposed the open-systems thermodynamic paradigm, which is based on three assumptions: first, that bipolarity is biological; second, that hypomania and mania are states of enhanced energy; and third, that biological and psychological energy are forms of physical energy. The third assumption restates the first law of thermodynamics, which restates Einstein's concept that energy is conserved. Creative processes are explained through the idea that irreversible processes, or "asymmetrically flowing processes," create order through fluctuation, resulting in new structures (creative products) (Sabelli et al. 1990). The theory is based on the concept that the individual is not a closed system, but rather an open system that interacts with the surrounding environment. In each individual, many processes are occurring simultaneously. As a component of an open system interacting with the environment, many biological and psychological processes appear to be far from equilibrium. In this theory, bipolar illness is viewed as a high-energy process that includes four types of abnormality: first, a failure of homeostasis; second, an increase in cyclicities; third, catastrophic switches and chaotic processes; and fourth, the formation of novel dissipative structures both normal (creativity) and pathological (delusional).

▶ CONCLUSION

The question as to the existence of an association of outstanding creativity and mental illness dates back to the days of Socrates (born in 469 B.C. in Athens, Greece) (Radioe 1969) and is only recently beginning to be tested by systematic scientific methodology. The question is difficult to approach in this manner for several reasons, including the lack of a consensual definition of creativity and the need for more creativity scales. Richard's (1993) theory of mood disorder, offering a compensatory advantage of a higher degree of creativity to first-degree relatives of bipolar patients, extends the hypothesized association to creative persons who are mentally healthy. One point is certain: some individuals of great creative skill suffer from bipolar disorder.

The significance of this association can be viewed both from an individual perspective and from a social perspective. When treating a bipolar individual who depends on his or her creativity to subsist, it must be kept in mind that mood-stabilizing agents might cause alterations in creative states that may vary with each individual. Some patients have become noncompliant with lithium therapy because of perceived alterations in their ability to be creative, and they respond well to having these issues addressed. It might be prudent in some cases to make reasonable medication adjustments, keeping in mind the risk-benefit ratio of pharmacotherapeutic treatment of bipolar disorder in each case. Some cognitive changes attributed to lithium treatment appear to be dose related.

To better serve the creative bipolar person, much investigative work is yet to be done. Studies of the effects of carbamazepine and valproic acid on creativity are yet to be undertaken. Studies of possible behavioral interventions may prove helpful. For example, patients may be able to plot and predict cycles and tailor their creative work to times of relative mood stability, just as Beethoven performed technical work in the summer by recognizing a pattern in his states. Studies of psychotherapeutic techniques that nurture creative accomplishment have been published (Kinney 1992; Ostwald 1992).

From a societal perspective, the question remains: does the association of mood disorder and creativity exist? If so, is it a causal relationship? As previously mentioned, although in the literature the association is predominantly accepted, it is not undisputed. Using modern research methodology, a consensual definition of creativity is needed as are more instruments in addition to the Lifetime Creativity Scale, both in adults and in children. Furthering the study of creativity and mood disorders in children (akin to existing studies of vulnerable children of mentally ill parents) might add a developmental perspective to this age-old question. Much work is yet to be done to better understand what might link bipolar disorder to creativity, the still mysterious human quality that characterizes the lifetime achievements of some individuals. These achievements reverberate to a societal level transcending time, place, and culture and move humanity forward to new levels of emotional, intellectual, and societal development.

▶ REFERENCES

Akiskal HS, Akiskal K: Reassessing the prevalence of bipolar disorders: clinical significance and artistic creativity. Psychiatry and Psychobiology 3:29–36, 1988

American Psychiatric Association: Diagnostic and Statistical Manual of Mental Disorders, 3rd Edition, Revised. Washington, DC, American Psychiatric Association, 1987

Andreasen NC: Creativity and mental illness: prevalence rates in writers and their first degree relatives. Am J Psychiatry 144:1288–1292, 1987

Andreasen NC: Dr. Andreasen replies (letter). Am J Psychiatry 141:908, 1988

Andreasen NJC, Canter A: The creative writer: psychiatric symptoms and family history. Compr Psychiatry 15:123–131, 1974

Andreasen NC, Glick ID: Bipolar affective disorder and creativity: implications and clinical management. Compr Psychiatry 29:207–217, 1988

Andreasen NJC, Powers PS: Creativity and psychosis: an examination of conceptual style. Arch Gen Psychiatry 32:70–73, 1975

Angier N: An old idea about genius wins new scientific support. The New York Times, October 12, 1993

Benson R: The forgotten treatment modality in bipolar illness: psychotherapy. Diseases of the Nervous System 36:634–638, 1975

Bond AH: Virginia Woolf: manic depressive psychosis and genius. an illustration of separation-individuation theory. J Am Acad Psychoanal 13:191–210, 1985

Bond AH: Virginia Woolf and Leslie Stephen: a father's contribution to psychosis and genius. J Am Acad Psychoanal 14:507–524, 1986

Caldwell AE: La Malinconia: final movement of Beethoven's quartet Op. 18 No. 6—a musical account of manic depressive states. J Am Med Wom Assoc 27:241–248, 1972

Corwin D: Letter to the editor. Am J Psychiatry 152:816, 1995

DeMoss K, Milich R, DeMers S: Gender, creativity, depression, and attributional style in adolescents with high academic ability. J Abnorm Child Psychol 21:455–467, 1993

Destaing F: Le soleil et l'orage ou la maladie de van Gogh. Nouvelle Presse Medicale 1:3141–3143, 1972

Fama PG, Thompson AC: Charles Meryon: a biographical and psychiatric reassessment. N Z Med J 78:448–455, 1973

Feighner JP, Robins E, Guze SB, et al: Diagnostic criteria for use in psychiatric research. Arch Gen Psychiatry 26:57–63, 1972

Feinstein SC: Why they were afraid of Virginia Woolf: perspectives on juvenile manic-depressive illness. Adolesc Psychiatry 8:332–343, 1980

Fromm-Reichmann F: The assets of the mentally handicapped: the interplay of mental illness and creativity. J Am Acad Psychoanal 18:47–72, 1990

George MS, Melvin JA, Mossman D: Mental illness and creativity (letter). Am J Psychiatry 145:908, 1988

Goodwin FK, Jamison KR: Manic-Depressive Illness. New York, Oxford University Press, 1990

Henry JH, Goodnick PJ: Mood symptoms of professional cheerleaders. New Research Program and Abstracts (NR84, 68), 144th Annual Meeting, American Psychiatric Association, New Orleans, LA, May 11–16, 1991

Henry WD: The personality of Oliver Cromwell. Practitioner 215:102–110, 1975

Hershman DJ, Lieb J: The Key to Genius: Manic-Depression and the Crea-
tive Life. Buffalo, NY, Prometheus Books, 1988
James J: Though this were madness, was there yet method in't? The New
York Times, August 7, 1994
Jamison KR: Mood disorders and patterns of creativity in British writers and
artists. Psychiatry 52:125–134, 1989
Jamison KR: Touched With Fire: Manic-Depressive Illness and the Artistic
Temperament. New York, Free Press, 1993
Jamison KR: Manic depressive illness and creativity. Sci Am 272:February
1995, pp 62–67
Jamison KR, Wyatt RJ: Vincent van Gogh's illness (letter). BMJ 304:577,
1992
Joseph RJ: John Ruskin: radical and psychotic genius. Psychoanal Rev
56:425–441, 1969
Juda A: The relationship between highest mental capacity and psychic ab-
normalities. Am J Psychiatry 106:296–307, 1949
Judd LL: Effect of lithium on mood, cognition, and personality function in
normal subjects. Arch Gen Psychiatry 36:860–865, 1979
Karlsson JL: Genetic association of giftedness and creativity with schizophrenia. Hereditas 66:177–182, 1970
Kauffman C, Grunebaum H, Cohler B, et al: Superkids: competent children
of psychotic mothers. Am J Psychiatry 136:1398–1402, 1979
Kinney DK: The Therapist as muse: greater roles for clinicians in fostering
innovation. Am J Psychother 46:434–453, 1992
Kocsis JH, Shaw ED, Stokes PE, et al: Neuropsychologic effects of lithium
discontinuation. J Clin Psychopharmacol 13:268–275, 1993
Lieb J, Hershman D: Isaac Newton: mercury poisoning or manic depres-
sion? Lancet 2:1479–1480, 1983
Ludwig AM: Creative achievement and psychopathology: comparison
among professions. Am J Psychother 46:330–354, 1992
Ludwig AM: Mental illness and creative activity in female writers. Am J
Psychiatry 151:1650–1656, 1994
Mack M, Knox BMW, McGalliard JC, et al (eds): The Norton Anthology of
World Masterpieces, Vol 2. New York, WW Norton, 1979
Marshall MH: Are there benefits of mental illness? Behavioral Neuropsychi-
atry 2:40–42, 1970
Marshall MH, Neumann CP, Robinson M: Lithium, creativity and manic-
depressive illness: review and prospectus. Psychosomatics 11:406–408,
1970
Miller L: Ego autonomy, creativity, and cognitive style: a neuropsychody-
namic approach. Psychiatr Clin North Am 11:383–397, 1988
Monroe RR: Creative brainstorms: a story of madness and genius. J Am
Acad Psychoanal 19:462–470, 1991

Myerson A, Boyle RD: The incidence of manic-depressive psychosis in certain socially important families. Am J Psychiatry 98:11–21, 1941

Ostwald PF: Psychotherapeutic facilitation of musical creativity. Am J Psychother 46:383–403, 1992

Post F: Creativity and psychopathology: a study of 291 world-famous men. Br J Psychiatry 165:22–34, 1994

Radioe B (ed): Plato: the last days of Socrates. Translated by Tredennick H. Aylesbury, England, Penguin Books, 1969

Ravin JG: Van Gogh's illness. Ohio State Medical Journal 77:600–702, 1981

Richards R: Everyday creativity, eminent creativity and psychopathology. Psychological Inquiry 4:212–217, 1993

Richards R, Kinney DK: Eminent and everyday creativity may be associated with milder mood disorders and states (letter). Compr Psychiatry 30:272–273, 1989

Richards R, Kinney DK: Mood swings and creativity. Creativity Research Journal 3:202–217, 1990

Richards R, Kinney DK, Benet M, et al: Assessing everyday creativity: characteristics of the lifetime creativity scales and validation with three large samples. J Pers Soc Psychol 54:476–485, 1988a

Richards R, Kinney DK, Lunde I, et al: Creativity in manic-depressives, cyclothymes, their normal relatives and control subjects. J Abnorm Psychol 97:281–288, 1988b

Rooney PJ, Buchanan WW, MacNeill AL: Robert Fergusson: poet and patient. Practitioner 219:402–407, 1977

Roth N: King George III and porphyria. Am J Psychiatry 123:866–871, 1967

Rothenberg A: Psychopathology and creative cognition. Arch Gen Psychiatry 40:937–942, 1983

Rothenberg A: Creativity and Madness. Baltimore, MD, Johns Hopkins University Press, 1990

Rothenberg A: Creativity and affective illness: an objection. Percept Mot Skills 80:161–162, 1995a

Rothenberg A: Creativity and mental illness (letter). Am J Psychiatry 152:815–816, 1995b

Sabelli HC, Carlson-Sabelli L, Javaid JI: The thermodynamics of bipolarity: a bifurcation model of bipolar illness and bipolar character and its psychotherapeutic applications. Psychiatry 53:346–368, 1990

Salzmann MM: George III and the mad-business (letter). BMJ 3:406, 1970

Schildkraut JJ: Mind and mood in modern art, II: depressive disorders, spirituality, and early deaths in abstract expressionist artists of the New York School. Am J Psychiatry 151:482–488, 1994

Schou M: Artistic productivity and lithium prophylaxis in manic-depressive illness. Br J Psychiatry 135:97–103, 1979

Schou M: Lithium perspectives. Neuropsychobiology 10:7–12, 1983

Shaw ED, Mann JJ, Stokes PE, et al: Effects of lithium carbonate on associative productivity and idiosyncrasy in bipolar outpatients. Am J Psychiatry 143:1166–1169, 1986

Wechsler D: Wechsler Adult Intelligence Scale—Revised. San Antonio, TX, Psychological Corporation, 1981

World Health Organization: Mental Disorders: Glossary and Guide to Their Classification in Accordance With the Ninth Revision of the International Classification of Diseases. Geneva, World Health Organization, 1978

CHAPTER 3

CHILD AND ADOLESCENT MANIA

Gary Sachs, M.D., and
Beny Lafer, M.D.

L ike patients with adult mania, the child or adolescent with
mania may have life-threatening symptoms. The young patient with mania is often harder to diagnosis and more difficult to treat than a typical adult patient. The transition from
childhood to adolescence brings a developing human from the phase
of development during which onset of mania is least likely to the developmental phase during which the vulnerability to onset of mania
is greatest. The variation in the expression of mania in early developmental phases compared with the adult form of bipolar illness has
important clinical and theoretical implications. An understanding of
mania across the life cycle may improve diagnosis and lead to improved outcome for all bipolar patients.

In this chapter, we consider the diagnosis and treatment of mania
during childhood and adolescence.

▶ Concept of Mood Disorder as Applied to Children

Theoretical considerations have long plagued research on childhood
mood disorders. In the past, many psychiatrists viewed relatively ma-
ture ego function as necessary for the development of depression and
mania (Koran 1975). According to this formulation, the limited ego

function of children protected them against major mood disorders. However, empirical studies have revealed that depression during childhood is surprisingly common. Systematic study of childhood mania has been sparse, but after Kraepelin's (1921) description of a 5-year-old patient with mania, additional cases gradually appeared in the psychiatric literature. Anthony and Scott (1960) reviewed the 28 published reports of childhood mania described between 1884 and 1960. The only three cases that met their stringent criteria for mania were of patients age 11 or in late childhood.

Although many psychiatrists continue to express skepticism about reports of full-blown mania prior to puberty, a growing literature has documented childhood cases meeting adult DSM-III-R (American Psychiatric Association 1987) and DSM-IV (American Psychiatric Association 1994) criteria for mania. Carlson, Weller, and others (Carlson 1983; Weinberg and Brumback 1976; Weller et al. 1986) have described cases in which children of preschool age demonstrate symptoms meeting criteria for mania and hypomania. Vranka et al. (1988) described 10 hospitalized children meeting DSM-III (American Psychiatric Association 1980) criteria for mania. All children (ages 6–12 years) in this series had mood-congruent psychotic features and were treated with lithium. All responded to lithium therapy with "substantial improvement," including complete resolution of psychotic features and euthymic mood.

Based on structured interview (Schedule for Affective Disorders and Schizophrenia for School-aged Children) with the mother, Wozniak et al. (1993) found that 17% of 183 children 12 years or younger who were consecutively referred for child psychiatry evaluation met criteria for mania or hypomania. Age at onset was before age 5 in 68% of the sample.

Children meeting the full criteria for mania are still considered rarities. Akiskal et al. (1985) examined 68 children and younger siblings of bipolar probands referred for psychiatric evaluation. In this sample, 4 of 10 prepubertal subjects met criteria for hypomania, but none were found to have "full-blown manic psychosis" before puberty. The mean age at onset of affective illness was 15.9 years.

The mixture of rapidly changing symptoms is likely to account for a lack of diagnostic consensus. Wozniak et al. (1993) reported that only 25% of prepubertal patients had discrete cycles and suggested that chronic course and irritable mood are the typical presentation in this age group. Strober et al. (1989) suggested that the prepubertal presentation of bipolar children is one of frequent brief episodes in which dysphoria and hypomanic symptoms are mixed. With the onset of puberty, Strober et al. saw the emergence of cyclical extremes of mania and depression.

Based on a systematic review of the literature on mania in childhood, Carlson (1990) also found differences in the phenomenology of mania associated with early versus late childhood. Mania occurring in children younger than 8 years old was more likely to be characterized by hyperactivity, irritability, emotional lability, and lack of discrete episodes. The presentation of mania in children between 9 and 12 years of age was more likely to demonstrate the classic features of adult mania (discrete episodes with euphoria, grandiosity, and paranoia).

The occurrence of discrete episodes is a central feature of adult mania. Therefore, it is not surprising that considerable debate remains about diagnosis of mania prior to puberty. Given the well-established observation that adult bipolar illness can follow a chronic course, it is difficult to justify the disregard of cases of mania described during early childhood as the result of simple misdiagnosis. Because there seems to be little doubt about the existence of hypomania in children, this population should be considered at risk for bipolar illness.

▶ DIAGNOSIS

The adoption of criteria-based diagnostic systems such as DSM-III and DSM-IV enhances our ability to interpret reports describing childhood mania. DSM-IV continues the convention of applying the same criteria to the diagnosis of mania in children as are used to diagnose adults. There are some mood disorder criteria, however, that are modified for application to children and adolescents. The diagnosis of dysthymia or cyclothymia requires that the duration of symptoms be at least 1 year for children or adolescents, whereas a 2-year duration is the minimum necessary to diagnose these disorders in adults. DSM-IV also permits a diagnosis of depression in children and adolescents if their mood state is irritable even in the absence of sadness or diminished ability to experience pleasure.

It is important to remain aware of the fact that the descriptive diagnostic criteria sets of DSM-IV provide a useful but somewhat arbitrary way of ensuring uniformity of syndromic diagnosis but do not constitute precise definitions for discrete psychiatric diseases. Within the DSM-IV criteria for mania, there is considerable room for etiologic heterogeneity and phenotypic heterogeneity. Etiologic heterogeneity refers to different causes producing similar presentation. Phenotypic heterogeneity refers to different presentations of the same etiology. Etiologic heterogeneity and phenotypic heterogeneity are important problems in the diagnosis of bipolar illness in both children and adults. Any disease that can produce mood episodes in the appropriate pattern to meet DSM-IV criteria for mania or hypomania is a bipolar illness. Because 1%–3% of the population has a bipolar illness, a similar percentage of children could be expected to be at least carriers of the same disease process. The question of greater concern to child psychiatry is whether the phenotypic expression of bipolar illness is sufficiently different during the early phase of development to warrant separate criteria for diagnosing mania prior to adulthood. Put a different way, the question is—does the use of adult criteria blind us to the presence of syndromes that represent markers for later development of mania?

Etiologic and phenotypic heterogeneity frame the debate about the significance of childhood bipolar illness. This debate is best put into context by considering clinical issues.

What Is the Significance of Symptoms Meeting Criteria for Mania in Childhood?

The recurrent reports of manic syndromes in children alter the focus of debate from the dispute of whether children exist who meet the adult criteria for mania, to the more interesting question of the diagnostic, hence prognostic significance of episodes meeting these criteria during childhood. Several possibilities exist.

- The adult (DSM-IV) definition mania is not appropriate for children. Symptoms diagnostic of mania in an adult might be normal during childhood. A child's certainty that he or she will be president of the United States might reasonably be accepted as normal, but an adult expressing such confidence would be regarded as grandiose. This argument finds it possible to consider even the most extreme or outrageous behavior to be within the norm for children.

- A child may have an extreme reaction to an overwhelming stress (e.g., death of a parent). This reaction accounts for a manic syndrome as resulting from a child's adjustment to overwhelming traumatic events.

- Children meeting DSM-IV criteria for mania actually have another psychiatric illness. This argument rests on the overlap in symptoms between mania and disorders such as attention-deficit/hyperactivity disorder (ADHD) or conduct disorder. As can be seen in Table 3–1, there is considerable overlap between mania and other diagnostic criteria for disorders presenting in childhood.

- Children meeting criteria for mania have a secondary mood disorder like secondary mood disorders observed in adult manic patients.

- Children meeting criteria for mania have a primary mood disorder distinct from that observed in adult manic patients.

- Children meeting the DSM-IV criteria for mania have the same illness as adults. This possibility suggests that the observed differences in the presentation of mania result from the interaction between the disease process and an evolving biological substrate.

Each of these possibilities is likely to account for some cases meeting formal criteria for mania during childhood. Although it is impossible to distinguish between them with complete certainty, it is important to recognize and consider these possibilities when children meet criteria for hypomania or mania.

▌ EPIDEMIOLOGY

Most epidemiological studies find the lifetime prevalence of mania to be about 1%. When bipolar type II and other forms of bipolar illness

Table 3–1. Comparison of DSM-IV mania, attention-deficit/hyperactivity disorder (ADHD), and conduct disorder

Mania	ADHD	Conduct disorder
A. A distinct period of abnormally and persistently elevated, expansive, or irritable mood, lasting at least 1 week (or any duration if hospitalization is necessary). B. During the period of mood disturbance, three (or more) of the following symptoms have persisted (four if the mood is only irritable) and have been present to a significant degree:	A. Either (1) or (2): (1) inattention: six (or more) of the following symptoms of inattention have persisted for at least 6 months to a degree that is maladaptive and inconsistent with developmental level: (2) hyperactivity-impulsivity: six (or more) of the following symptoms of hyperactivity-impulsivity have persisted for at least 6 months to a degree that is maladaptive and inconsistent with developmental level:	A repetitive and persistent pattern of behavior in which the basic rights of others or major age-appropriate societal norms or rules are violated, as manifested by the presence of three (or more) of the following criteria in the past 12 months, with at least one criterion present in the past 6 months:
1) inflated self-esteem or grandiosity 2) decreased need for sleep 3) more talkative than usual or pressure to keep talking	1) often has difficulty awaiting turn 2) often talks excessively 3) often blurts out answers before questions have been completed 4) often interrupts or intrudes on others	1) often bullies, threatens, or intimidates others 2) often initiates physical fights

4) flight of ideas or subjective experience that thoughts are racing

5) distractibility (i.e., attention too easily drawn to unimportant or irrelevant external stimuli)

6) increase in goal-directed activity (either socially, at work or school, or sexually) or psychomotor agitation

5) often does not follow through on instructions and fails to finish schoolwork, chores, or duties in the workplace

6) often has difficulty organizing tasks and activities

7) often fails to give close attention to details or makes careless mistakes in schoolwork, work, or other activities

8) often has difficulty sustaining attention in tasks or play activities

9) often loses things necessary for tasks or activities

10) is often forgetful in daily activities

11) is often easily distracted by extraneous stimuli

12) often does not seem to listen when spoken to directly

13) often leaves seat in classroom or in other situations in which remaining seated is expected

3) has used a weapon that can cause serious physical harm to others

4) has been physically cruel to people

5) has been physically cruel to animals

(continued)

Table 3–1. Comparison of DSM-IV mania, attention-deficit/hyperactivity disorder (ADHD), and conduct disorder *(continued)*

Mania	ADHD	Conduct disorder
7) excessive involvement in pleasurable activities that have a high potential for painful consequences	14) often avoids, dislikes, or is reluctant to engage in tasks requiring sustained mental effort (e.g., schoolwork or homework)	6) has stolen while confronting a victim 7) has forced someone into sexual activity 8) has deliberately engaged in fire setting with the intention of causing serious damage 9) has deliberately destroyed others' property 10) has broken into someone else's house, building, or car 11) often lies to obtain goods or favors or to avoid obligations 12) has stolen items of nontrivial value without confronting a victim 13) often stays out at night despite parental prohibitions, beginning before age 13 years 14) has run away from home overnight at least twice while living in parental or parental surrogate home (or once without returning for a lengthy period) 15) is often truant from school beginning before age 13 years

are included, the prevalence increases to between 2% and 3%. A similar prevalence may apply to children and adolescents. Thomsen et al. (1992) used the nationwide psychiatric case registry in Denmark to identify 23 boys and 13 girls admitted with a diagnosis of manic-depressive psychosis before the age of 15. Based on the population at risk, a 1.2% prevalence was calculated with a mean age at first admission of 12.7 years.

The task of determining the onset of bipolar illness in a sample of children is complicated. A substantial proportion of children diagnosed as depressed are likely to have bipolar illness. Geller et al. (1994) reported longitudinal follow-up of 79 children diagnosed with major depression. In this sample, 31.7% developed bipolarity (10 mania, 15 hypomania) over the 2- to 5-year follow-up period.

What Is the Incidence of Bipolar Disorder During Childhood and Adolescence?

Kraepelin's (1921) data are often cited as showing the rarity of mania before puberty. Among 903 patients diagnosed with manic-depressive insanity, Kraepelin found that only 0.4% had onset of their first episode before reaching age 10 years. Kraepelin found that in patients 15 years old or younger, more than 75% of the mood episodes included mania (pure mania or phases of mania alternating with depression).

As indicated earlier, Wozniak et al. (1993) found mania and hypomania to be common (17%) and readily identifiable in children referred to the child psychiatry clinic. Few studies have addressed the prevalence of mania among children and adolescents in the general population. In one of the only studies to examine a community sample of adolescents ($N = 150$), Carlson and Kashani (1988) found that 20% endorsed four or more manic symptoms on the Diagnostic Interview for Children and Adolescents. In contrast to the adult bipolar population, where the proportions of males and of females are roughly even, studies that sample affectively ill children have found a high proportion of males (Dwyer and DeLong 1987; Thomsen et al. 1992; Wozniak et al. 1993).

What Is the Period of Greatest Risk for
Onset of Bipolar Illness?

Bipolar illness appears to be an illness with onset during the first two decades of life. The age at onset can be defined in a variety of ways. The impact of using the first episode approach versus first hospitalization can be dramatic. Winokur et al. (1980) applied both definitions to determine onset in 61 patients. The proportion of patients with onset of illness between ages 10 and 19 changed from 9.8% using first hospitalization to 34.4% using age at first episode. Whichever definition is used, late adolescence (ages 15–19) appears to be a period of high vulnerability for onset of bipolar illness (Kraepelin 1921; Loranger and Levine 1978; Sachs 1990; Sachs et al. 1994; Winokur et al. 1980).

Sachs et al. (1994) used a specially modified version of the Structured Clinical Interview for DSM-III-R to determine the age at onset in 52 bipolar probands. This methodology indicated that bipolar illness is a disease most often rooted in youth. Onset of illness was reported by age 15 years in 50% and by age 21 years in 75% of the subjects (see Figure 3–1). Consistent with Wozniak et al.'s (1993) data, a substantial number of bipolar patients met criteria for onset of full major affective episode before age 12 years. Like most prior studies, the incidence of mania before puberty was low, but nearly one-third of cases included a subsyndromal episode before the age of 10. The majority of diagnosable childhood episodes met criteria for depression.

Similarly, Akiskal et al. (1979) reported that 86% of cyclothymic patients come to clinical attention during their late teens or early 20s. On evaluation, these patients "revealed that not infrequently the actual age of onset of the disorder was buried in the vague past of very early adolescence" (p. 533). As can be seen in Figure 3–1 and Figure 3–2, the risk of onset rises steeply during adolescence.

The generally consistent finding that the majority of cases have onset between ages 10 and 30 establishes this as a period of greatest risk. The data in Loranger and Levine (1978) (obtained by chart review) suggested that the vulnerability to onset of bipolar illness is more constant across the life cycle. Overall, the data suggest a relationship be-

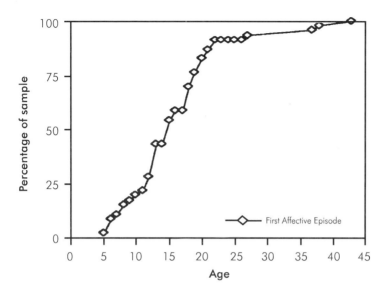

Figure 3–1. Age at onset of bipolar illness.
Source.   Adapted from Sachs GS, Lafer B, Thibault AB, et al., poster
presented at 147th annual meeting of the American Psychiatric
Association, Phildelphia, PA, May 21–26, 1994.

tween onset of bipolar illness and the developmental processes occurring between the peripubertal phase and early adulthood.

What Are the Characteristics of Children Who Will
Develop Bipolar Illness Later in Life?

Few studies of children at risk for bipolar illness have employed ac-
ceptable methods including structured diagnostic assessment and a
comparison group. The studies (see Table 3–2) designed to compare
the lifetime prevalence of psychopathology in children of bipolar probands (top-down design) with control subjects have consistently
found higher rates of both affective and nonaffective psychopathology
in children of bipolar probands. In the largest such study, Grigoroiu-
Serbanescu et al. (1989) used blind raters and structured interviews
to determine DSM-III-R diagnoses in 72 children of bipolar probands
and 72 children of control subjects. Children of bipolar probands had

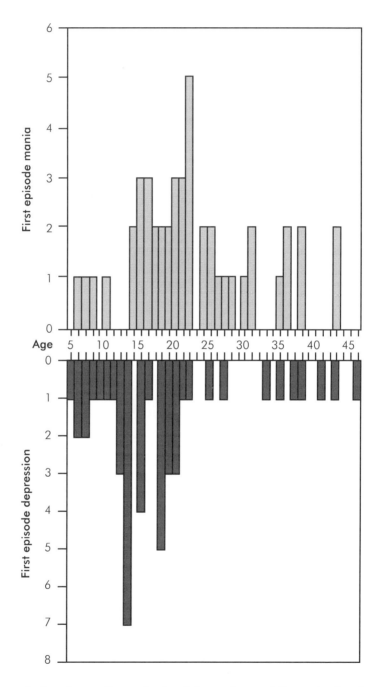

Figure 3–2.   Age at first episode of depression and first episode of mania.

significantly higher rates of psychopathology (61% versus 25%), particularly ADHD (21% versus 7%), anxiety disorder (12% versus 4%), personality disorders (12% versus 3%), and unipolar depression (8% versus 1%). Several factors related to the proband's bipolar illness were predictive of severity of psychopathology in the children, including age at onset of bipolar illness, number of episodes manic or mixed, and number of episodes depressed.

A few studies have provided data addressing the question of early versus late onset of bipolar illness. Taylor and Abrams (1973) stratified bipolar probands on the basis of onset of affective illness before or after age 30 years. Risk of affective illness was 3.5 times greater in the first-degree relatives of early-onset probands (EOP).

Based on study of bipolar probands and their children, Sachs et al. (1994) suggested that age at onset of the proband's mood disorder and the development of anxiety disorders, disruptive behavior disorders, and elimination disorders in early childhood may be factors identifying those children at greatest risk to develop bipolar mood disorder. As part of this study, a cohort of more than 40 bipolar children in 30 families was identified. Pilot results using structured interview methods with blind independent raters (Structured Clinical Interview for DSM-III-R, Schedule for Affective Disorders and Schizophrenia for School-Aged Children, Family Interview for Genetic Studies) showed that those children of probands with early (age ≤ 18 years) onset of mood disorder were significantly more likely to have serious psychopathology than children of probands with onset of mood disorder at age 19 years or later (Sachs et al. 1993). Characterization of these children and their parents included several striking findings that, if replicated, may allow identification of children at risk for serious psychopathology.

- Overall, EOPs met criteria for significantly more comorbid diagnoses (mean, 4.58 ± 2.9) than late-onset probands (mean, 0.65 ± 0.9) with a 2.44 times higher risk for anxiety disorders ($P < .02$).
- Among probands, the EOP group accounted for all observed cases of alcohol abuse, drug abuse, separation anxiety, social phobia, generalized anxiety disorder, overanxious disorder, ADHD, conduct disorder, and enuresis.

Table 3–2. Studies of lifetime prevalence of psychopathology in children of bipolar probands (top-down design)

Investigator	N	Any psychiatric diagnosis		Mood disorder		Comments
		%	n	%	n	
O'Connell et al. 1979	Mothers, 8; fathers, 4; daughters, 9; sons, 13		10		2	
Kuyler 1980	Parents, 27; children, 49	45		8		
Waters and Marchenko-Bouer 1980	Mothers, 8; fathers, 8; children, 48			42 (daughters), 13 (sons)		
LaRoche 1981	Mothers, 5; fathers, 5; children, 17	6		—	—	
Kron et al. 1982	Parents, 18; children, 31	52		25		
Decina et al. 1983	Mothers, 11; fathers, 7; sons, 14; daughters, 17	52	16	26	8	6% ($n = 2$) were diagnosed with ADHD
Waters et al. 1983	Parents, 17; sons, 24; daughters, 29	57	30	45	24	21% were diagnosed with bipolar I disorder

Study	Sample					Findings
Akiskal et al. 1985	Parents, 67; children, 68	100		100		57% were diagnosed with bipolar I disorder
Klein et al. 1985	Parents, 24; sons, 19; daughters, 18	43	16	38	14	27% ($n = 10$) were diagnosed with bipolar I disorder; 5% ($n = 2$) were diagnosed with any anxiety disorder; 11% ($n = 4$) were diagnosed with any disruptive disorder[a]
Hammen et al. 1987	Mothers, 9; sons, 5; daughters, 7	92	11	67	8	? were diagnosed with bipolar I disorder; 38% ($n = 5$) were diagnosed with any anxiety disorder; 33% ($n = 4$) were diagnosed with any disruptive disorder; 8% ($n = 1$) were diagnosed with ADHD[b]
LaRoche et al. 1987	Mothers, 17; fathers, 4; sons, 25; daughters, 12	24	9	16	6	5% ($n = 2$) were diagnosed with any anxiety disorder
Zahn-Waxler 1988	Mothers, 4; fathers, 3; sons, 7	?	?	43	3	? ($n = 7$) were diagnosed with any anxiety disorder; 43% ($n = 3$) were diagnosed with any disruptive disorder

(continued)

Table 3–2. Studies of lifetime prevalence of psychopathology in children of bipolar probands (top-down design) *(continued)*

Investigator	N	Any psychiatric diagnosis		Mood disorder		Comments
		%	n	%	n	
Grigoroiu-Serbanescu et al. 1989	Mothers, 28, fathers, 19; sons, 34, daughters, 38	61	44	10	7	1% (n = 1) were diagnosed with bipolar I disorder; 12% (n = 9) were diagnosed with any anxiety disorder; 14% (n = 10) were diagnosed with any disruptive disorder; 21% (n = 15) were diagnosed with ADHD

Note. ADHD = attention-deficit/hyperactivity disorder. ≥ = assigned number not known.
[a]"Any anxiety disorder" includes panic, phobic, and generalized anxiety disorders. "Any disruptive disorder" includes conduct disorder and antisocial personality.
[b]"Any disruptive disorder" includes ADHD, conduct disorder, and substance abuse.

- Children of EOPs were significantly more likely to receive at least one diagnosis ($P < .02$).
- All observed cases of separation anxiety, simple phobia, social phobia, obsessive-compulsive disorder, overanxious disorder, and enuresis were children of EOPs. The children of EOPs had a 4.2 times higher risk for anxiety disorders ($P < .25$).
- The risk of depression and ADHD in children was nearly the same in both groups.

Nearly all prior studies have suggested that early age at onset occurs in families with high loading for affective illness (Kutcher and Marton 1991; McMahon et al. 1994; Rice et al. 1987; Taylor et al. 1981; Weissman et al. 1984a, 1984b).

Childhood History of Adult Probands

Sachs et al.'s (1994) study of the childhood history of adult bipolar patients has revealed some common patterns seen over the life cycle of these patients (see Figure 3–2).

- Preschool years may be marked by anxiety, elimination disorders, and sleep disorders. Among adult bipolar patients in the study sample, 50% met criteria for an anxiety disorder before the age of 10.
- Prepubertal school-age children frequently meet criteria for disruptive behavior disorders as well as overanxious disorder and panic attacks.
- It is common for adult bipolar patients to date the onset of subsyndromal mood symptoms, dysthymia, and cyclothymia to the years just before or after puberty. Although episodes meeting the full criteria for mania are described as early as age 5, the median age at onset for full affective episodes is in adolescence. Interestingly, Sachs et al.'s (1994) sample shows the median age at onset for depression, substance abuse, and mania to be 16, 18, and 21, respectively.

The significance of comorbid psychopathology, particularly the nonaffective symptoms that occur before the onset of actual mood episodes, is still a matter of speculation. The higher than expected rates of other diagnostic entities seen in bipolar patients may represent a common vulnerability to separate diseases. It is also possible that the early nonaffective symptomatology represents a precursor of the affective illness. It this were the case, such nonaffective illness might provide an opportunity to identify children at risk.

It is easy to accept the idea that many of the children who manifest depression, dysthymia, or cyclothymia will eventually suffer mania or hypomania and should be offered treatment for their mood disorder even before meeting criteria for diagnosis of bipolar illness. For instance, among those meeting criteria for cyclothymia, there is a 15%–50% risk for subsequent development of bipolar I or bipolar II disorder. The relationship between neuropsychiatric abnormalities, bipolar illness, and nonaffective antecedent conditions remains unclear. However, given the similarity between EOPs and their children in the pattern of early nonaffective psychopathology, it seems likely that children of EOP meeting criteria for anxiety, elimination, or disruptive behavior disorders are at high risk for early development of mood disorder. Children with a history of significant birth trauma or abnormality on neuropsychiatric testing should also be considered at high risk. Furthermore, the data from Sachs et al. (1994) suggest children of EOPs may be at much higher risk for substance abuse. The apparent progression of symptoms across development is consistent with the kindling hypothesis and offers the possibility that effective treatment of anxiety disorders might modify the course of illness. Programs aimed at prevention might have little impact on future course unless they reach children before the age of risk for substance abuse.

▶ DIFFERENTIAL DIAGNOSIS

Differentiation of bipolar illness from other psychiatric and medical conditions rests on making the diagnosis of mania. Unfortunately, a variety of obstacles appear to lessen the likelihood that bipolar children and adolescents will be diagnosed. Carlson et al. (1994) compared the diagnosis made by the admitting clinician to the diagnosis made by structured interview, then compared both methods to the consensus diagnosis 6 months after an index hospital admission. Excellent agreement was found between clinicians and structured interview for adults. However, for adolescents, there was significant disagreement; the diagnosis made by structured interview was more likely to agree with the best-estimate diagnosis made at 6 months. This study demonstrated that symptoms of mania are not difficult to elicit but that in younger patients there is a tendency for clinicians to fail in eliciting or recognizing mania. Thus mania is systematically underdiagnosed in young patients.

Unfortunately, the criteria for mania have substantial overlap with several common conditions. As can be seen in Table 3–1, a young patient with 3 or more symptoms of mania would be very likely to meet multiple criteria for ADHD and or conduct disorder. The diagnosis of ADHD requires a period of 6 months during which at least 6 of 14 symptoms are present to a significant degree. A patient whose symptoms of mood elation included pressured speech, flight of ideas, and distractibility could easily meet 10 of the ADHD symptoms. Conduct disorder requires only 3 associated symptoms, but a patient with mood elevation and excessive involvement in pleasurable activities that have high potential for painful consequences could potentially explain 10 symptoms of conduct disorder. Where differential diagnosis is not possible, patients might be best understood as having both illnesses.

Disruptive Behavior Disorder—ADHD

The difficulty in differentiating ADHD and mania during childhood and adolescence suggests a close relationship between these disorders. Biederman et al. (1991) found high rates of affective disorders among first-degrees relatives of probands with attention-deficit disorder. The rate of affective disorder in the relatives was similar for relatives of probands with attention-deficit disorder without a history of comorbid mood disorder (28%) and relatives of probands with attention-deficit disorder plus a mood disorder (25%). The frequency of affective disorder was significantly higher in both groups than in relatives of control subjects.

Symptoms of both ADHD and mania can coexist and overlap (e.g., psychomotor component, impulsivity, distractibility, and shortened attention span). Wozniack et al. (1993) found 90% of children with bipolar illness also met criteria for ADHD, but only 19% of children in an ADHD sample met criteria for mania or hypomania. However, the symptoms of ADHD may start as early as age 2–3 years and tend to continue in a chronic fashion. Gittleman (1985) found no excess of affective illness in a follow-up of hyperactive children. Manic children tend to have later age at onset, pressured speech, flight of ideas, as well as psychotic symptoms that are not typically present in ADHD (see Table 3–1). Bipolar disorder is typically more episodic and may be characterized by rapid mood swings and periods of superior academic performance.

Schizophrenia

The unsupported but strongly held belief that schizophrenia is the most common psychosis in young people hampers recognition of mania in adolescents and older children. Joyce (1984) found that 72% of young patients with a manic episode versus 24% of older patients with a manic episode were given a diagnosis of schizophrenia. Similarly, Werry (1991) found more than half of adolescents presenting with mania were initially misdiagnosed as schizophrenic. A youthful psychotic patient may be diagnosed as schizophrenic instead of manic because the incidence of atypical mood features and psychosis is higher in younger populations (Ballenger et al. 1982). Unfortunately, the belief continues that thought disorder, grandiosity, bizarre delusions, and hallucinations are pathognomonic of schizophrenia. Although the acute florid psychotic presentation of mania in adolescence often resembles schizophrenia, family history, premorbid function, and the longitudinal course are useful in the differentiation of bipolar disorder and schizophrenia.

Personality Disorder

The features of conduct disorder in childhood and antisocial personality disorder in later adolescence include behaviors common in mania (impulsivity, deceit, shoplifting, substance abuse, and aggressiveness) (see Table 3–1). As pointed out by Carlson (1990), the common co-occurrence of ADHD and conduct disorder further complicates the distinction between these disorders and bipolar illness. The lying, stealing, and fighting commonly seen in children with conduct disorder tend to have a more chronic course and are rarely associated with psychotic symptomatology. Additional factors that may be useful in the differential diagnosis are family history, premorbid personality, history of phobia and anxiety disorder, and history of full depressive episodes.

Substance Abuse

DSM-IV recognizes that a manic episode can be induced by drug use as well as drug abuse. Stimulants and hallucinogens, in particular amphetamines, cocaine, and phencyclidine (PCP), can produce a syndrome much like mania even in individuals with no predisposition to bipolar disorder. In addition, the role of caffeine in producing symptoms typical of hypomania is often overlooked. Adolescents, particularly at times when preparing for school exams, are prone to overstimulation by caffeine and may suffer dysphoria on discontinuation of high caffeine intake. The insomnia produced by stimulant use may in itself precipitate mania.

The distinction between drug-induced mania and primary mania/ mixed mania, not substance-induced, is largely based on a history of drug use. Young bipolar patients are probably more prone to drug abuse than their peers and are likely to have mood symptoms prior to their drug use. Careful history sometimes reveals that drug use in this population is an attempt at self-medication. Here, stimulants are typically used to sustain a period of mood elevation or avoid depression at the termination of a hypomanic or manic episode. This pattern of substance abuse appears secondary to a primary mood disorder.

Medical Conditions

Episodes of mania should be distinguished from episodes of mood disorder due to a general medical condition. Although most of these conditions are extremely rare during childhood and adolescence, the clinician should be particularly attentive to ruling out those that are most prevalent (multiple sclerosis, temporal lobe epilepsy, and systemic lupus erythematosus) in the young population.

▶ CONCLUSION

Manic-depressive illness afflicts 1%–2% of the adult population and may be expressed in a large portion of patients before they reach adulthood. Along with acute episodes of depression and mania, bipolar illness is frequently complicated by violence, suicide, substance abuse, interpersonal conflict, and high rates of academic and vocational disability. The impact of this illness is heightened by its tendency to strike during developmentally sensitive periods. Thus, children and adolescents suffering from bipolar illness face additional burdens due to developmental, social, and educational disruption. Furthermore, early age at onset is associated with more severe acute symptoms, poor response to treatment, and poor long-term prognosis.

As has been seen with depression, expectation plays a significant role in the frequency of diagnosis. It is likely that mania and bipolar mood disorders are more common than suggested by older literature. Children with cyclothymia, hypomania, and mania are likely to have a recurrent course and may benefit from early diagnosis and treatment. Risk factors such as having a first-degree relative with early-onset bipolar illness, early onset of psychopathology (including nonaffective disorders), history of birth trauma, or neurological deficits may help clarify the diagnosis or identify patients for whom preventive measures should be considered.

▶ REFERENCES

Akiskal HS, Khani MK, Scott-Strauss A: Cyclothymic temperamental disorders. Psychiatr Clin North Am 2:527–554, 1979

Akiskal H, Downs J, Jordan P, et al: Affective disorders in referred children and younger siblings if manic-depressives. Arch Gen Psychiatry 42:996–1003, 1985

American Psychiatric Association: Diagnostic and Statistical Manual of Mental Disorders, 3rd Edition. Washington, DC, American Psychiatric Association, 1980

American Psychiatric Association: Diagnostic and Statistical Manual of Mental Disorders, 3rd Edition, Revised. Washington, DC, American Psychiatric Association, 1987

American Psychiatric Association: Diagnostic and Statistical Manual of Mental Disorders, 4th Edition. Washington, DC, American Psychiatric Association, 1994

Anthony JC, Scott P: Manic-depressive psychosis in childhood. J Child Psychol Psychiatry 1:53–72, 1960

Ballenger JC, Reus VI, Post RM: The "atypical" clinical picture of adolescent mania. Am J Psychiatry 139:602–606, 1982

Biederman J, Faraone S, Keenan K, et al: Evidence of familial association between attention deficit disorder and major affective disorders. Arch Gen Psychiatry 48:633–642, 1991

Carlson G: Bipolar affective disorders in childhood and adolescence, in Affective Disorders in Childhood and Adolescence. Edited by Cantwell D, Carlson G. New York, Spectrum Publications, 1983, pp 61–83

Carlson G: Annotation: child and adolescent mania—diagnostic considerations. J Child Psychol Psychiatry 31:331–341, 1990

Carlson G, Kashani J: Manic symptoms in a referred adolescent population. J Affect Disord 15:219–226, 1988

Carlson GA, Fenning S, Bromet EJ: The confusion between bipolar disorder and schizophrenia in youth: where does it stand in the 1990s? J Am Acad Child Adolesc Psychiatry 33:453–460, 1994

Dwyer JT, DeLong GR: A family history study of twenty probands with childhood manic depressive illness. J Am Acad Child Adolesc Psychiatry 26:176, 1987

Geller B, Fox LW, Clark KA: Rate and predictors of prepubertal bipolarity during followup of 6- to 12-year-old depressed children. J Am Acad Child Adolesc Psychiatry 33:461–468, 1994

Gittelman R, Mannuzza S, Shenker R, et al: Hyperactive boys almost grown up, I: psychiatric status.Arch Gen Psychiatry 42:937–947, 1985

Grigoroiu-Serbanescu M, Christodorescu D, Jipescu I, et al: Psychopathology in children aged 10–17 of bipolar patients: psychopathology rate and correlates of the severity of psychopathology. J Affect Disord 16:167–179, 1989

Joyce PR: Age of onset in bipolar affective disorder and misdiagnosis as schizophrenia. Psychol Med 14:145–149, 1984

Koran LM: The reliability of clinical methods, data and judgments. N Engl J Med 293:642–646, 1975

Kraepelin E: Manic-Depressive Insanity and Paranoia (1895). Translated by Barclay RM. Edited by Robertson GM. New York, Arno Press, 1976

Kutcher S, Marton P: Affective disorders in first degree relatives of adolescent onset bipolars, unipolars, and normal controls. J Am Acad Child Adolesc Psychiatry 30:75–78, 1991

Loranger A, Levine P: Age of onset of bipolar affective illness. Arch Gen Psychiatry 39:1245–1248, 1978

McMahon FJ, Stine OC, Chase GA, et al: Influence of clinical subtype, sex, and lineality on age at onset of major affective disorder in a family sample. Am J Psychiatry 151:210–215, 1994

Rice J, Reich T, Andreasen NC, et al: The familial transmission of bipolar illness. Arch Gen Psychiatry 44:441–447, 1987

Sachs G: Use of clonazepam for bipolar affective disorder. J Clin Psychiatry 51 (5 suppl):31–34, 1990

Sachs G, Conklin A, Lafer B, et al: Psychopathology in children of late versus early onset bipolar probands. Paper presented at the annual meeting of American Academy of Child and Adolescent Psychiatry, San Antonio, TX, 1993

Sachs GS, Lafer B, Thibault AB, et al: Childhood psychopathology in 40 adult bipolar probands. Paper presented at the annual meeting of American Academy of Child and Adolescent Psychiatry, Philadelphia, PA, 1994

Strober M, Hanna G, McCracken J: Handbook of Child Psychiatric Diagnosis. Edited by Last CG, Hersen M. New York, Wiley, 1989, pp 299–319

Taylor M, Abrams R: Manic states: a genetic study of early and late onset affective disorder. Arch Gen Psychiatry 28:656–658, 1973

Taylor MA, Redfield J, Abrams R: Neuropsychological dysfunction in schizophrenia and affective disease. Biol Psychiatry 16:467–478, 1981

Thomsen PH, Moller LL, Dehlholm B, et al: Manic-depressive psychosis in children younger than 15 years: a register-based investigation of 39 cases in Denmark. Acta Psychiatr Scand 85:401–406, 1992

Vranka TM, Weller RA, Weller EB, et al: Lithium treatment of manic episodes with psychotic features in prepubertal children. Am J Psychiatry 145:1557–1559, 1988

Weinberg WA, Brumback RA: Mania in childhood: case studies and literature review. Am J Dis Child 130:380–385, 1976

Weissman M, Wickramaratne P, Merikangas K, et al: Onset of major depression in early adulthood: increased familial loading and specificity. Arch Gen Psychiatry 41:1136–1143, 1984a

Weissman M, Gersho E, Kidd K, et al: Psychiatric disorders in the relatives of probands with affective disorders: the Yale University-National Institute of Mental Health collaborative study. Arch Gen Psychiatry 41:13–21, 1984b

Weller RA, Tucker S, Weller EB, et al: Prepubertal mania: has it been underdiagnosed? J Affect Disord 11:151–154, 1986

Werry JS: Childhood and adolescent schizophrenic, bipolar, and schizoaffective disorders: a clinical and outcome study. J Am Acad Child Adolesc Psychiatry 30:457–465, 1991

Winokur A, March V, Mendels J: Primary affective disorder in relatives of patients with anorexia nervosa. Am J Psychiatry 137:695–698, 1980

Wozniak J, Biederman J, Kiely K, et al: Prepubertal mania revisited. Paper presented at the annual meeting of American Academy of Child and Adolescent Psychiatry, San Antonio, TX, 1993

CHAPTER 4

ALCOHOL

Barbara J. Mason, Ph.D., and
Raymond L. Ownby, M.D., Ph.D.

T he relation between alcohol use and bipolar disorders is complex, and similarities in their presentations can create confusion. Differences between the two can be obscured by
confusion of specific symptoms with complete syndromes, changes
in diagnostic criteria used in research, and the time in each disorder's
progression when patients are studied. Many bipolar patients abuse
or are dependent on alcohol. Evaluating alcohol use in bipolar patients is important—alcohol use and bipolar disorders occur together
at greater than chance frequency, and both are associated with increased rates of suicide. In this chapter, we review recent research on
the relationship of the two disorders.

▶ RATES OF COMORBID ALCOHOL USE AND BIPOLAR DISORDERS

The Epidemiologic Catchment Area (ECA) study data show that the
prevalence of bipolar disorder in the United States is about 1%,
whereas that of alcohol use disorders is about 14% (Brady and Sonne
1995; Helzer and Pryzbeck 1988; Regier et al. 1990). Helzer and
Pryzbeck (1988) used ECA data to calculate the odds ratio for mania
co-occurring with alcoholism at 6.2. This ratio was higher than the
ratio for any other DSM axis I diagnosis. ECA data show a prevalence
of 31.5% for alcohol dependence in bipolar I subjects (odds ratio 5.5)

and a prevalence of alcohol dependence of 20.8% in bipolar II subjects (odds ratio 3.1). The prevalence of alcohol abuse, by contrast, in bipolar I subjects was 14.7% (odds ratio 3.0), and the prevalence of alcohol abuse in bipolar II subjects was 18.4% (odds ratio 3.9) (Regier et al. 1990). More recently, Nelson et al. (1995) showed higher rates of alcoholism in patients with mood disorders, but they did not address the issues of mood disorder subtypes or the comorbidity of the two disorders. Because unipolar and bipolar mood disorders are probably genetically distinct (Winokur et al. 1995a), this failure is regrettable.

ECA analyses that show a higher than chance co-occurrence of alcohol use with bipolar disorder in the general community has been replicated in studies of treatment-seeking alcoholics. Estimates of the prevalence of bipolar disorder in alcoholism treatment samples range from 1.9% to 4% (Hesselbrock et al. 1985; Ross et al. 1988; Lydiard et al. 1987). Similarly, much higher rates of alcoholism are found in patients treated for bipolar disorder than in the general population, ranging from 5% to 58% (Estroff et al. 1985; Freed 1969; Keller et al. 1993; Miller et al. 1989; Morrison 1974; Reich et al. 1974; Winokur et al. 1969; Zisook and Schuckit 1987). Studies in different settings are thus consistent in reporting elevated rates of comorbid alcohol use and bipolar disorders.

▶ Genetic Factors

The co-occurrence of alcohol use and bipolar disorders suggests the possibility of an underlying biological or genetic predisposition. Support for this theory would be provided by increased rates of alcoholism in relatives of patients with mania. D. W. Goodwin et al. (1973) did not find increased rates of mood disorders in adopted-away sons of alcoholics; James and Chapman (1975) did not find increased rates of alcohol use disorders in families of bipolar patients. Ingraham and Wender (1992) studied the risk for development of alcoholism in persons related to those with mood disorders. They found elevated rates of both mood disorders and alcoholism in adopted-away children of persons with mood disorders alone. Ingraham and Wender, however, did not differentiate among various mood disorders in this sample, making it difficult to draw conclusions.

In a more definitive study, Winokur et al. (1993) studied 189 bipolar patients from the National Institute of Mental Health collaborative study on the psychobiology of depression. They found higher rates of alcoholism in the families of the bipolar patients than in the families of unipolar patients, even when alcoholism in the probands was controlled. This difference, however, was not significant, and a later study showed no relation between family history of alcoholism and bipolar disorder (Winokur et al. 1995b). A consensus now exists that alcohol use disorders are not part of the spectrum of bipolar disorders; these disorders are transmitted independently.

▶ Diagnostic Issues

The overlap between symptoms of alcohol use and bipolar disorders presents a diagnostic challenge whether the disorders occur separately or in combination. Increased alcohol intake, for example, can result from developing tolerance to alcohol (a diagnostic criterion for alcohol dependence) or from increased activity in a manic episode. Conversely, psychiatric symptoms such as grandiosity, irritability, or expansiveness can arise during a manic episode or alcohol intoxication. Other symptoms, such as insomnia, psychomotor agitation, or anxiety, may be symptoms of a hypomanic or manic episode or alcohol withdrawal. Symptoms of one disorder can thus mask or confuse the presentation of the other. Especially relevant are data that show that alcohol use may precipitate a bipolar disorder that then persists independent of alcohol use (Winokur et al. 1994).

Clinical evaluation of bipolar patients should routinely include inquiry about alcohol use and its sequelae. Alcohol intoxication can be ruled out by patient or observer report, by the smell of alcohol on the patient's breath, or by assay of alcohol in the patient's breath or blood. Alcohol withdrawal symptoms will abate in response to benzodiazepines. Accurate diagnosis of alcohol use disorders in bipolar patients can be more challenging. Diagnosis may be impeded by unreliability in their history giving and by reluctance of the clinician to ask about patients' alcohol use. Additional assessment strategies can include use of a collateral informant designated by the patient; systematic inquiry using standardized diagnostic criteria; obtaining a family history of each disorder; and learning about medical, legal, employment, and relationship problems related to these disorders. An elevation (greater than 30 units) of γ-glutamyltransferase (GGT) is a sensitive, commonly available laboratory indicator of heavy drinking (Rosman and Lieber 1990).

DSM-IV (American Psychiatric Association 1994) includes diagnostic criteria for alcohol-related disorders that present with mood disorder symptoms. An alcohol-induced mood disorder, with manic features, with onset during intoxication (or withdrawal) can be distinguished from a primary manic episode: manic symptoms result from the physiological effects of alcohol during intoxication with alcohol or withdrawal from alcohol. Full criteria for a manic episode need not be met for this diagnosis, although manic symptoms must be more intense than the behaviors often associated with alcohol intoxication or withdrawal. They also must be sufficiently severe as to cause distress, impair functioning, or require clinical attention.

An alcohol-induced manic episode does not count in meeting criteria for bipolar I disorder (these criteria require the occurrence of at least one manic or hypomanic episode). If alcohol use does not fully account for the episode, or if the manic symptoms continue independently after alcohol-related symptoms resolve (about a month), then the manic episode could count toward the diagnosis of bipolar I disorder. A "false-positive" diagnosis of alcohol abuse could occur in bipolar patients. Drinking during a manic episode could result in the harmful social sequelae (damaging consequences to vocational or social functioning) included in the diagnostic criteria for alcohol abuse. When these sequelae are accompanied by evidence of tolerance, withdrawal, or compulsive alcohol-seeking behavior related to alcohol, a DSM-IV diagnosis of alcohol dependence is unequivocal, no matter what other mood disorder symptoms are present.

▶ PRIMARY VERSUS SECONDARY DISORDERS

Schuckit (1986) and others emphasize the importance of deciding whether an alcohol use or mood disorder is primary (occurs before another disorder) or secondary (occurs after another disorder has begun). Alcohol use, for example, may result in symptoms of clinical depression, whereas some have seen alcohol use as an attempt by depressed individuals to self-medicate. The person's clinical course is hypothesized to follow the typical pattern of the primary disorder. Discriminating between primary and secondary disorders is possible based on chronology of occurrence; the disorder that appeared first is primary. Schuckit reported that among patients he has studied, clinical course is likely to follow that of the primary disorder. Primary bipolar disorder with secondary alcohol abuse, for example, would suggest that a patient's drinking might have been an attempt at self-medication. The course of the illness would be expected to follow that of bipolar disorder. Conversely, primary alcohol dependence with a secondary manic episode would suggest that manic symptoms stem from physical effects of alcohol. Here the illness' course would follow that of alcohol dependence.

When alcohol and mood disorders occur together, they cannot be assessed from ECA study data, because they show the age at which the first symptom of a disorder appeared rather than age at onset of the full syndrome. Presence of a disorder was determined as the occurrence of sufficient symptoms to meet criteria over the life course. A mood disorder symptom might occur first, even though the full syndrome of alcohol dependence was present before the complete syndrome of major depression. Reports about occasional occurrences of isolated symptoms, sometimes years apart, do not provide enough information to decide whether disorders are comorbid. The higher prevalence of alcohol dependence than of alcohol abuse, comorbid with bipolar disorders in the ECA data, fails to support a self-medication explanation for co-occurrence of alcohol use disorders in bipolar patients. Another study that did not support this hypothesis is that of Strakowski et al. (1992); the authors reported that among their sample of first-admission manic patients, onset of alcohol use disorder preceded onset of mania in all but one of their patients with comorbidity.

Strakowski et al. (1992) prospectively studied age at onset and comorbidity in 41 consecutive first-hospital admissions for bipolar disorder. All presented with manic or mixed symptoms. Alcohol dependence was the most common comorbid diagnosis, affecting 24.4% of these patients. The onset of substance abuse preceded first hospitalization by more than 1 year in all but one subject. The authors noted that prodromal affective symptoms may have predated or been concurrent with the onset of substance abuse, but this possibility could not be reliably determined from the data. The relation of the two disorders in these patients is thus unclear.

Winokur et al. (1994) showed that patients with primary or secondary alcohol use disorders may represent distinct subtypes. They followed a group of bipolar patients for 10 years. Patients whose alcohol use disorder preceded mood symptoms had fewer exacerbations of their bipolar disorder in the follow-up period than did those whose drinking developed after their mood disorders. The course of alcohol use disorders in this sample confirmed Schuckit's (1986) argument. Patients with primary alcohol use disorders were much more likely to continue to have alcohol problems over 10 years. Those whose drinking problem was secondary were more likely to stop drinking over the same period.

Roy et al. (1991) studied 249 alcoholic men at the Laboratory of Clinical Studies, National Institute on Alcohol Abuse and Alcoholism (NIAAA). They divided these men into two groups: those whose heavy drinking began either before or after age 20 years (early versus late onset). Significantly more of the men in the early-onset group had lifetime histories of hypomanic disorder (9% versus 2%), of bipolar disorder (9% versus 3%), and of suicide attempts. The men with an early onset of drinking also endorsed more Schedule for Affective Disorders and Schizophrenia items assessing characteristics of antisocial personality than did men whose heavy drinking began after age 20 years. No significant differences were found between women with an early versus a late onset of heavy drinking ($N = 90$). These data show that age at onset of heavy drinking may define groups of male alcoholics who are different in important ways, including their risk for developing a secondary bipolar disorder.

▶ LITHIUM AND ALCOHOLISM

Similarities in symptoms and the successful treatment of bipolar disorder with lithium led to interest in using lithium to treat alcoholism. Lithium might act on underlying mood disorders in alcoholics or by directly affecting alcohol consumption in alcoholics without mood disorders. Early support for using lithium to treat alcoholism came from a study that showed reductions in voluntary alcohol consumption in lithium-treated rats (Ho and Tsai 1976). Further support came from a study of alcoholics that found that lithium blocked some effects of alcohol, such as the sensation of intoxication and the desire to continue drinking (Judd and Huey 1984). Drinking behavior outside a laboratory is not as responsive to lithium treatment. Early clinical trials of lithium with alcohol-dependent patients had mixed results, and dropout rates were high.

Fawcett and colleagues (Fawcett 1989; Fawcett et al. 1984, 1987) conducted a 12-month placebo-controlled lithium trial in alcohol-dependent patients. They found that compliance with treatment was a strong predictor of outcome, no matter which treatment patients were assigned to. Lithium treatment reduced the risk of relapse to drinking only during the first month of this 12-month study. All outcomes in this study were independent of the presence of comorbid depressive disorder.

The largest, most rigorously controlled, and most recent, lithium in alcoholism study found no support for lithium as a treatment for alcoholism (Dorus et al. 1989). Patients were separated into depressed and nondepressed categories and randomly assigned to 1 year of double-blind treatment with lithium or placebo. No differences were found between lithium and placebo treatment in either the depressed or nondepressed groups on several outcome measures.

Early reports of successful treatment of alcoholic dependence with lithium have been attributed to the inclusion in these studies of patients with unrecognized manic-depressive illness. Nagel et al. (1991) described a syndrome of irritability, grandiosity, increased sociability, hypersexuality, and loquaciousness in about half their inpatients after detoxification. This syndrome resembles hypomania, and Nagel et al. hypothesized that it might be treated with lithium. In a small pilot study, patients with a personal or family history of bipolar disorder were excluded. The study then assessed response of this syndrome to double-blind treatment with lithium or placebo. They found significant decreases in hypomanic symptoms in the lithium-treated group after 2 weeks of treatment. These authors argued that lithium's effects on mood may have a time-limited impact on alcoholism. They proposed that lithium's initial mood-stabilizing effects decrease patients' return to drinking in the early recovery period. Lithium treatment may not prevent longer term relapses that could be related to psychosocial factors as well as biological predisposition. Nagel et al. suggested that a brief normalization of mood may be a useful intervention when it is part of other rehabilitative efforts such as psychotherapy and education. Without mood stabilization, these other efforts may not benefit some patients during the period immediately following detoxification.

The Nagel et al. (1991) study showed that hypomania during early recovery may respond to lithium. Much additional research is needed on treatment of bipolar patients who also have alcohol use disorders. No controlled clinical trials have been done in alcohol-dependent patients with comorbid bipolar I disorder, although this would be the group for whom lithium treatment would be most appropriate. Studies should also investigate whether alcohol abuse alters the lithium pharmacokinetics. Bipolar patients who are alcohol dependent are often noncompliant with lithium, thus reducing the effectiveness of and increasing the dangers associated with this treatment. Strategies for enhancing compliance should be further developed. It is unclear whether alcoholic bipolar patients are ambivalent about taking lithium due to the drug-free philosophy of Alcoholics Anonymous (AA) and other self-help groups. Does this affect their compliance with treatment? Assessing whether predictor variables can be found that define subtypes of patients who are differentially responsive to treatment would be useful. For example, Wolpe et al. (1993) reported a profile of variables in mixed dual-diagnosis inpatients that predicted noncompliance with aftercare treatment. These variables included a presenting complaint of cocaine dependence, more erratic pattern of privilege loss and gain during the inpatient stay, and discharge diagnosis of depression. Other variables might be found to make clinicians better able to assess patients for likelihood of noncompliance.

Alcoholic bipolar patients treated with lithium should be informed of potential interaction effects between alcohol and lithium. Alcohol has additive, occasionally synergistic, effects with lithium that can affect judgment and driving. Increased thirst can lead to increased alcohol consumption. F. K. Goodwin and Jamison (1990) found liver damage that resulted from insidious and often unnoticed increases in drinking. Verifying a patient's drinking status from a friend or relative, repeat liver function tests (GGT, alanine aminotransferase [ALT], aspartate aminotransferase [AST]), and lithium plasma levels may be especially important in managing alcoholic patients with bipolar disorder who are being treated with lithium.

Potential Pharmacotherapies

On a more theoretical note, Brady and Lydiard (1992) reviewed the literature on kindling in alcoholism and in bipolar disorder. They argued that a comparison of lithium with an antikindling agent, such as valproate or carbamazepine, would be useful with patients with comorbid alcoholism and bipolar disorder. Post et al. (1984) proposed that bipolar disorder may be a kindling-like phenomenon. The course of the disorder is characterized by increasingly short periods of remission between episodes of illness, and later episodes are less dependent on environmental causes. In a similar vein, Brown et al. (1986) noted that alcoholics with more prior withdrawals from alcohol use were more likely to experience seizures during subsequent withdrawals. They hypothesized that progressive changes in the central nervous system may accrue during repeat episodes of alcohol abuse and withdrawal. Providing additional support for this hypothesis, Malcolm et al. (1989) found that carbamazepine was as effective as oxazepam in treating alcohol withdrawal.

More recently, however, in a 10-year follow-up study, Winokur et al. (1994) showed that the course of bipolar disorder may not represent a kindling phenomenon. In a prospective longitudinal study, they found that patients with rapid cycling did not maintain this pattern; over time, their episodes became less rather than more frequent. For other patients, the frequency of mood disorder exacerbations also became less rather than more frequent. Both findings are inconsistent with the kindling hypothesis of bipolar disorder. Winokur et al. also showed (discussed earlier) that the frequency of alcohol use disorders declined with time. Although secondary alcoholics were more likely to remit than were primary alcoholics, the overall frequency of alcohol use disorders decreased over the 10-year period. This finding is inconsistent with a kindling hypothesis of alcohol use disorders.

Valproate has been widely used in recent years as a mood-stabilizing agent, and is effective in the management of mania (Bowden et al. 1994). Given this use plus its known antikindling properties, valproate is a logical candidate for treating comorbid bipolar and alcohol use disorders. Brady et al. (1994) reported the effective use of valproate in two patients with manic symptoms and alcohol abuse. Both patients' mood symptoms improved with valproate use, and they maintained abstinence from alcohol at follow-up. In a later report, Brady et al. (1995) showed similar therapeutic effects in a group of substance-abusing persons, some of whom used alcohol exclusively. They speculated that valproate may reduce both substance craving and mood symptoms.

Kresyun et al. (1991) reported greater suppression of alcohol consumption in alcohol-dependent rats treated with the semihydrated lithium salt of pyridine-3-carboxylic acid (Lithonit), than with lithium carbonate or lithium chloride. These authors reported that, unlike the latter two compounds, the therapeutic efficacy of Lithonit consistently correlated with alcohol dehydrogenase and catalase activity stabilization and with the concentration of nicotinamide coenzymes and lipid peroxides. Lithonit may have potential utility as a new drug for alcoholic bipolar patients, although clinical trials have not been reported.

Finally, clozapine may be effective in reducing symptoms of mania (Zarate et al. 1995). Zarate et al. showed that patients with manic symptoms were more likely to respond to clozapine than were schizophrenic patients without clear mood symptoms. Although clozapine may thus be considered in treatment of manic patients, enthusiasm for this treatment in patients with comorbid alcohol use disorders must be tempered by knowledge of one of clozapine's possible adverse effects, the development of seizures.

▶ GENERAL TREATMENT CONSIDERATIONS

The importance of early identification and effective treatment of comorbid alcoholism and bipolar disorder was confirmed in a study of features associated with suicide attempts among participants in a maintenance therapy in recurrent depression protocol (Bulik et al. 1990).

Comorbid alcoholism or bipolar II disorder were among the five features used in a logistic regression analysis that correctly classified 77% of suicide attempters over this 4-year protocol (67 attempted suicide and 163 did not). Further supporting the need for effective intervention for these comorbid patients, Tohen et al. (1990) reported that history of alcoholism was a predictor of an unfavorable outcome in mania in a 4-year posttreatment follow-up study.

Liskow et al. (1982) stressed that although it may be appealing to our sense of parsimony to consider excessive drinking as a symptom of mood disorder that will cease when it is controlled, in practice this usually does not occur. Patients with comorbid disorder thus require the same commitment to abstinence as do alcoholics without mood disorders.

Integrated Treatment Approach to Comorbidity

The *Eighth Special Report to the U.S. Congress on Alcohol and Health* (National Institute on Alcohol Abuse and Alcoholism 1993) reviewed the recent literature on organizational barriers to treatment of patients with alcoholism and comorbid psychiatric disorders. The data reviewed suggested that diagnosis and treatment are frequently suboptimal because psychiatric and alcoholism treatment services are usually administered by separate agencies and provided by different staff members, a problem compounded by the lack of professionals trained to treat both disorders (Sellman 1989).

Our mental health system is oriented to treating single rather than multiple disorders. Bipolar patients with comorbid alcohol use disorders may be less likely to be referred for treatment of the alcoholism and to receive less treatment than nonalcoholic peers (Solomon 1986; Solomon and Davis 1986). The NIAAA report described how comorbid patients can be caught in a therapeutic catch-22, in which they cannot enter the mental health service system until they stop drinking, and cannot enter alcoholism treatment until their bipolar disorder is controlled. Studies suggest that specialized treatments for comorbid patients could bypass many such problems (Jerrell and Ridgely 1995; Lehman et al. 1989) and that standard therapeutic approaches to alcoholism treatment may be less effective for comorbid patients (Osher and Kofoed 1989). Osher and Kofoed proposed integrated treatment programs for comorbid patients that include the following features: strategies to engage and retain patients in treatment, persuasion about the relation of alcohol abuse to psychiatric disorder, and concomitant treatment of both disorders to avoid any conflict between treatment modalities.

Methods to Increase Compliance With Treatment

In studies of lithium and alcoholism, Fawcett and colleagues (Fawcett 1989; Fawcett et al. 1984, 1987) showed that compliance with treatment is an important predictor of outcome for many alcoholics, no matter the treatment assignment. This evidence suggests that strategies to enhance compliance may be particularly important in this population. In a similar way, compliance with treatment is closely related to rehospitalization among patients with mental disorders, including bipolar disorder (Casper and Regan 1993; Goldberg et al. 1995). Drinking may affect patients' ability or desire to comply with a prescribed medication regimen. Compliance may be increased by involving a close friend or relative designated by the patient to witness the taking of medication at a set time of the day, verify drinking status at regular intervals, and inform the treatment provider when a significant relapse occurs. Drug plasma levels offer another important source of compliance data and should be obtained regularly. Alcoholics frequently strive to maintain their jobs despite decline in functioning in other areas. Therefore, a contract with the patient specifying a work-related contingency, such as Employee Assistance Program reporting, may serve as a motivator for treatment compliance and abstinence.

Informing patients and their significant others about the properties and common side effects of medication they are taking may also increase compliance. We have found it helpful to give comorbid patients a "fact sheet" regarding their medication to read and keep, and we refer to it at regular intervals. The fact sheet includes a statement that the drug is not addicting, habit forming, or mood altering; describes potential interactions with alcohol; lists common side effects; gives their physician's name and 24-hour emergency phone number; instructs patients to call their physician if they are having problems with their medication; and lists potential effects of discontinuing or reducing medication precipitously and without medical advice.

Psychoeducational Strategies

Patients and their significant others should be educated about the disease models of both alcoholism and bipolar disorder and about how one disorder can interact with the other. For example, alcohol can alter sleep patterns and induce pathological mood changes, which in turn can exacerbate or precipitate an episode of bipolar disorder. Patients with alcoholism and comorbid bipolar disorder therefore should be strongly cautioned to abstain from drinking. Bipolar patients with a family history of alcoholism should be advised about the increased risk for alcoholism, although they may not currently meet criteria for an alcohol use disorder.

Self-help groups in the community (e.g., the Manic Depressive Support Group, AA, Al-Anon, Rational Recovery) can be helpful in reinforcing the disease model and in offering coping strategies and fellowship. Rational Recovery is a nonreligious self-help group that may appeal to alcoholics who are put off by the "higher power" component of AA. However, the fragility and lack of social assurance of comorbid patients may make them more resistant than are noncomorbid alcoholics to group modalities.

The Treatment Branch of NIAAA has developed manuals for three alcoholism-specific individual psychotherapies as part of a multicenter matching study of patient variables and therapy characteristics. The coping skills of cognitive-behavioral therapy may be particularly effective for a broad range of patients. This structured therapy focuses on identifying cues that prompt a patient to drink and developing strategies for avoiding or coping with these situations without drinking (Kadden et al. 1993; O'Malley et al. 1992). Patients are also given homework reviewed with the therapist in their next session. The coping skills approach may be helpful during the early outpatient phase of treatment in recently stabilized comorbid patients, although patients presenting with both alcoholism and bipolar disorder probably require inpatient treatment. Assessing suicide potential is critical in such patients. The cue recognition components of the therapy may be applied to recognizing triggers associated with the emergence of affective symptoms as well as drinking behavior.

▶ SUMMARY

The cost of comorbid alcoholism and bipolar disorder is extremely high to both the individual and society, yet little is known about effective treatments for such patients. This situation is particularly unfortunate given the morbidity and mortality associated with these illnesses. Furthermore, the complexity of genetic and environmental factors causally associated with alcoholism make it unlikely that any single treatment approach will be equally effective for all comorbid patients. Matching studies may give us future guidelines about treatments that are efficacious for subgroups of patients with a certain pattern of characteristics. However, the data currently available show that integrating pharmacotherapy with behavioral and psychosocial treatments is associated with an optimal outcome.

Comorbid alcoholism and bipolar disorder, by definition, are associated with marked impairment in social and occupational functioning, and potentially harmful behavior to self and others. Clearly, although pharmacotherapy may be integral to attenuating an episode and maintaining a symptom-free state, medication alone would not be sufficient to treat the associated psychosocial sequelae. Psychosocial and behavioral strategies are needed to help patients avoid relapse. These strategies would help the patient manage psychosocial stressors and develop impulse control and interpersonal skills. They would also help the patient to recognize cues that signal a new episode of illness and then to seek treatment before a full-scale relapse.

▶ REFERENCES

American Psychiatric Association: Diagnostic and Statistical Manual of Mental Disorders, 4th Edition. Washington, DC, American Psychiatric Association, 1994
Bowden CL, Brugger AM, Swann AC, et al: Efficacy of divalproex vs lithium and placebo in the treatment of mania. JAMA 271:918–924, 1994
Bulik CM, Carpenter LL, Kupfer DJ, et al: Features associated with suicide attempts in recurrent major depression. J Affect Disord 18:29–37, 1990

Brady KT, Lydiard RB: Bipolar affective disorder and substance abuse. J Clin Psychopharmacol 12 (suppl 1):17S–22S, 1992

Brady KT, Sonne SC: The relationship between substance abuse and bipolar disorder. J Clin Psychiatry 56 (suppl 3):19–24, 1995

Brady KT, Sonne S, Lydiard RB: Valproate treatment of comorbid panic disorder and affective disorders in two alcoholic patients (letter). J Clin Psychopharmacol 14:81–82, 1994

Brady KT, Sonne SC, Anton R, et al: Valproate in the treatment of acute bipolar affective episodes complicated by substance abuses: a pilot study. J Clin Psychiatry 56:118–121, 1995

Brown ME, Anton RF, Malcolm R, et al: Alcoholic detoxification and withdrawal seizures: clinical support for a kindling hypothesis. Biol Psychiatry 43:107–113, 1986

Casper ES, Regan JR: Reasons for admission among six profile subgroups of recidivists of inpatient services. Can J Psychiatry 38:657–661, 1993

Dorus W, Ostrow DG, Anton R, et al: Lithium treatment of depressed and nondepressed alcoholics. JAMA 262:1646–1652, 1989

Estroff TW, Dackis CA, Gold MS, et al: Drug abuse and bipolar disorders. Int J Psychiatry Med 15:37–40, 1985

Fawcett J: Valproate use in acute mania and bipolar disorder: an international perspective. J Clin Psychiatry 50 (suppl):10–12, 1989

Fawcett J, Clark DC, Gibbons RD, et al: Evaluation of lithium therapy for alcoholism. J Clin Psychiatry 45:494–499, 1984

Fawcett J, Scheftner W, Clark D, et al: Clinical predictors of suicide in patients with major affective disorders: a controlled prospective study. Am J Psychiatry 144:35–40, 1987

Freed EX: Alcohol abuse by manic patients. Psychol Rep 25:280, 1969

Goldberg JF, Harrow M, Grossman LS: Recurrent affective syndromes in bipolar and unipolar mood disorders at follow-up. Br J Psychiatry 166:382–385, 1995

Goodwin DW, Schulsinger F, Hermansen L, et al: Alcohol problems in adoptees raised apart from alcoholic biological parents. Arch Gen Psychiatry 28:233–243, 1973

Goodwin FK, Jamison KR: Manic-Depressive Illness. New York, Oxford University Press, 1990

Helzer JE, Pryzbeck TR: The co-occurrence of alcoholism with other psychiatric disorders in the general population and its impact on treatment. J Stud Alcohol 49:219–224, 1988

Hesselbrock MN, Meyer RE, Keener JJ: Psychopathology in hospitalized alcoholics. Arch Gen Psychiatry 42:1050–1055, 1985

Ho AKS, Tsai CS: Effects of lithium on alcohol preference and withdrawal. Ann N Y Acad Sci 273:371–377, 1976

Ingraham LJ, Wender PH: Risk for affective disorder and alcohol and other drug abuse in the relatives of affectively ill adoptees. J Affect Disord 26:45–52, 1992

James NM, Chapman CJ: A genetic study of bipolar affective disorder. Br J Psychiatry 126:449–456, 1975

Jerrell JM, Ridgely MS: Evaluating changes in symptoms and functioning of dually diagnosed clients in specialized treatment. Psychiatric Services 46:233–238, 1995

Judd LL, Huey LY: Lithium antagonizes ethanol intoxication in alcoholics. Am J Psychiatry 141:1517–1521, 1984

Kadden RM, Carroll K, Donovan D, et al: Cognitive behavioral coping skills program: a clinical research protocol for therapists treating individuals with alcohol dependence or abuse (NIAAA Monogr Ser). Washington, DC, National Institute on Alcohol Abuse and Alcoholism, 1993

Keller MB, Lavori PW, Coryell W, et al: Differential outcome of pure manic, mixed/cycling, and pure depressive episodes in patients with bipolar illness. JAMA 255:3138–3142, 1993

Kresyun VL, Aryaev VL, Kostev FI: Chronic alcohol dependence: efficiency of lithium salts therapy. Lithium 2:163–166, 1991

Lehman AF, Meyers CP, Corty E: Assessment and classification of patients with psychiatric and substance abuse syndromes. Hosp Community Psychiatry 40:1019–1025, 1989

Liskow B, Mayfield D, Thiele J: Alcohol and affective disorder: assessment and treatment. J Clin Psychiatry 43:144–147, 1982

Lydiard RB, Howell EF, Ballenger JC, et al: Prevalence of anxiety and mood disorders in hospitalized alcoholics. Presented at the annual meeting of the American College of Neuropsychopharmacology, San Juan, Puerto Rico, December 1987

Malcolm R, Ballenger JC, Sturgis ET, et al: Double-blind controlled trial comparing carbamazepine to oxazepam treatment of alcohol withdrawal. Am J Psychiatry 146:617–621, 1989

Miller FT, Busch F, Tanenbaum JH: Drug abuse in schizophrenia and bipolar disorder. Am J Drug Alcohol Abuse 15:291–295, 1989

Morrison JR: Bipolar affective disorder and alcoholism. Am J Psychiatry 131:1130–1133, 1974

Nagel K, Adler LE, Bell J, et al: Lithium carbonate and mood disorder in recently detoxified alcoholics: a double-blind, placebo-controlled pilot study. Alcoholism: Clinical and Experimental Research 15:978–981, 1991

National Institute on Alcohol Abuse and Alcoholism: Eighth Special Report to the U.S. Congress on Alcohol and Health. Rockville, MD, U.S. Department of Health and Human Services, 1993

Nelson E, Rice J, Rochberg N, et al: Affective illness in family members and matched controls. Acta Psychiatr Scand 91:146–151, 1995

O'Malley SS, Jaffe AJ, Change G, et al: Naltrexone and coping skills therapy for alcohol dependence. Arch Gen Psychiatry 49:881–887, 1992

Osher FC, Kofoed LL: Treatment of patients with psychiatric and psychoactive substance abuse disorders. Hosp Community Psychiatry 40:1025–1030, 1989

Post RM, Rubinow DR, Ballenger JC: Conditioning, sensitization, and kindling: implications for the course of affective illness, in Neurobiology of Mood Disorders. Edited by Post RM, Ballenger JC. Baltimore, MD, Williams & Wilkins, 1984, pp 432–466

Regier DA, Farmer ME, Rae DS, et al: Comorbidity of mental disorders with alcohol and other drug abuse: results from the Epidemiologic Catchment Area (ECA) study. JAMA 264:2511–2518, 1990

Reich LH, Davies RK, Himmelhoch JM: Excessive alcohol use in manic-depressive illness. Am J Psychiatry 131:83–86, 1974

Rosman AS, Lieber CS: Biochemical markers of alcohol consumption. Alcohol Health and Research World 14:210–218, 1990

Ross HE, Glaser FB, Germanson T: The prevalence of psychiatric disorders in patients with alcohol and other drug problems. Arch Gen Psychiatry 45:1023–1031, 1988

Roy A, DeJong J, Lamparski D, et al: Mental disorders among alcoholics. Arch Gen Psychiatry 48:423–427, 1991

Schuckit MA: Genetic and clinical implications of alcoholism and affective disorder. Am J Psychiatry 143:140–147, 1986

Sellman D: Services for alcohol and drug dependent patients with psychiatric comorbidity. N Z Med J 102:390, 1989

Solomon P: Receipt of aftercare services by problem types: psychiatric, psychiatric/substance abuse and substance abuse. Psychiatr Q 58:180–188, 1986

Solomon P, Davis JM: The effects of alcohol abuse among the new chronically mentally ill. Soc Work Health Care 11:65–74, 1986

Strakowski SM, Tohen M, Stoll AL, et al: Comorbidity in mania at first hospitalization. Am J Psychiatry 149:554–556, 1992

Tohen M, Waternaux CM, Tsuang MT: Outcome in mania. Arch Gen Psychiatry 47:1105–1111, 1990

Winokur G, Clayton PJ, Reich T: Manic Depressive Illness. St. Louis, MO, CV Mosby, 1969

Winokur G, Coryell W, Endicott J, et al: Further distinctions between manic-depressive illness (bipolar disorder) and primary depressive disorder (unipolar depression). Am J Psychiatry 150:1176–1181, 1993

Winokur G, Coryell W, Akiskal HS, et al: Manic-depressive (bipolar) disorder: the course in light of a prospective ten-year follow-up of 131 patients. Acta Psychiatr Scand 89:102–110, 1994

Winokur G, Coryell W, Akiskal HS, et al: Alcoholism in manic-depressive (bipolar) illness: familial illness, course of illness, and the primary-secondary distinction. Am J Psychiatry 152:365–372, 1995a

Winokur G, Coryell W, Keller M, et al: A family study of manic-depressive (bipolar I) disease. Arch Gen Psychiatry 52:367–373, 1995b

Wolpe PR, Gorton G, Serota R, et al: Predicting compliance of dual diagnosis inpatients with aftercare treatment. Hosp Community Psychiatry 44:45–49, 1993

Zarate CA, Tohen M, Baldessarini RJ: Clozapine in severe mood disorders. J Clin Psychiatry 56:411–417, 1995

Zisook S, Schuckit MA: Male primary alcoholics with and without family histories of affective disorder. J Stud Alcohol 48:337–344, 1987

CHAPTER 5

GENETICS

Sylvia G. Simpson, M.D., and
J. Raymond DePaulo Jr., M.D.

T he last decade has produced a dramatic increase in knowledge regarding the genes and genetic mechanisms involved in many familial diseases. However, despite a century of clinical research supporting a genetic contribution to bipolar disorder (beginning with Kraepelin [1895/1976]), the last decade has produced several genetic linkage studies of bipolar disorder, several of which have been recanted or "reevaluated" (Baron et al. 1993; Kelsoe et al. 1989) and only two have been convincingly replicated. Thus, the field is still awaiting a replicated linkage finding. In this chapter, we present a brief review of the methodology of genetic studies and attempt to answer the following questions: What types of genetic studies of bipolar disorder have been done and what do we know from them about the genetic causes of bipolar disorder? What are the issues that complicate bipolar genetics? What new molecular technologies and analytic methods are being employed to elucidate the genetic underpinnings of bipolar disorder? How are they likely to affect the search for genes for bipolar disorder?

▶ METHODOLOGY OF LINKAGE STUDIES

Genetic linkage studies consist of several components: clinical assessment and diagnosis, deoxyribonucleic acid (DNA) analysis, and genetic analysis based on the clinical and laboratory data.

Clinical Assessment and Diagnosis

The family study method of directly interviewing family members with a semistructured interview instrument is preferred. All psychopathology must be carefully described, because delineating a Mendelian subtype(s) of the illness may depend on a discriminatory characteristic such as early age at onset. Best-estimate diagnoses (Leckman et al. 1982) for all interviewed family members are made by one or more senior psychiatrists based on data from an interview such as the Schedule for Affective Disorders and Schizophrenia, Lifetime Version (SADS-L) (Endicott and Spitzer 1978), on hospital and outpatient treatment records, and on information from family informants. Diagnoses are made in accordance with accepted diagnostic criteria such as the Research Diagnostic Criteria (Spitzer et al. 1975).

Establishing the phenotype is critical to the success of any genetic study. This process involves 1) a decision as to which conditions constitute the affected phenotype and 2) the ability to diagnose these conditions accurately.

A decision must be made as to whether only "core" diagnoses will constitute the affected phenotype or whether spectrum disorders will also be included. The exclusion of spectrum disorders decreases sensitivity but increases the specificity (Kendler 1988). Reliability and validity of the diagnoses are related issues. The formulation of diagnostic criteria has been associated with a substantial increase in the reliability of the direct assessment of affective disorders. However desirable, reliability does not ensure the validity of diagnoses. Neither does the decline in reliability seen in some diagnoses make them invalid for genetic analysis (Faraone and Tsuang 1994).

Diagnosing an unaffected individual as affected (false positive) decreases the power of the linkage analysis. Thus, the diagnosticians should use a high threshold for calling a case in these studies. The use of an "uncertain phenotype" classification allows some difficult cases to be excluded from the analyses; they should be followed up at regular intervals to determine whether their status becomes clear after repeated assessments. For the same reason, every attempt must be made to screen out nongenetically caused cases, known as phenocopies. Diagnosing as unaffected someone who actually has the gene (false negative) usually results from lack of expression of the gene (incomplete penetrance). This can be more easily accounted for by employing an estimate of penetrance in the analysis.

DNA Analyses

Genetic markers. The early genetic studies used phenotypic trait markers and classical protein markers for which the chromosomal location of the gene was known—for example, color blindness, glucose-6-phosphate dehydrogenase (G6PD) deficiency, and the Xq blood group—all of which are located on the X chromosome. These markers were supplanted by the use of DNA markers called restriction fragment length polymorphisms (RFLPs) (Botstein et al. 1980). RFLPs, which are produced by digestion of DNA by restriction endonucleases, are easily detected and greatly increased the number of potential markers. Since then, simple sequence repeat markers, from dinucleotide repeats such as CA up to pentanucleotide repeats, have been found to be more polymorphic/informative than most RFLPs as well as more abundant and more evenly spaced throughout the genome (Litt and Luty 1989; Weber and May 1989). The use of polymerase chain reaction (Mullis and Faloona 1987; Saiko et al. 1988) technology to type these DNA polymorphisms consumes less DNA and is faster than standard blotting and hybridization. Newer methods of detecting variations in DNA sequences that may further speed up these analyses are being explored.

DNA marker maps. The first DNA marker map of the human genome, published in 1987 by Donis-Keller et al., included 393 RFLP markers. A second-generation human linkage map of dinucleotide markers was developed at Genethen (France) (Weissenbach et al. 1992). This map was followed by the Cooperative Human Linkage Center (CHLC) genetic map, with 5,840 loci at a marker density of 0.7 centimorgan (Murray et al. 1994). Sequence-tagged sites (STS) are the bases of a map that provides radiation hybrid coverage of 99% *and* physical coverage of 94% of the human genome (Hudson et al. 1995). Now a gene map of more than 1,600 human genes is available, unifying existing genetic and physical maps with the nucleotide and protein sequence databases (Schuler et al. 1996).

Cytogenetic studies. An old technique used to check for chromosomal abnormalities, karyotyping can provide clues as to the chromosomal location of genes for disease if a particular deletion or translocation occurs in individuals affected with the disorder of interest. A technique known as fluorescence in situ hybridization (FISH) can detect specific chromosomal abnormalities (Weigant et al. 1991). Human chromosome painting (Speicher et al. 1996), an advance on the FISH method, has the capacity to analyze all the human chromosomes in a single hybridization experiment.

Genetic Association and Linkage Analytic Methods

Advances in molecular technology have led to a shift in emphasis from the mathematical estimation of recurrence risks and patterns of transmission (segregation analyses) to association and linkage studies.

Association studies compare marker allele frequencies in affected individuals with those in control subjects. In population association studies, the control subjects must be demographically similar to the patients, particularly in ethnicity, because allele frequencies may vary across ethnic groups. One way of controlling for ethnicity is to do family association studies, using the parents' nontransmitting alleles as the comparison genotypes and calculating a haplotype relative risk (Falk and Rubenstein 1987; Ott 1989). A positive association, if confirmed, would be followed up with linkage studies to determine whether the marker represented a locus conferring susceptibility to or linkage with the illness.

In linkage analysis, evidence for or against a hypothesized location of a disease gene is obtained by following the distribution of the disease phenotype and of a genetic marker among family members. If the marker and disease phenotype cosegregate so frequently that the odds against the cosegregation being due to chance exceed 95%, then they are considered to be "linked." The likelihood of linkage is measured by the LOD score, the logarithm to the base 10 of the odds ratio of the probability of linkage to the probability of no linkage. A LOD score of 3, which represents odds of 1,000 to 1 favoring linkage, is the 95% confidence level used when testing one marker locus and one disease gene locus. More stringent criteria have been suggested for modern studies employing genome-wide maps (Lander and Kruglyak 1995).

Additional methods of genetic analyses are now being employed. Computerized simulation studies, based on family phenotypes, are used to suggest models of inheritance for likelihood linkage studies. Two important applications of simulation studies are power analysis, an evaluation of the capabilities of a given family set to detect linkage if linkage exists, and determination of the P value associated with an apparent finding of linkage, given the absence of linkage (Ott 1991).

Nonparametric (model-free) methods such as sibling pair analyses (Penrose 1935) are widely used for studies of complex genetic traits such as diabetes mellitus, schizophrenia, and bipolar disorder. The affected sibling-pair method is based on identity by descent (Suarez 1978); the relevant observation is how frequently two affected offspring share copies of the same parental marker. Kruglyak and Lander (1995) and Kruglyak et al. (1996) have recently devised computer programs (MAPMAKER/SIBS and GENEHUNTER) for multipoint sib-pair and other affected relative-pair analyses of quantitative traits that make maximum use of the genetic information in the pedigree. The affected pedigree member (APM) method uses pairs of affected relatives other than siblings in the analysis (Risch 1994) but relies on identity by state (Bishop and Williamson 1990). Identity by state means that the relatives share an allele, but the method does not ensure that they both inherited the allele from the same parent. Thus, higher rates of false-positive findings are expected with traditional APM analyses. Recently, analyses based on identity by descent have been adapted to affected relative pairs (Kruglyak et al. 1996).

The traditional linkage study methods have yielded the greatest success for rare Mendelian disorders for which the mode of inheritance was known and the phenotype was clearly specified, as in cystic fibrosis (Kerem et al. 1989; Riordan et al. 1989; Rommens et al. 1989). Psychiatric diseases are more prevalent and appear to have more complicated forms of inheritance. Seemingly contradictory findings have emerged from early linkage studies of bipolar affective disorder.

▶ Genetic Findings in Bipolar Disorder

Family Studies

Controlled family studies by Dunner et al. (1976), Gershon et al. (1982), and Coryell et al. (1985) demonstrated dramatically increased rates of affective disorders in family members of affectively ill probands, compared with family members of probands who have other psychiatric disorders or no psychiatric disorder. Twin studies (Bertelsen et al. 1977) found greater concordance for affective disorders among monozygotic than among dizygotic twins. Adoption studies (Mendlewicz and Rainer 1977) showed that affective disorders were more common in adopted children whose biological parents had the illness, regardless of the health status of the adoptive parents. Although there is considerable evidence for an important genetic contribution to the etiology of bipolar disorder, knowledge regarding the mode(s) of transmission is lacking.

Segregation Studies

Segregation analysis allows one to test the goodness-of-fit of a postulated genetic model to the data. A general model, incorporating estimates of disease frequency, age-dependent penetrance, and so on, is generated and compared with the postulated model. Single major locus dominant and recessive, X-linked, polygenic, and mixed models can be evaluated. Different levels of affected status can be tested in separate analyses.

Spence et al. (1995) found that a single major locus was the best fit to the data when both bipolar I and II probands and relatives were included as affected in a segregation analysis of bipolar families. As the affected phenotype was broadened, either for the probands or the relatives, the power to reject other models relative to the single major locus model was reduced. A similar analysis was done on a subset of 212 bipolar I and bipolar II families from the National Institute of Mental Health Collaborative Depression Study (Spence et al. 1994). The results were similar to the previous study with a single major locus providing the best fit to the data, regardless of whether the relatives were defined as ill with bipolar I/bipolar II or bipolar I/II plus recurrent depression.

Linkage Studies

X-chromosome markers. The early bipolar linkage studies using phenotypic markers suggested that some bipolar families with no male-to-male transmission had an X-linked single-gene disorder. Reich et al. (1969) showed cosegregation of color blindness and affective illness in two North American pedigrees. Positive LOD scores for color blindness or G6PD were reported in several subsequent samples (del Zompo et al. 1984; Mendlewicz and Fleiss 1974), as well as a report of no linkage to color blindness (Gershon et al. 1979).

In more recent studies using DNA markers on Xq, Mendlewicz et al. (1987) reported linkage of bipolar disorder to the F9 locus in 10 Belgian families, and a positive LOD score for the same marker locus was noted in a British pedigree (Gill et al. 1992). Gejman et al. (1990) and Van Broeckhoven et al. (1991) were unable to confirm linkage to DNA markers in that region in either North American or Belgian pedigrees. Similarly, in studies with DNA markers in the color blindness or G6PD region, no linkage was found to that region in North American and Belgian families (Berrettini et al. 1990; Van Broeckhoven et al. 1991).

In 1987, Baron et al. reported finding linkage of bipolar disorder to either G6PD deficiency or color blindness in five Israeli families. Three families were later extended and reexamined. Several changes in psychiatric diagnosis were found, which were attributed primarily to recent illness onset, and there were some discrepancies with the earlier G6PD data. Multipoint linkage analysis was carried out using DNA markers spanning the Xq27-28 region. In 1993, Baron et al. reported that the LOD scores in two of the pedigrees had dropped to negative values, indicating no evidence of linkage; the LOD score in the third pedigree was 2.09, below the level of significance.

An association of bipolar disorder and a dinucleotide repeat polymorphism at the monoamine oxidase A locus at Xp11.3 has been reported (Lim et al. 1994). The strength of the association is weak but significant and may suggest that alleles at the monoamine oxidase A locus contribute to susceptibility to bipolar disorder rather than being a major determinant (Greenberg 1993).

Chromosome 11 markers.   In 1987, Egeland et al. reported finding linkage in an Old Order Amish family with bipolar disorder to RFLP markers for the insulin gene and H-ras oncogene, which flank the locus for tyrosine hydroxylase on the short arm of chromosome 11. Since the initial study, however, clinical follow-up on members of the Old Order Amish core pedigree has revealed that two previously unaffected individuals subsequently became ill (Kelsoe et al. 1989). These two recombinants dropped the LOD score below the level of significance. Genetic reevaluation of the core pedigree that included 10 members who had previously been incompletely genotyped decreased the LOD score even further, as did extending two branches of the family. In retrospect, it appears from the extended pedigree that there was probably more than one gene for bipolar disorder in the founders' generation.

A candidate-gene strategy has been widely used in linkage studies. Because noradrenergic and dopaminergic neurotransmission have been implicated in psychiatric disorders, investigators have continued to look for linkage between bipolar disorder and genes for tyrosine hydroxylase and the dopamine D_4 receptor, which are both located at 11p15.5 (Craig et al. 1985; Gelernter et al. 1992), and the dopamine D_2 receptor, which is located at 11q22-23 (Grandy et al. 1989).

There are conflicting findings from association studies for the tyrosine hydroxylase gene on chromosome 11. Leboyer et al. (1990) reported an association between bipolar disorder and two loci on chromosome 11, within or near the tyrosine hydroxylase gene. In a smaller United States sample, Todd and O'Malley (1989) found no association for two marker loci in the tyrosine hydroxylase gene, as was the case in a second larger sample (Todd et al. 1996).

Reports of translocations involving 11q22-23 have also fueled interest. A family in which affective disorder is cosegregating with a balanced 9/11 chromosomal translocation has been reported (Smith et al. 1989). In addition, there is a report of a family with multiple major mental illnesses (schizophrenia, schizoaffective disorder, and recurrent major depression) who have a balanced translocation involving 11q21 and 11q43 (St. Clair et al. 1990).

Other chromosomes reported to be linked to bipolar disorder. Several reports suggested that there might be linkage of bipolar disorder (Smeraldi et al. 1978; Turner and King 1981) and unipolar disorder (Weitkamp et al. 1981) with the human leukocyte antigen region on chromosome 6p. However, there were methodological problems with some of the studies, and the reports lacked statistical significance and were not consistent with each other. Other investigators were unable to find any evidence of linkage to the human leukocyte antigen region (Goldin and Gershon 1983; Targum et al. 1979).

Straub et al. (1994) reported data using short-sequence repeat polymorphisms in their set of 42 extended bipolar families. Although they have studied only a few families at many loci, they have reported a significant LOD score for one large family on chromosome 21q22. Affected sib pair-analyses in another set of 22 bipolar pedigrees (Detera-Wadleigh et al. 1996) provided support for a locus for bipolar disorder on 21q.

More recently, Berrettini et al. (1994) found evidence of linkage between bipolar disorder and pericentromeric loci on chromosome 18 in 22 families. In a set of 28 unilineal bipolar I families, Stine et al. (1995) reported some evidence for linkage on 18p, which overlapped with the finding by Berrettini et al. (1994), as well as evidence for linkage for a region of 18q. Most of the linkage evidence comes from families with paternal transmission of the illness and from marker alleles transmitted on the paternal chromosome.

Three other groups have since reported weak support for an 18q locus for bipolar disorder (Coon et al. 1996; DeBruyn et al. 1996; Freimer et al. 1996). A new study of a series of 30 bipolar families (F. J. McMahon, P. J. Hopkins, M. G. McInnis, S. Shaw, L. Cardon, S. G. Simpson, D.F. MacKinnon, O.C. Stine, R. Sherrington, D. A. Meyers, and J. R. De-Paulo, "Linkage of bipolar affective disorder to chromosome 18q: confirmation in a new pedigree series," unpublished data, 1997) found confirmatory evidence for a locus on 18q, although the susceptibility gene is not well localized. The parent-of-origin effect remains but is less than in the original sample of 28 families (Stine et al. 1995).

▌ Possible Novel Mechanisms of Inheritance

Clinical analysis has suggested other possible mechanisms of inheritance that are now being investigated.

In a subset of 34 unilineal bipolar families, McInnis et al. (1993) found evidence for anticipation, a phenomenon in which there is an increase in disease severity or decrease in age at onset in succeeding generations. In several disorders, including Huntington's disease, fragile X, and myotonic dystrophy, anticipation correlates with the expansion of trinucleotide repeat sequences. In the bipolar families, intergenerational pair-wise comparisons showed onset 8.9–13.5 years earlier ($P < .001$) and illness episode frequency 1.8–3.4 times greater ($P < .001$) in the probands' than in the parents' generation. These findings may implicate genes with expanding trinucleotide repeats in the genetic etiology of bipolar affective disorder.

In the same family study, McMahon et al. (1995) found evidence of a maternal effect in the transmission of bipolar disorder, which was replicated by Gershon et al. (1996). McMahon et al. (1995) found a higher than expected frequency of affected mothers ($P < .04$), a 2.3- to 2.8-fold increased risk of illness for maternal relatives ($P < .006$), and a 1.3- to 2.5-fold increased risk of illness for the offspring of affected mothers ($P < .017$). In seven enlarged bipolar pedigrees, fathers repeatedly failed to transmit the affected phenotype to daughters or sons. If these findings are confirmed in an epidemiologic sample, they would indicate the need for molecular studies of mitochondrial DNA (mtDNA) and imprinted DNA in patients with bipolar I disorder.

These seemingly contradictory findings point out some of the major problems involved in doing linkage analyses in the major psychiatric disorders, particularly the affective disorders.

Lack of Clear-Cut Mendelian Patterns of Inheritance

The lack of clear-cut Mendelian patterns of inheritance has impeded LOD score linkage studies in bipolar disorder. Although not precluding the possible existence of a single locus with a very large effect, the general familial pattern of psychiatric diseases appears consistent with multiple, common interacting genes, also known as epistasis (Risch 1994). Failure to replicate any of the reported linkages for bipolar disorder has raised doubts about the existence of Mendelian (single gene) forms of the disorder. Only recently, however, have genome-wide scans using evenly spaced informative DNA markers been conducted, so single gene forms have not been excluded.

Because the mechanism(s) of inheritance of bipolar disorder is unknown, likelihood linkage analyses using different genetic models are being conducted, as well as nonparametric ("model-free") analyses.

Heterogeneity

Heterogeneity, the phenomenon of a single phenotype being caused by any one of several mutations, creates a major problem for linkage analyses, because evidence in favor of linkage to a particular locus in several of the families may be canceled out by evidence against linkage at that locus in other families in which bipolar illness is associated with a different locus.

The traditional approach used to deal with heterogeneity has been to study one large family. Using one large family, one may be able to find one locus associated with the condition but it involves a great deal of work to find one, possibly rare, locus. Experience with the Old Order Amish family has shown that even this approach is fallible.

An alternative approach to the problem of heterogeneity is to study a set of small families with multiple affected individuals. This has become feasible, given the advent of denser marker maps (Hudson et al. 1995) and the development of computer programs such as MAP-MAKER/SIBS and GENEHUNTER (Kruglyak et al. 1996) that make maximum use of the genetic information in the pedigrees.

Assortative Mating

Assortative mating (Gershon et al. 1973; Merikangas and Spiker 1982), another major problem encountered in linkage studies, refers to the marriage of two individuals with major affective disorders more often than would be expected by chance. This phenomenon results in bilineal families (i.e., those with affective disorders in both parental lines). Assortative mating may introduce two different disease genes into a family and presents a problem for linkage studies, which are efficient at detecting only one disease locus per family. For this reason, the selection and study of unilineal families, those that have affective illness in only one parental line, should be the best strategy for detecting single gene forms of the illness, if they do exist. On the other hand, the fact that many families are bilineal for affective disorder raises the possibility that, for offspring to be affected, there must be a contribution from both parental lines.

The definition of bilineality varies. Some would use it to describe only affected-by-affected matings (Hodge 1992), whereas others would also designate as bilineal those families that have one unaffected parent if that parent has an affected sibling or parent (Simpson et al. 1992). Although bilineal families contribute some information to a linkage analysis, it is usually significantly less than that from unilineal families. Based on a simulation study of three-generation families, Hodge estimated that the drop in maximum LOD score was approximately 50% from purely unilineal data sets to extremely bilineal ones. It is essential that the existence of bilineality in families be known so that this can be taken into consideration in the analyses. For this reason, it is preferable to directly interview first-degree relatives of the unaffected as well as the affected parent, in addition to gathering family history data from several informants.

Phenotype Establishment

Establishing the phenotype is critical to the success of any linkage study. Most linkage studies of bipolar disorder have included bipolar I and II, schizoaffective disorder/bipolar, and recurrent major depression as part of the affected phenotype. Support for the inclusion of bipolar II as part of the bipolar phenotype has come from a segregation analysis (Spence et al. 1993) and an age-at-onset analysis of familial affective disorders (McMahon et al. 1994). The inclusion of recurrent unipolar disorder as part of the affected phenotype is problematic because depression appears to be more etiologically and clinically heterogeneous than bipolar disorder and may contribute many false positives; on the other hand, exclusion of recurrent unipolar persons or designating them as "phenotype unknown" entails a substantial loss of information. Blacker and Tsuang (1993) estimated that 65%–74% of familial cases of unipolar disorder are "genetically bipolar."

Reliability of the clinical diagnoses is crucial in genetic studies. Severe cases are easily and reliably diagnosed; however, mildly affected relatives are much more difficult to diagnose because there is no clear separation between mildly affected and unaffected individuals.

Replication

Lack of replication has plagued linkage studies in affective disorders. This problem may in part be due to the variability among studies in types and numbers of families studied, in clinical assessment, and in types and numbers of DNA markers used; it may also be partially due to haste to publish any positive findings. Risch (1990) stated that "a uniformly positive study followed by a uniformly negative study using an ethnically similar population is more evidence for non-replication than genetic heterogeneity" (p. 6).

▶ FUTURE DIRECTIONS FOR GENETIC LINKAGE STUDIES

Because findings to date indicate that the genetics of bipolar illness are much more complicated than had been appreciated, more study families are being recruited and new strategies are being employed. Most researchers are using a genome-wide survey as their primary approach rather than just looking at candidate genes. New technologies and methods of analysis are also being brought to bear on the problem. As previously mentioned, polymerase chain reaction and automated sequencers have greatly increased the speed of genotyping. Simple sequence repeats provide a tremendous resource of new DNA markers. New technologies such as genome mismatch screening (Nelson et al. 1993) and representational difference analysis (Lisitsyn et al. 1993) are based on cloning the regions of similarity (genome mismatch screening) or difference (representational difference analysis) between two genomes and do not rely on conventional DNA markers. These new methodologies show promise of being quicker and less expensive than standard genetic techniques but as yet have not been adapted for the study of human disease.

Several collaborations have been developed to facilitate the recruitment and study of the large numbers of families that are needed for research on psychiatric disorders. The National Institute of Mental Health has funded a genetics initiative for bipolar disorder as well as for schizophrenia and Alzheimer's disease. For the bipolar and schizophrenia studies, new diagnostic instruments—the Diagnostic Interview for Genetic Studies and the Family Interview for Genetic Studies—were developed and reliability tested (Nurnberger et al. 1994). The four centers studying bipolar disorders will collect a total of 265 families, which should increase the likelihood of finding other loci that are linked to bipolar disorders. Another collaboration for the study of bipolar disorder and schizophrenia is being funded by the European Science Foundation. The National Institute of Mental Health and European Science Foundation collaborations are collecting similar clinical data, so that one group could attempt to replicate a finding by the other group. The Dana Foundation is funding a collaboration between Johns Hopkins University and Stanford University and the Cold Spring Harbor Laboratory to further advance research on bipolar genetics. The Genome Project, a massive federally funded project whose mission is to sequence the entire human genome, will facilitate the mapping and isolation of genes and will lead to cloning of genes to determine the gene products.

The genetics of bipolar disorder have proved much more complicated than had been anticipated. Risch and Botstein (1996) concluded that the hypothesis that there is a single major locus accounting for the majority of inherited bipolar illness has by now been rejected and that it is unlikely that any single study will have sufficient power to produce a definite result. Risch and Botstein (1996) suggested that a simultaneous evaluation of all the available data with unique methods of analyses might be helpful in two ways: in eliminating some of the simpler genetic models for bipolar disorder and in defining the most promising chromosomal regions for follow-up.

▶ References

Baron M, Risch N, Hamburger R, et al: Genetic linkage between X-chromosome markers and bipolar affective illness. Nature 325:783–787, 1987

Baron M, Freimer NF, Risch N, et al: Diminished support for linkage between manic depressive illness and X-chromosome markers in three Israeli pedigrees. Nat Genet 3:49–55, 1993

Berrettini WH, Goldin LR, Gelernter J, et al: X-chromosome markers and manic-depressive illness. Arch Gen Psychiatry 47:366–373, 1990

Berrettini WH, Ferraro TN, Goldin LR, et al: Chromosome 18 DNA markers and manic-depressive illness: evidence for a susceptibility gene. Proc Natl Acad Sci U S A 91:5918–5921, 1994

Bertelsen A, Harvald B, Hauge M, et al: A Danish twin study of manic depressive disorders. Br J Psychiatry 130:330–351, 1977

Bishop DT, Williamson JA: The power of identity-by-state methods for linkage analysis. Am J Hum Genet 46:254–265, 1990

Blacker D, Tsuang MT: Unipolar relatives in bipolar pedigrees: are they bipolar? Psychiatric Genetics 3:5–16, 1993

Botstein D, White R, Skolnick M, et al: Construction of a genetic linkage map in man using restriction fragment length polymorphisms. Am J Hum Genet 32:314–331, 1980

Coon H, Hoff M, Holik J, et al: Analysis of chromosome 18 DNA markers in multiplex pedigrees with manic depression. Biol Psychiatry 39:689–696, 1996

Coryell W, Endicott J, Andreasen NC, et al: Bipolar I, bipolar II, and non-bipolar major depression among the relatives of affectively ill probands. Am J Psychiatry 142:817–821, 1985

Craig SP, Buckle VJ, Lamouroux A, et al: Localization of the human tyrosine hydroxylase gene to chromosome 11p15. Cytogenet Cell Genet 42:29–32, 1986

DeBruyn a, Souery D, Mendelbaum K, et al: Linkage analysis of families with bipolar illness and chromosome 18 markers. Biol Psychiatry 39:679–688, 1996

del Zompo M, Bochetta A, Goldin LR, et al: Linkage between X-chromosome markers and manic-depressive illness: two Sardinian pedigrees. Acta Psychiatr Scand 70:282–287, 1984

Detera-Wadleigh SD, Badner JA, Goldin LR, et al: Affected sib-pair analyses reveal support of prior evidence for a susceptibility locus for bipolar disorder on 21q. Am J Hum Genet 58:1279–1285, 1996

Donis-Keller H, Green P, Helms C, et al: A genetic linkage map of the human genome. Cell 51:319–337, 1987

Dunner DL, Gershon ES, Goodwin FK: Heritable factors in the severity of affective illness. Biol Psychiatry 11:31–42, 1976

Egeland JA, Gerhard DS, Pauls DL, et al: Bipolar affective disorders linked to DNA markers on chromosome 11. Nature 325:783–787, 1987

Endicott J, Spitzer RL: A diagnostic interview: The Schedule for Affective Disorders and Schizophrenia. Arch Gen Psychiatry 35:837–844, 1978

Falk CT, Rubenstein P: Haplotype relative risks: an easy way to construct a proper control sample for risk calculations. Ann Hum Genet 51:227–233, 1987

Faraone SV, Tsuang MT: Measuring diagnostic accuracy in the absence of a "gold standard." Am J Psychiatry 151:650–657, 1994

Freimer NB, Reus Vi, Escamilla MA, et al: Genetic mapping using haplotype, association and linkage methods suggests a locus for sever bipolar disorder (BPI) at 18q22-23 Nat Genet 12:436–441, 1996

Gejman PV, Detera-Wadleigh E, Martinez MM, et al: Manic depressive illness not linked to factor IX region in an independent series of pedigrees. Genomics 8:648–655, 1990

Gelernter J, Kennedy JL, Van Tol HHM, et al: The D4 dopamine receptor (DRD4) maps to distal 11p close to HRAS. Genomics 13:208–210, 1992

Gershon ES, Dunner DL, Sturt L, et al: Assortative mating in the affective disorders. Biol Psychiatry 7:63–74, 1973

Gershon ES, Targum SD, Matthysse S, et al: Color blindness not closely linked to bipolar illness. Arch Gen Psychiatry 36:1423–1430, 1979

Gershon ES, Hamovit S, Guroff JJ, et al: A family study of schizoaffective, bipolar I, bipolar II, unipolar, and normal control probands. Arch Gen Psychiatry 39:1157–1167, 1982

Gershon ES, Badner JA, Detera-Wadleigh SD, et al: Maternal inheritance and chromosome 18 allele sharing in unilineal bipolar illness pedigrees. Am J Med Genet 67:202–207, 1996

Gill M, Castle D, Duggan C: Cosegregation of Christmas disease and major affective disorder in a pedigree. Br J Psychiatry 160:112–114, 1992

Goldin LR, Gershon ES: Association and linkage studies of genetic marker loci in major psychiatric disorders. Psychiatric Developments 4:387–418, 1983

Grandy DK, Litt M, Allen L, et al: Human dopamine D2 receptor gene is located on chromosome 11 at q22-q23 and identifies Taq1 RFLP. Am J Hum Genet 45:778–785, 1989

Greenberg DA: Linkage analysis of "necessary" disease loci versus "susceptibility" loci. Am J Hum Genet 52:135–143, 1993

Hodge SE: Do bilineal pedigrees represent a problem for linkage analysis? Genet Epidemiol 9:191–206, 1992

Hudson TJ, Stein LD, Gerety SS, et al: An STS-based map of the human genome. Science 270:1945–1954, 1995

Kelsoe JR, Ginns EI, Egeland JA, et al: Re-evaluation of the linkage relationship between chromosome 11p loci and the gene for bipolar affective disorder in the Old Order Amish. Nature 342:238–243, 1989

Kendler KS: The impact of varying diagnostic thresholds on affected sib pair linkage analysis. Genet Epidemiol 5:407–419, 1988

Kerem B, Rommens JM, Buchanan JA, et al: Identification of the cystic fibrosis gene: genetic analysis. Science 245:1066–1073, 1989

Kraepelin E: Manic-Depressive Insanity and Paranoia (1895). Translated by Barclay RM. Edited by Robertson GM. New York, Arno Press, 1976

Kruglyak L, Lander ES: Complete multipoint sib-pair analysis of qualitative and quantitative traits. Am J Hum Genet 57:439–454, 1995

Kruglyak L, Daly MJ, Reeve-Daly MP, et al: Parametric and non-parametric linkage analysis: a unified multipoint approch. Am J Hum Genet 58:1347–1363, 1996

Lander E, Botstein D: Strategies for studying heterogeneous genetic traits in humans by using a linkage map of restriction fragment length polymorphisms. Proc Natl Acad Sci U S A 83:7353–7357, 1986

Lander ES, Kruglyak L: Genetic dissection of complex traits: guidelines for interpreting and reporting linkage results. Nat Genet 11: 241–247, 1995

Leboyer M, Malafosse A, Boularand S, et al: Tyrosine hydroxylase polymorphisms associated with manic-depressive illness (letter). Lancet 335:1219, 1990

Leckman JF, Sholomskas D, Thompson W, et al: Best estimate of lifetime psychiatric diagnosis: a methodological study. Arch Gen Psychiatry 39:879–883, 1982

Lim LC, Powell JF, Murray R, et al: Monoamine oxidase A gene and bipolar affective disorder (letter). Am J Hum Genet 54:1122–1124, 1994

Lisitsyn N, Lisitsyn N, Wigler M: Cloning the difference between two complex genomes. Science 259:949–951, 1993

Litt M, Luty JA: A hypervariable microsatellite revealed by in vitro amplification of a dinucleotide repeat within the cardiac muscle actin gene. Am J Hum Genet 44:397–401, 1989

McInnis MG, McMahon FJ, Simpson SG, et al: Anticipation in bipolar affective disorder. Am J Hum Genet 53:385–390, 1993

McMahon FJ, Chase GA, Simpson SG, et al: Clinical subtype, sex, and lineality influence onset age of major affective disorder in a family sample. Am J Psychiatry 151:210–215, 1994

McMahon FJ, Stine OC, Meyers DA, et al: Patterns of maternal transmission in bipolar affective disorder. Am J Hum Genet 56:1277–1286, 1995

Mendlewicz J, Fleiss JL: Linkage studies with X-chromosome markers in bipolar (manic-depressive) and unipolar (depressive) illness. Biol Psychiatry 9:261–294, 1974

Mendlewicz J, Rainer JD: Adoption study supporting genetic transmission in manic-depressive illness. Nature 268:327–329, 1977

Mendlewicz J, Simon P, Sevy S, et al: Polymorphic DNA marker on X-chromosome and manic depression. Lancet 1:1230–1232, 1987

Merikangas KR, Spiker DG: Assortative mating among in-patients with primary affective disorder. Psychol Med 12:753–764, 1982

Mullis KB, Faloona FA: Specific synthesis of DNA in vitro via a polymerase-catalyzed chain reaction. Methods Enzymol 155:335–350, 1987

Murray JC, Buetow KH, Weber JL, et al: A comprehensive human linkage map with centimorgan density. Science 265:2049–2054, 1994

Nelson SF, McCusker JH, Sander MA, et al: Genomic mismatch scanning: a new approach to genetic linkage mapping. Nat Genet 4:11–18, 1993

Nurnberger JI, Blehar MC, Kaufmann CA, et al: Diagnostic interview for genetic studies: rationale, unique features, and training. Arch Gen Psychiatry 51:849–859, 1994

Ott J: Statistical properties of the haplotype relative risk. Genet Epidemiol 6127–6130, 1989

Ott J: Analysis of Human Genetic Linkage, Revised Edition. Baltimore, MD, Johns Hopkins University Press, 1991

Penrose LS: The detection of autosomal linkage in data which consist of pairs of brothers and sisters of unspecified parentage. Annals of Eugenics 6:133–138, 1935

Reich T, Clayton P, Winokur G: Family history studies, V: the genetics of mania. Am J Psychiatry 125:1358–1369, 1969

Riordan JR, Rommens JM, Kerem B, et al: Identification of the cystic fibrosis gene: cloning and characterization of complementary DNA. Science 245:1066–1073, 1989

Risch N: Genetic linkage and complex diseases, with special reference to psychiatric disorders. Genet Epidemiol 7:3–16, 1990

Risch N: Mapping genes for psychiatric disorders, in Genetic Studies in Affective Disorders. Edited by Papalos DF, Lachman HM. New York, Wiley, 1994, pp 47–61

Risch N, Botstein D: A manic-depressive history. Nat Genet 12:351–353, 1996

Rommens JM, Iannuzzi MC, Kerem B, et al: Identification of the cystic fibrosis gene: chromosome walking and jumping. Science 245:1059–1065, 1989

Saiko RK, Gelfand DH, Stoffel S, et al: Primer-directed enzymatic amplification of DNA with a thermostable DNA polymerase. Science 239:487–491, 1988

Schuler GD, Boguski MS, Stewart EA, et al: A gene map of the human genome. Science 274:540–546, 1996

Simpson SG, Folstein SE, Meyers DA, et al: Assessment of lineality in bipolar I linkage studies. Am J Psychiatry 149:1660–1665, 1992

Smeraldi E, Negri F, Melica AM, et al: HLA system and affective disorders: a sibship study. Tissue Antigens 12:270–274, 1978

Smith M, Wasmuth JD, McPherson C, et al: Cosegregation of an 11q22.3-9p22 translocation with affective disorder: proximity of the dopamine D2 receptor gene relative to the translocation breakpoint. Am Soc Hum Genet Annual Meeting, Abstract 0864, 1989

Spence MA, Flodman PL, Sadovnik AD, et al: Bipolar disorder: evidence for a major locus. Am J Hum Genet 60:370–376, 1995

Spence MA, Flodman P, Sadovnik AD, et al: Reanalysis of the NIMH collaborative bipolar family data: results of complex segregation analyses (Poster 957), American Society of Human Genetics Annual Meeting, Montreal, Canada, October 18–22, 1994

Speicher MR, Ballard SG, Ward DC: Karyotyping human chromosomes by combinatorial multifluor FSH. Nat Genet 12:368–375, 1996

Spitzer RL, Endicott J, Robins E: Research Diagnostic Criteria for a Selected Group of Functional Disorders. New York, Biometrics, 1975

St. Clair D, Blackwood D, Muir W, et al: Association within a family of a balanced autosomal translocation with major mental illness. Lancet 336:13–16, 1990

Stine OC, Xu J, Koskela R, et al: Evidence for linkage of bipolar disorder to chromosome 18 with a parent-of-origin effect. Am J Hum Genet 57:1384–1394, 1995

Straub RE, Lehner T, Luo Y, et al: A possible vulnerability locus for bipolar affective disorder on chromosome 21q22.3. Nat Genet 8:291–296, 1994

Suarez BK: The affected sib pair IBD distribution for HLA-linked disease susceptibility genes. Tissue Antigens 12:87–93, 1978

Targum SD, Gershon ES, Van Eerdewegh M, et al: Human leukocyte antigen system not closely linked to or associated with bipolar manic-depressive illness. Biol Psychiatry 14:615–636, 1979

Todd RD, O'Malley KL: Population frequencies of tyrosine hydroxylase restriction fragment length polymorphisms in bipolar affective disorder. Biol Psychiatry 25:626–630, 1989

Todd RD, Lobos EA, Parsicor A, et al: Manic-depression illness and tyrosine hydroxylase markers. Lancet 347:1634, 1996

Turner WJ, King S: Two genetically distinct forms of bipolar affective disorder? Biol Psychiatry 16:417–439, 1981

Van Broeckhoven C, de Bruyn A, Raeymaekers P, et al: Linkage analysis of families with manic depressive illness with markers from chromosome X and 11 (abstract). Am J Hum Genet 49 (suppl):362, 1991

Weber JL, May PE: Abundant class of human DNA polymorphisms which can be typed using the polymerase chain reaction. Am J Hum Genet 44:388–396, 1989

Weigant J, Ried T, Nederlof PM, et al: In situ hybridization with fluoresce-inated DNA. Nucleic Acids Research 19:3237–3241, 1991

Weissenbach J, Gyapay G, Dib C, et al: A second-generation linkage map of the human genome. Nature 359:794–801, 1992

Weitkamp LR, Stancer HC, Persad E, et al: Depressive disorders and HLA: a gene on chromosome 6 that can affect behavior. N Engl J Med 305:1301–1306, 1981

SECTION

2

Biology

CHAPTER 6

SEROTONIN

Paul J. Goodnick, M.D.

There have been many theories over the years on the neuro-chemical etiology of manic-depressive or bipolar disorder, as well as of mania in particular. Among them are 1) that there is excess norepinephrine or dopamine in mania, and depleted norepi-nephrine or dopamine in depression (Post 1980); 2) that there is ex-cess norepinephrine with depleted acetylcholine in mania, and excess acetylcholine with depleted norepinephrine in depression (Janowsky et al. 1973); and 3) that manic and depressive mood swings are "per-mitted" by serotonin (5-hydroxytryptamine; 5-HT) depletion (Prange et al. 1973). The "permissive" hypothesis suggests that ma-nia is then followed by norepinephrine excess; depression is followed by norepinephrine depletion.

In this chapter, evidence is reviewed regarding urinary, blood, and cerebrospinal fluid (CSF) levels of 5-HT; its precursor—tryptophan; and its metabolite—5-hydroxyindoleacetic acid (5-HIAA). Also re-viewed is platelet 5-HT uptake and content and neuroendocrine studies on serotonin pathways in bipolar disorder. It will be seen that in many studies, results for both manic and depressed patients are quite similar to each other and different from nonpsychiatric control subjects. This is followed by a discussion on how treatment of mania and bipolar disorder can be related to effects of therapeutic agents on serotonin.

▶ Biochemical Parameters

Urine

Although changes induced by lithium have been studied (Linnoila et al. 1984; Rudorfer et al. 1985), total urinary 5-HT and 5-HIAA have not been studied in bipolar disorder in comparison with nonpsychiatric control subjects or other groups. This is because much of the measured serotonin in urine comes from the peripheral nervous system.

Blood

Four reports on combined groups of bipolar and unipolar depressed patients (Garfinkel et al. 1976; Moller et al. 1976; Niskanen et al. 1976; Wirz-Justice et al. 1975) have found no differences from control subjects in plasma total or free tryptophan. There have been no published studies on mania.

CSF

There have been 13 published studies, not including those on probenecid-induced accumulations, that have attempted to contrast levels of the metabolite 5-HIAA among manic patients, depressed patients, and nonpsychiatric control subjects. Of great interest is that the relationship of results of manic and depressive patients in relation to control subjects agreed in 10 of 13 studies (77%) (see Table 6–1). One study has been completed on eight euthymic medication-free bipolar patients (Berrettini et al. 1985); these patients showed a mean level of 5-HIAA (pmol/mL) of 92.3 ± 41.4, in contrast to a mean level of 72.3 ± 21.3 in 25 nonpsychiatric control subjects. The most recent confirmatory data on 5-HT similarity between manic and depressed patients comes from the National Institute on Mental Health Collaborative Study Protocol (Swann et al. 1994). In CSF 5-HIAA, in terms of concentration relative to control subjects, mixed manic patients (1.35) were practically equal to agitated depressed patients (1.45), and pure manic patients (0.90) were similar to nonagitated depressed patients (1.05).

Table 6–1. Cerebrospinal fluid 5-HIAA and its relation to control subjects (± SEM)

Study	Mania N	+/0/−	Depression N	+/0/−
Ashcroft et al. 1966	4	0	24	−
Bowers et al. 1969	8	−	8	−
Roos and Sjöström 1969	19	+	17	+
Coppen et al. 1972	18	−	31	−
Wilk et al. 1972	6	−	5	−
Goodwin et al. 1973	16	0	58	0
Sjöström 1973	15	+	23	+
Ashcroft et al. 1976	11	0	9	+
Banki 1977	10	−	71	−
Vestergaard et al. 1978	4	+	28	0
Koslow et al. 1983	9M	0	49M	0
	5F	+	43F	+
Gerner et al. 1984	13	0	38	0
Swann et al. 1994[a]	9	0	27	0

[a]National Institute of Mental Health Collaborative Study ("pure manics" versus "nonagitated bipolar depression").

Platelet Serotonin Studies

Platelet 5-HT content. Platelet 5-HT content has been reported in only two studies (Stahl et al. 1983; Wirz-Justice and Puhringer 1978). Wirz-Justice and Puhringer reported that this measure was greater in seven bipolar depressed patients (2.67) than in 43 control subjects (1.94, $P < .01$). Furthermore, in a few of these bipolar patients that were followed during hypomania, platelet 5-HT was also reported to be higher than in control subjects. Stahl et al. replicated these results in that levels found in 11 bipolar depressed patients were significantly greater than in 66 control subjects or in 14 unipolar depressed patients.

Platelet serotonin uptake.   Platelet serotonin uptake has been studied in five reports (Arora and Meltzer 1980; Meagher et al. 1990;
Meltzer et al. 1981, 1983; Stahl et al. 1983). Overall, for uptake V_{max}
in these studies,

- Levels in bipolar depressed patients were lower than those in control subjects in four of four studies.
- Levels in manic patients were lower than those in control subjects
  in two of three studies.
- Levels in unipolar depressed patients were higher than those in
  control subjects in one of two studies.

Platelet ^{3}H-imipramine binding.   Platelet ^{3}H-imipramine binding
has been considered to be related to the 5-HT receptor binding site
in human platelets (Paul et al. 1981). There have been five studies with
results related to bipolar disorder (Baron et al. 1986; Berrettini et al.
1982; Mellerup et al. 1982; Suranyi-Cadotte et al. 1983; Wood et al.
1983). Detail is supplied in Table 6–2, but overall measures of B_{max}
indicated that manic patients on lithium are similar to control subjects,
and that bipolar euthymic and bipolar depressed patients have lower
values than control subjects.

   Although the initial study appeared to show that "manic-melancholic"
patients had a mean B_{max} greater than control subjects, this was probably due to the fact that unipolar patients were included in the study
group. Berrettini et al.'s (1982) results were probably effected by lack
of sufficient washout, as lithium effects may persist up to 3 weeks after
discontinuation (Goodnick et al. 1984).

   Suranyi-Cadotte et al. (1983) from the same group attempted to
show that schizoaffective manic patients have a B_{max} value similar to
control subjects; this result may have been influenced by lithium's
effect on reuptake (Goodnick 1990); further, this schizoaffective manic
group may be biologically somewhat different from a manic group.

**Adenosine-phosphate–augmented 5-HT–induced platelet aggre-
gation response.**   The adenosine-phosphate–augmented 5-HT–
induced platelet aggregation response has been investigated in 6 manic
and 10 depressed patients and contrasted with that of 10 control subjects

Table 6–2. Platelet ^{3}H-imipramine binding in bipolar disorder (B_{max}) (fmol/mg protein)

Study	Mania SD	N	Bipolar SD	N	Control subjects SD	N
Mellerup et al. 1982						
Bipolar + unipolar			1190 ± 230^a	19	1010 ± 280	33
Berrettini et al. 1982						
Off lithium 2 weeks			450 ± 151^b	12	440 ± 168	12
Wood et al. 1983			467 ± 35^a	7	658 ± 33	17
			Unipolar (no lithium)		675 ± 49	8
Suranyi-Cadotte et al. 1983						
On lithium	609 ± 70	4			658 ± 33	17
Baron et al. 1986			754 ± 250^b	33	944 ± 344	58
			Unipolar		821 ± 316	34

[a]Depressed. [b]Euthymic.

(McAdams and Leonard 1992). The measured aggregation response (slope of aggregation curve * s–1 ± SEM) was significantly less ($P <$ .005) in both manic patients ($0.53 \pm .03$) and depressed patients ($0.44 \pm .01$) than in control subjects ($0.78 \pm .02$).

Serotonin-Induced Platelet Calcium Mobilization

5-HT–induced intracellular calcium (Ca^{+2}) increase in platelets has been found to be a reliable indicator of 5-HT$_2$ receptor function (Kagaya et al. 1990; Kusumi et al. 1991). The time course of this mobilization is a rapid peak within 10 seconds, followed by a prolonged plateau phase. Platelets from manic patients have been found to display a greater peak amplitude as well as an enhancement of the plateau phase of Ca^{+2} response to serotonin (Okamoto et al. 1994). Peak net response to 5-HT was also found to be greater in platelets from bipolar depressed patients and melancholic major depression patients than from nonmelancholic depressed patients and control subjects (Kusumi et al. 1994).

Neuroendocrine Studies

Cortisol response to 5-hydroxytryptophan (5-HTP). The cortisol response to 5-HTP has been studied in manic patients, euthymic bipolar patients, depressed patients, and control subjects. As shown in Table 6–3, when 200 mg of tryptophan is administered orally, the cortisol response is elevated over control subjects in all three groups (Goodnick 1985; Goodnick et al. 1987; Meltzer et al. 1984a).

Buspirone-induced prolactin release. An initial test of buspirone-induced prolactin release showed a nonsignificant difference between manic patients and control subjects (Yatham 1994). Buspirone is a putative 5-HT_{1A} agonist whose effect to stimulate prolactin release is attenuated by metergoline or methysergide (Gregory et al. 1990). The lack of robust findings in this case could have been effected by diagnostic criteria (DSM-III-R [American Psychiatric Association 1987]) used instead of the Research Diagnostic Criteria (Spitzer et al. 1978) used in the previous studies), buspirone's similarity to 5-HTP, and buspirone's lack of specificity to 5-HT (i.e., buspirone may interact with dopamine pathways) (Traber and Glaser 1987).

Fenfluramine-induced changes in plasma cortisol and prolactin. Yatham and Block (1994) reported no difference between DSM-III-R manic patients and control subjects in a paradigm of 60 mg fenfluramine-induced changes in plasma cortisol and prolactin. However, this result is also impaired by lack of specificity, to a degree. Fenfluramine may release more than just 5-HT; it is related chemically to the amphetamines and has led to abuse.

Postmortem Studies

Earlier postmortem studies have at times reported findings of decreased 5-HT and 5-HIAA in brains of depressed patients and of those who have committed suicide (Bourne et al. 1968; Pare et al. 1969), although not consistently (Crow et al. 1984; Korpi et al. 1986). However, none of these studies focused on bipolar disorder. Young et al. (1994) studied nine autopsied brains with medical records sufficient

Table 6–3. Neuroendocrinology of mania

Studies	Mania		Euthymic		Depressed		Control subjects	
	SD	N	SD	N	SD	N	SD	N
5-HTP/cortisol studies								
Meltzer et al. 1984a, 1984b	9.0 ± 7.1	16			7.9 ± 7.4	31	3.0 ± 3.2	62
Goodnick 1985	7.1 ± 8.2	15					3.8 ± 4.2	16
	11.0 ± 6.6	3						
Goodnick et al. 1987			15.2 ± 2.4	3			5.2 ± 8.0	5
Buspirone/prolactin studies								
Yatham 1994 (approx)[a]	13	11					30	11

Note. 5-HTP = 5-hydroxytryptophan.
[a] Approximate prolactin level, estimated from graph without specifics.

to establish independent diagnosis of DSM-III-R bipolar affective disorder by two independent research psychiatrists. Although 5-HT levels did not differ significantly from control subjects in any of eight brain regions studied, 5-HIAA levels were significantly lower than in control subjects in frontal cortex (0.052 versus 0.113, $P = .001$) and in parietal cortex (0.054 versus 0.147, $P = .003$). A similar trend was found in the caudate nucleus.

Summary of Biochemical Parameters

Thus, from available biochemical results, it appears that manic patients, bipolar euthymic patients, and bipolar depressed patients are similar with respect to levels of CSF 5-HIAA, platelet 5-HT content and uptake, cortisol response to 5-HTP, and postmortem 5-HIAA concentrations. In terms of relationship to control subjects, CSF 5-HIAA for bipolar disorder is generally undetermined. However, platelet 5-HT content is elevated, platelet 5-HT V_{max} and ^{3}H-imipramine B_{max} are reduced, cortisol response to 5-HTP is elevated, and postmortem brain 5-HIAA is reduced. If less serotonin is produced and released by the central nervous system in bipolar disorder, then content would increase, uptake would be reduced, and postsynaptic sensitivity to 5-HT agonists would be enhanced. Thus, these results are generally consistent with the reduced 5-HT utilization in bipolar disorder that might be predicted by the "permissive" hypothesis of manic-depression.

▶ SEROTONIN BIOCHEMISTRY AND TREATMENT OF BIPOLAR DISORDER

Tryptophan

If serotonin deficiency is at least partially responsible for the cycling found in patients with bipolar disorder, surmounting this deficiency should, it is hoped, both reduce severity of mania and bipolar depression and help to prevent recurrences. To this end, L-tryptophan (LTP) has been used as both a primary and adjunctive treatment in mania and depression. There have been numerous reports on the use of LTP in the treatment of depression in 170 patients with mixed results, possibly related to lack of differentiation between bipolar and unipolar depressive patients (Goodwin and Jamison 1990). Van Praag (1983) showed that the precursor 5-HTP, in seven open studies at a dose of 50–600 mg/day for 7–35 days, produced improvement in 191 of 350 (55%) depressed patients. Similarly, in five double-blind studies of a dose of 50–3,250 mg/day 5-HTP for 1–24 days, 46 of 71 (65%) depressed patients showed improvement.

There have also been five reports on the use of LTP in the treatment of mania and three on its use in the prophylaxis of bipolar disorder. Of the five double-blind studies in mania, four (Brewerton and Reus 1983; Chouinard et al. 1985; Murphy et al. 1974; Prange et al. 1974) indicated that LTP was beneficial, and in only one (Chambers and Naylor 1978) did it fail. A summary of these studies is provided in Table 6–4.

There have been three reports on LTP's prophylactic use (Beitman and Dunner 1982; Chouinard et al. 1979; Landry et al. 1991). In six cases, the addition of 2–12 g/day led to significant increased mood stabilization. Landry et al. found in a 1-year, crossover, double-blind, randomized maintenance study of "drug-resistant" bipolar patients that there was a lower rate of relapse (6.4% over 6 months) for patients

Table 6–4. L-tryptophan (LTP) treatment of mania

Study	N	Design	Dose (g)	Days	Result
Prange et al. 1973	10	Double-blind, crossover	6	14	LTP > carbamazepine; 3/5 LTP #1 improved
Murphy et al. 1974	10	Double-blind, crossover	9.6	20	70% improved
Chambers and Naylor 1978	10	Double-blind, placebo	6	14	LTP = placebo
Brewerton and Reus 1983	9	Double-blind, placebo	9	21	LTP > placebo
Chouinard et al. 1985	24	Randomized	12	14	LTP > placebo

on a combination of lithium plus LTP than on lithium plus placebo (14.9% over 6 months).

Thus, LTP, the precursor of serotonin, has been used successfully in both the treatment and prophylaxis of bipolar disorder. Although the information is of clear biochemical and theoretical interest, it is unfortunate that due to onset of eosinophilia-myalgia syndrome associated not with LTP per se, but with the ingestion of a chemical constituent associated with specific tryptophan-manufacturing conditions of one company (Belongia et al. 1990), LTP has become unavailable for clinical use in the United States.

Lithium

Lithium has long been established as the treatment of choice for mania and the prophylaxis for bipolar disorder since its properties were discovered by Cade in 1949 and developed by Schou, Baastrup, Fieve, and Gershon (Johnson 1984). Many hypotheses and biological findings affect the explanation of lithium's unique ability to treat and prevent relapse of two seemingly opposite conditions: mania and depression (see Ownby and Goodnick, Chapter 12, this volume). However, among these findings, lithium has been found to have a significant effect on measures of serotonin in urine, blood, CSF, and the brain (Goodnick 1987, 1990) (Table 6–5). It appears that many of lithium's initial effects offset conditions of serotonin synaptic depletion and increase postsynaptic 5-HT effects as rapidly as possible by decreasing urinary turnover with elevating CSF 5-HIAA, increasing platelet 5-HT content with decreasing 5-HT reuptake, and enhancing postsynaptic sensitivity to 5-HTP. Later, during prophylaxis, particu-

Table 6–5.   Lithium and serotonin

Parameter	Acute treatment		Prophylaxis	
	Change (%)	Studies	Change (%)	Studies
Platelet 5-HT content	+22	1	−34	1
Platelet 5-HT uptake	−24	4	+60	5
5-HTP-cortisol (peak-baseline)	+30	2	−49	3

Note.   5-HTP = 5-hydroxytryptophan.

larly after 6 months when prophylaxis is established, these effects are then reversed, bringing the biological indices of bipolar patients closer to those of nonpsychiatric control subjects (Goodnick 1990). The negative results reported for urinary 5-HT/5-HIAA turnover, platelet measures, and neuroendocrine challenges in volunteers (Glue et al. 1986; Manji et al. 1991; Rudorfer et al. 1985) may be due to the inherent hypothesized central nervous system differences between bipolar patients and nonpsychiatric control subjects.

▶ Conclusion

The biochemistry of mania and bipolar disorder includes a major, perhaps "permissive," role for serotonin perturbation in the abnormalities that have been reported in metabolite studies, platelet investigations, neuroendocrine challenge tests, and postmortem results. These results are complemented both by support for a therapeutic role in bipolar disorder for serotonin precursors (LTP and 5-HTP) and by results explaining lithium's therapeutic and prophylactic role in bipolar disorder (on at least a partial basis) by effects of serotonin function on these same measures.

▶ References

American Psychiatric Association: Diagnostic and Statistical Manual of Mental Disorders, 3rd Edition, Revised. Washington, DC, American Psychiatric Association, 1987

Arora R, Meltzer HY: Lithium and serotonin uptake by platelets. Br J Psychiatry 137:396–397, 1980

Ashcroft GW, Crawford TBB, Eccleston D, et al: 5-Hydroxyindole compounds in the cerebrospinal fluid of patients with psychiatric or neurologic diseases. Lancet 2:1049–1052, 1966

Ashcroft GW, Dow R, Yates C: Significance of lumbar CSF metabolite measurements in affective illness, in CNS and Behavioral Pharmacology. Edited by Tuomisto J, Paasonen M. Helsinki, Finland, University of Helsinki, 1976, pp 277–284

Banki CM: Correlation between cerebrospinal fluid amine metabolites and psychomotor activity in affective disorders. J Neurochem 28:255–257, 1977

Baron M, Barkai A, Gruen R, et al: Platelet [³H]imipramine binding in affective disorders: trait versus state characteristics. Am J Psychiatry 143:711–717, 1986

Beitman B, Dunner DL: L-tryptophan in the maintenance treatment of bipolar II manic-depressive illness. Am J Psychiatry 139:1498–1499, 1982

Belongia EA, Hedberg CW, Gieich GJ, et al: An investigation of the cause of the eosinophilia-myalgia syndrome associated with tryptophan use. N Engl J Med 323:357–365, 1990

Berrettini WH, Nurnberger JI Jr, Post RM, et al: Platelet ³H-imipramine binding in euthymic bipolar patients. Psychiatry Res 7:215–219, 1982

Berrettini WH, Nurnberger JI Jr, Scheinin M, et al: Cerebrospinal fluid and plasma monoamines and their metabolites in euthymic bipolar patients. Biol Psychiatry 20:257–269, 1985

Bourne HR, Bunney WE, Coburn RW, et al: Noradrenaline, 5-hydroxytryptamine, and 5-hydroxyindoleacetic acid in hindbrain in suicidal patients. Lancet 2:805–808, 1968

Bowers MB, Henninger GR, Gerbode FA: Cerebrospinal fluid 5-HIAA and HVA in psychiatric patients. Int J Neuropharmacol 8:155–162, 1969

Brewerton TD, Reus VI: Lithium carbonate and L-tryptophan in the treatment of bipolar and schizoaffective disorders. Am J Psychiatry 140:757–760, 1983

Chambers CA, Naylor GJ: A controlled trial of L-tryptophan in mania. Br J Psychiatry 132:555–559, 1978

Chouinard G, Jones BD, Young SN, et al: Potentiation of lithium by tryptophan in a patient with bipolar illness. Am J Psychiatry 136:719–720, 1979

Chouinard G, Young SN, Annable L: A controlled clinical trial of L-tryptophan in acute mania. Biol Psychiatry 20:546–557, 1985

Coppen A, Prange AJ Jr, Whybrow PC, et al: Abnormalities of indoleamines in affective disorders. Arch Gen Psychiatry 26:474–478, 1972

Crow TJ, Cross AJ, Cooper SJ, et al: Neurotransmitter receptors and monoamine metabolites in the brains of patients with Alzheimer-type dementia and depression, and suicides. Neuropharmacology 23:1561–1569, 1984

Garfinkel PE, Warsh JJ, Stancer HC, et al: Total and free plasma tryptophan in patients with affective disorders: effects of a peripheral decarboxylase inhibitor. Arch Gen Psychiatry 33:1462–1466, 1976

Gerner RH, Fairbanks L, Anderson GM, et al: CSF neurochemistry in depressed, manic, and schizophrenic patients compared with that of normal controls. Am J Psychiatry 141:1533–1540, 1984

Glue PW, Cowen PJ, Nutt DJ, et al: The effect of lithium on 5-HT mediated neuroendocrine responses and platelet 5-HT receptors. Psychopharmacology 90:398–402, 1986

Goodnick PJ: Effect of long-term lithium on the 5-HTP–induced cortisol response in bipolar patients. Abstracts of 40th annual meeting of the Society of Biological Psychiatry, Dallas, Texas 1985. Biol Psychiatry, 1985, No. 89, p 135

Goodnick PJ: Serontonergic mechanisms of lithium action. Mt Sinai J Med 54:182–187, 1987

Goodnick PJ: Effects of lithium on indices of 5-HT and catecholamines in the clinical context. Lithium 1:65–73, 1990

Goodnick PJ, Arora RC, Jackman H, et al: Neurochemical changes during discontinuation of lithium prophylaxis, II: alterations in platelet serotonin function. Biol Psychiatry 19:891–898, 1984

Goodnick PJ, Fieve RR, Schlegel A: Clinical, biochemical, and neuroendocrine effects of lithium discontinuation. Psychopharmacol Bull 23:510–513, 1987

Goodwin FK, Jamison KR: Manic-Depressive Illness. New York, Oxford University Press, 1990

Goodwin FK, Post RM, Dunner DL, et al: Cerebrospinal fluid amine metabolites in affective illness: the probenecid technique. Am J Psychiatry 130:73–79, 1973

Gregory CA, Anderson IM, Cowen PJ: Metergoline abolishes the prolactin response to buspirone. Psychopharmacology 100:383–384, 1990

Janowsky DS, El-Yousef MK, Davis JM, et al: Antagonistic effects of physostigmine and methylphenidate in man. Am J Psychiatry 130:1370–1376, 1973

Johnson FN: The History of Lithium Therapy. London, England, MacMillan Press Ltd, 1984

Kagaya A, Mikuni M, Kusumi I, et al: Serotonin-induced acute desensitization of serotonin$_2$ receptors in human platelets via a mechanism involving protein kinase. J Pharmacol Exp Ther 255:305–311, 1990

Korpi ER, Kleinman JE, Goodman SI, et al: Serotonin and 5-hydroxyindoleacetic acid in brains of suicide victims. Arch Gen Psychiatry 43:594–600, 1986

Koslow SH, Maas JW, Bowden CL, et al: CSF and urinary biogenic amines and metabolites in depression and mania: a controlled, univariate analysis. Arch Gen Psychiatry 40:999–1010, 1983

Kusumi I, Koyama T, Yamashita I: Effects of various factors on serotonin-induced Ca^{+2} response in human platelets. Life Sci 48:2405–2412, 1991

Kusumi I, Koyama T, Yamashita I: Serotonin-induced platelet intracellular calcium mobilization in depressed patients. Psychopharmacology 113:322–327, 1994

Landry P, Chouinard G, Primeau F: Lithium-tryptophan combination in the maintenance treatment of bipolar affective illness. Lithium 2:135–140, 1991

Linnoila M, Miller TL, Bartko J: Five antidepressant treatments in depressed patients. Arch Gen Psychiatry 41:688–692, 1984

Manji HK, Hsiao JK, Risby ED, et al: The mechanisms of action of lithium, I: effects on serotoninergic and noradrenergic systems in normal subjects. Arch Gen Psychiatry 48:505–512, 1991

McAdams C, Leonard BE: Changes in platelet aggregatory responses to collagen and 5-hydroxytryptamine in depressed, schizophrenic and manic patients. Int Clin Psychopharmacol 7:81–85, 1992

Meagher JB, O'Halloran A, Carney PA, et al: Changes in platelet 5-hydroxytryptamine uptake in mania. J Affect Disord 19:191–196, 1990

Mellerup ET, Plenge P, Rosenberg R: ^{3}H-imipramine binding sites in platelets from psychiatric patients. Psychiatry Res 7:221–227, 1982

Meltzer HY, Arora RC, Baber R, et al: Serotonin uptake in blood platelets of psychiatric patients. Arch Gen Psychiatry 38:1322–1326, 1981

Meltzer HY, Arora RC, Goodnick PJ: Effect of lithium carbonate on serotonin uptake in blood platelets of patients with affective disorders. J Affect Disord 5:215–221, 1983

Meltzer HY, Umberkoman-Witta B, Robertson A, et al: Effect of 5-hydroxytryptophan on serum cortisol levels in major affective disorders, I: enhanced response in depression and mania. Arch Gen Psychiatry 41: 366–374, 1984a

Meltzer HY, Lowy M, Robertson A, et al: Effect of 5-hydroxytryptophan on serum cortisol levels in major affective disorders, III: effect of antidepressants and lithium carbonate. Arch Gen Psychiatry 41:391–397, 1984b

Moller SE, Kirk L, Fremming KH: Plasma amino acids as an index for subgroups in manic-depressive psychosis: correlation to effect of tryptophan. Psychopharmacology (Berlin) 49:205–213, 1976

Murphy DL, Baker M, Goodwin FK, et al: L-tryptophan in affective disorders: indoleamine changes and differential clinical effects. Psychopharmacologia 34:11–20, 1974

Niskanen P, Huttunen M, Tamminen T, et al: The daily rhythm of plasma tryptophan and tyrosine in depression. Br J Psychiatry 128:67–73, 1976

Okamoto Y, Kagaya A, Shinno H, et al: Serotonin-induced calcium mobilization is enhanced in mania. Life Sci 56:327–332, 1994

Pare CMB, Yeung DPH, Price K, et al: 5-Hydroxytryptamine, noradrenaline, and dopamine in brainstem, hypothalamus, and caudate nucleus of controls and of patients committing suicide by coal gas poisoning. Lancet 2:133–135, 1969

Paul SM, Rehavi M, Skolnick P, et al: Depressed patients have decreased binding of tritiated imipramine to platelet serotonin "transporter." Arch Gen Psychiatry 38:1315–1317, 1981

Post RM: Biochemical theories of mania, in Mania: An Evolving Concept. Edited by Belmaker RH, van Praag HM. New York, Spectrum Publications, 1980, pp 217–266

Prange AJ Jr, Sisk JL, Wilson IC: Balance, permission, and discrimination among amines: a theoretical consideration of l-tryptophan in disorders of movements and affects, in Serotonin in Affective Disorders. Edited by Barchas J, Usdin E. New York, Academic Press, 1973, pp 539–548

Prange AJ Jr, Wilson IC, Lynn CW, et al: L-tryptophan in mania: contributions to a permissive hypothesis of affective disorders. Arch Gen Psychiatry 30:56–62, 1974

Roos BE, Sjöström R: 5-Hydroxyindoleacetic acid (and homovanillic acid) levels in the cerebrospinal fluid after probenecid application in patients with manic-depressive psychosis. Pharmacologia Clinica 1:153–155, 1969

Rudorfer MV, Karoum F, Ross RJ: Differences in lithium effects in depressed and healthy subjects. Clin Pharmacol Ther 37:66–71, 1985

Sjöström R: 5-Hydroxyindoleacetic acid and homovanillic acid in cerebrospinal fluid in manic-depressive psychosis and the effect of probenecid treatment. Eur J Clin Pharmacol 6:75–80, 1973

Spitzer RL, Endicott J, Robins E: Research Diagnostic Criteria: rationale and reliability. Arch Gen Psychiatry 35:773–782, 1978

Stahl SM, Woo DJ, Mefford IN, et al: Hyperserotonemia and platelet serotonin uptake and release in schizophrenia and affective disorders. Am J Psychiatry 140:26–30, 1983

Suranyi-Cadotte BE, Wood PL, Schwartz G, et al: Altered platelet ^{3}H-imipramine binding in schizoaffective and depressive disorders. Biol Psychiatry 18:923–927, 1983

Swann AC, Stokes PE, Secunda SK, et al: Depressive mania versus agitated depression: biogenic amine and hypothalamic-pituitary-adrenocortical function. Biol Psychiatry 35:803–813, 1994

Traber J, Glaser T: 5-HT$_{1A}$ receptor anxiolytics. Trends Pharmacol Sci 8:432–437, 1987

Van Praag HM: Serotonin precursors in the treatment of depression, in Serotonin in Biological Psychiatry. Edited by Ho BT, Schooler JC, Usdin E. New York, Raven, 1983, pp 259–286

Vestergaard P, Sorensen T, Hoppe E, et al: Biogenic amine metabolites in cerebrospinal fluid of patients with affective disorders. Acta Psychiatr Scand 58:88–96, 1978

Wilk S, Shopsin B, Gershon S, et al: Cerebrospinal fluid levels of MHPG in affective disorders. Nature 235:440–441, 1972

Wirz-Justice A, Puhringer W: Increased platelet serotonin in bipolar depression and hypomania. J Neural Transm 42:55–62, 1978

Wirz-Justice A, Puhringer W, Hole G, et al: Monoamine oxidase and free tryptophan in human plasma: normal variations and their implications for biochemical research in affective disorders. Pharmakopsychiatr Neuropsychopharmakol 8:310–317, 1975

Wood PL, Suranyi-Cadotte B, Schwartz G, et al: Platelet ³H-imipramine binding and red blood cell choline in affective disorders: indications of heterogenous pathogenesis. Biol Psychiatry 18:715–719, 1983

Yatham LN: Buspirone induced prolactin release in mania. Biol Psychiatry 35:553–556, 1994

Yatham LN, Block M: Fenfluramine challenge in mania, in New Research Program and Abstracts, 147th annual meeting of the American Psychiatric Association, Philadelphia, PA, May 21–26, 1994, p 100 (#NR174)

Young LT, Warsh JJ, Kish SJ, et al: Reduced brain 5-HT and elevated NE turnover and metabolites in bipolar affective disorder. Biol Psychiatry 35:121–127, 1994

CHAPTER 7

CATECHOLAMINES

Virginia M. V. Buki, M.D., and
Paul J. Goodnick, M.D.

T he etiology and pathophysiology of mania are still unclear. Many hypotheses and theories have been formulated. In this chapter, we explore the catecholamine hypothesis, first formulated by Schildkraut (1965), implying that catecholamine levels are elevated in mania and decreased in depression.

▶ BIOCHEMICAL THEORY

Behavioral Anatomy

The relationship between neurotransmitters, mood, and behavior was first suspected in the 1950s when increased catecholamines were observed in urine. At the same time, other investigators found that iproniazid, a monoamine oxidase inhibitor (MAOI), caused excited behavior (Kety et al. 1971). Later it was found out that these two substances affected norepinephrine (NE) levels in the brain. Woodward et al. (1979) considered the possibility that NE could function as a modulating agent rather than cause a direct action on the neuronal membrane. Martin and Reichlin (1987) described the locations of NE, serotonin, and dopamine (DA) in the brain stem. NE is found in the locus ceruleus, serotonin in the raphe nucleus, and DA in the substantial nigra. Epinephrine is found in very small concentrations in the medulla and hypothalamus. At the hypothalamic level, DA is located in the median eminence and arcuate nuclei. The tuberoinfundibular

119

tract represents the connection between the arcuate nuclei (containing DA) and the median eminence in the hypothalamus. Studies on the modulatory action of NE were reviewed by Leckman and Maas (1984) and showed that there is a connection between the strategic location of NE cell distribution in the brain and the diffuse responses elicited when these nuclei were stimulated. Schildkraut (1965) suggested that biogenic amines could induce their modulatory action in a hormone-like fashion. Kety et al. (1971) considered that a decrease in serotonin level would create a predisposition toward affective disorders. Mania and hypomania could appear as a consequence of increased adrenergic activity. The views of Prange et al. (1973) coincided with this permissive hypothesis of indoleamines over catecholamines. However, they further proposed that the deficiency in serotonin would lay the groundwork for affective disorders to appear and that increased or decreased levels of catecholamines would determine the arrival of the clinical manifestations of mania or depression.

▶ STUDIES OF CATECHOLAMINES AND METABOLITES

Relationship of Metabolite Levels to Psychiatric Diagnosis

After studies on the relationship between catecholamines and behavior, the focus of attention shifted to the measurement of these catecholamines and their metabolites (DA: homovanillic acid [HVA]; NE: 3-methoxy-4-hydroxyphenylglycol [MHPG]) in cerebrospinal fluid (CSF), plasma, and urine and their relation to differential diagnosis.

Historical Review of Research in Metabolite Studies

Greenspan et al. (1970) conducted the earliest studies of urinary MHPG in humans as an index of central noradrenergic activity. That study concluded that in all nine hypomanic patients, NE, epinephrine, their metabolites normetanephrine (N) and metanephrine (MET), MHPG, and HVA were higher in the hypomanic state.

Since that time, as summarized in Tables 7–1 through 7–6, these studies have indicated increased urinary MHPG in 12 of 19 studies, increased plasma MHPG in 5 of 6 studies, and increased CSF MHPG in 6 of 8 studies. Furthermore, manic patients have been found to have elevated urinary DA and HVA (1 in 1 study), urinary NE (6 in 6), plasma NE (1 in 1), and CSF NE (3 in 3). CSF HVA has been found to be elevated in manic patients in 7 of 11 studies. Replication attempts done after probenecid have not been successful.

We now consider the more recent studies. In an attempt to differentiate 10 bipolar manic patients from 10 paranoid schizophrenic patients, diagnosed according to Research Diagnostic Criteria (RDC) (Spitzer et al. 1978), Mason et al. (1991) found that 24-hour urine collections (μg/day) showed significantly higher mean levels ($P < .03$) for both NE and epinephrine in bipolar patients (60 μg/day and 21 μg/day, respectively) than in schizophrenic patients (36 μg/day and 13 μg/day, respectively).

Table 7–1. Cerebrospinal fluid (CSF) norepinephrine (NE) and vanillyl-mandelic acid (VMA) and urinary VMA in mania

Investigator	Parameter	Comments
Schildkraut 1965	urinary VMA: ↑	In hypomanic patients
Jimerson et al. 1977	CSF VMA: no change	Compared with non-depressed psychiatric patients and control subjects
Greenspan et al. 1970	urinary VMA: ↑	In hypomanic patients
Post and Goodwin 1978	CSF NE: ↑	Manic patients compared with depressed patients
Post et al. 1978a	CSF NE: ↑	Manic patients compared with depressed patients and control subjects at borderline and after probenecid-induced accumulation
Post et al. 1980	CSF NE: ↑	Manic patients at bed rest

Table 7–2.   Urinary 3-methoxy-4-hydroxyphenylglycol (MHPG) in mania

Investigator	Urinary MHPG	Comments
Greenspan et al. 1970	↑	Manic versus depressed patients
Bond et al. 1972	↑	Manic versus depressed patients
Bunney et al. 1972	NS	
Ebert et al. 1972	↑	Control subjects: S/P 4-hour activity
Jenner and Sampson 1972	↑	Manic versus depressed patients (long)
De Leon-Jones et al. 1973	↑	Manic versus depressed patients; end of the manic episode
Post et al. 1973	↑	Control subjects: S/P 4-hour activity
Goode et al. 1973	↑ ↓	Did not replicate findings
Goodwin and Beckmann 1975	↑	Manic versus bipolar depressed patients
Post et al. 1976	↑	
Wehr 1977	NS	
Casper et al. 1977	↑	Manic versus depressed patients
Post et al. 1977	↑	Manic versus depressed patients
Post et al. 1977	↑ ↓	No correlation with increased motor activity
Koslow et al. 1983	NS	
Muscettola et al. 1984	NS	
Leckman and Maas 1984	↑	
Swann et al. 1994	↑	Manic versus depressed patients

Note.   NS = not significant; long = longitudinal case switches of individuals; SP = status post.

Using RDC, Sharma et al. (1994) studied CSF and plasma MHPG among four diagnostic groups but found no significant differences. The respective results (sample size, CSF, plasma) reported were schizophrenia (30, 8.8, 2.5), depression (19, 9.2, 2.2), mania (8, 9.7, 2.6), and schizoaffective (13, 9.4, 2.4).

Swann et al. (1994) reported results of biological investigations on

Table 7-3. Plasma 3-methoxy-4-hydroxyphenylglycol (MHPG) findings in mania

Investigator	Plasma MHPG	Comments
Halaris 1978	↑	Levels were higher at the peak of mania
Jimerson et al. 1981	↑	Manic patients compared with control subjects without a psychiatric diagnosis
Berrettini et al. 1985	↑	Positive correlation in manic patients but not in control subjects
Adler et al. 1990	↑	Positive correlation with sensory gating in manic patients
Swann et al. 1990b	NS	Compared stress-related with autonomous episodes
Baker et al. 1990	↑	Positive correlation with sensory gating

Note. NS = not significant.

8 patients with mixed mania, 11 patients with pure mania, 20 patients with agitated bipolar depression, and 27 patients with nonagitated bipolar depression. They found that CSF levels relative to control subjects for both MHPG and HVA had the following respective sequence: mixed manic patients (1.5, 1.25), pure manic patients (1.15, 1.0), agitated bipolar depressed patients (1.15, 0.8), and nonagitated bipolar depressed patients (1.05, 0.9). Similarly, urinary NE relative to control subjects had the following order: mixed manic patients (3.1), pure manic patients (1.75), agitated bipolar depressed patients (1.25), and nonagitated bipolar depressed patients (1.12).

Young et al. (1994) suggested that increased NE turnovers/metabolism may be an important biochemical disturbance in bipolar affective disorder. Their study on postmortem brains of bipolar patients elicited the following major findings about catecholamines: 1) markedly increased NE turnover over control subjects as indicated by MHPG/NE ratio in frontal ($+107\%$, $P = .003$), temporal ($+103\%$, $P < .04$), and occipital ($+64\%$, $P < .01$) cortices; and 2) decreases in DA turnover compared with control subjects as indicated by HVA/DA ratios in the occipital cortex (-64%, $P < .01$).

Table 7–4. Cerebrospinal fluid (CSF) 3-methoxy-4-hydroxyphenylglycol (MHPG) in mania

Investigator	CSF MHPG	Comments
Post et al. 1973	↑	Manic versus depressed patients
Shopsin et al. 1973	↑	Manic versus depressed patients
Goodwin et al. 1973	↓	In manic patients, after furasic acid
Ashcroft et al. 1976	↑	Manic versus retarded patients but not agitated depressed patients
Vestergaard et al. 1978	NS	Manic versus depressed patients and control subjects (small sample)
Gerner et al. 1984	↑	In manic patients versus control subjects
Koslow et al. 1983	↑	In manic patients compared with depressed patients and control subjects
Swann et al. 1994	↑	Manic versus depressed patients

Note. NS = not significant.

Interactions of Catecholamines With Other Systems

In addition to having a role in the specific etiology of the symptoms or syndrome of mania, catecholamines may interact with other nervous or hormonal system pathways. For example, an interesting hypothesis was formulated by Whybrow and Prange (1981), who indicated that increased thyroid activity would increase β-adrenergic response to catecholamines and lead to manic symptoms.

Risch and Janowsky (1984) reflected on the modulatory action of NE with acetylcholine and its influence on affective states. Silverstone (1985) proposed that DA had a similar role in the pathogenesis of mania. Silverstone also looked at the relationship of DA with γ-amino-butyric acid (GABA) systems and concluded that DA also acts in close relationship with both of these systems in the onset of mania.

Role of Precursors in Onset of Mania

The possible mechanisms of action for different drugs have been used to help explain the pathogenesis of mania with relation to catecho-

Table 7–5. Urinary homovanillic acid (HVA), dopamine (DA), norepinephrine (NE), epinephrine (E), normetanephrine (NM),
and metanephrine (MET) studies and plasma NE and
E studies in mania

Investigator	Parameter	Comments
Ström-Olsen and	Urinary NE: ↑	
Weil-Malherbe 1958	Urinary E: ↑	During manic
Greenspan et al. 1970	Urinary HVA: ↑	In hypomanic patients
	Urinary NE, urinary E, urinary NM, urinary MET: ↑	
Bunney et al. 1972	Urinary DA: ↑	During manic episode
	Urinary NE: ↑	Prior to manic
	Urinary E: ↑	During manic
Post et al. 1977	Urinary NE: ↑	Prior to manic
Koslow et al. 1983	Urinary NE: ↑	Manic patients
Maas et al. 1984	Plasma NE, plasma E: ↑	During manic episode
Swann et al. 1990a	Urinary NE: ↑[a]	
	Urinary NM, urinary MET: ↑	
Swann et al. 1994	Urinary NE, urinary E, urinary NM: ↑	Compared to depressed
	Urinary MET	Manic = depressed

[a]In stress-related manic episodes compared with autonomous episodes.

lamines. Several studies have been done regarding mania induced by
the DA precursor, L-dopa, in predisposed patients (Goodwin et al.
1970; Murphy et al. 1971; Van Praag and Korf 1975). The doses and
rate of illness were 4–12.5 g/day with a combined rate of mania of
11/12 or 92%. Other researchers have reported on mania induced by
amphetamines and piribedil (Gerner et al. 1976; Jimerson et al. 1977;
Post et al. 1978b).

Role of Mood Stabilizers

Mania responds to medications such as lithium and carbamazepine.
The exact mechanism of action of these medications remains undeter-

Table 7–6. Cerebrospinal fluid (CSF) homovanillic acid (HVA) in mania

Investigator	CSF HVA	Comments
Roos and Sjöström 1969	NS	Manic patients versus control subjects
Sjöström and Roos 1972	↑	Manic patients versus control subjects
Wilk et al. 1972	NS	Manic patients versus control subjects
Sjöström 1973a	↑	Manic patients versus control subjects
Goodwin et al. 1973	NS	Manic patients versus control subjects
Banki 1977	↑	Manic patients versus control subjects
Vestergaard et al. 1978	↑	Manic patients versus control subjects (small sample)
Koslow et al. 1983	↑	Manic patients versus depressed women
Gerner et al. 1984	NS	Just a trend to increased
Tandon et al. 1988	↑	Manic patients versus depressed patients
Swann et al. 1994	↑	Manic patients versus depressed patients
Roos and Sjöström 1969	NS	Different onsets compared with control subjects[a]
Sjöström and Roos 1972	↓	Manic patients compared with depressed patients[a]
Goodwin et al. 1973	NS	Manic patients compared with control subjects[a]
Sjöström 1973b	NS	Manic patients compared with control subjects[a]

Note. NS = not significant.
[a]After probenecid-induced accumulations.

mined, but studies concerning their effect on catecholamines have been done. In particular, studies on lithium's mechanism of action have shed light on the pathogenesis of mania.

Greenspan et al. (1970) showed that 2–4 weeks of lithium administration led to changes in urinary MHPG (µg/24 hour) depending on patient state: manic patients showed reductions from 2,780 to 2,190 (−21%); euthymic bipolar patients showed little change from 2,595 to 2,485 (−4%); and depressed bipolar patients showed increases from 1,480 to 1,883 (+27%). Later that year, Messiha et al. (1970) partly replicated these results with regard to urinary DA (µg/24 hour): manic patients had reductions from 1,120 to 460 (−59%), whereas depressed bipolar patients had increases from 700 to 830 (+19%). In contrast, Linnoila et al. (1983), in studies of urinary NE and DA in depressed patients, found that lithium reduced the turnover of both MHPG (nmol/24 hour) from 7.5 to 4.7 (−37%) and DA (μmol/24 hour) from 4.46 to 4.20 (−6%). This result may be explained by the findings of Beckmann et al. (1975), who found that only those bipolar depressed patients who responded to lithium had increases in urinary MHPG (mg/24 hour) from 0.87 to 1.12 (+29%), whereas nonresponders fell from 1.52 to 1.16 (−24%). Corona et al. (1982) reported that 4 weeks of lithium led to significant increases in plasma NE (nanomoles/mL) in bipolar depressed patients from 0.15 to 0.19 (+27%). Wilk et al. (1972) showed that lithium administration to two manic patients produced reductions in CSF MHPG (no/mL) from 35 to 12 (−66%). Similarly, Bowers and Henninger (1977) showed that 3 weeks of lithium therapy led to changes in CSF HVA (no/mL) according to mood state: reductions in five manic patients (151.6–133.6, −12%) and increases in six bipolar depressed patients (133.7–149.5, +12%). Sharma et al. (1994) reported that in seven RDC manic patients, the administration of lithium at a mean dose of 1,242.8 mg/day for 5 weeks led to a mean fall in CSF MHPG from 7.8 to 6.3 ($P <$ .05). Thus, lithium has in general been shown to decrease levels of MHPG in manic patients and increase levels in bipolar depressed patients, particularly in responders. These results are in agreement with predictions based on the permissive theory of bipolar disorder (Prange et al. 1973).

Belmaker et al. (1982) discussed findings that at a molecular level, lithium prevents antagonist-supersensitivity in the β-adrenergic system. Bunney and Garland-Bunney (1987), in reviewing different mechanisms of lithium action, focused on lithium's role in blocking behavioral manifestations of development of postsynaptic supersensitive DA receptors. In a review of all human studies on lithium acute and long-term influences on measures of catecholamines and serotonin, Goodnick (1990) concluded that acute lithium administration acts through both catecholamines and serotonin to treat both mania and depression but that long-term prophylaxis appears to act through lithium influence on serotonin alone.

In contrast to lithium, Post et al. (1984) observed that carbamazepine caused decrements in CSF NE levels in mania patients. However, this study also noted that CSF HVA levels were not altered by carbamazepine in manic patients. Thus, carbamazepine's antimanic effects may occur via another pathway. This possibility may also explain the clinical differences between lithium and carbamazepine; for example, that carbamazepine may be more effective than lithium in treatment of rapid-cycling bipolar patients and of dysphoric or mixed manic patients (Post 1990; Post and Rubinow 1989).

▶ MOLECULAR THEORIES OF MANIA

Wehr et al. (1980) studied circadian rhythms of catecholamines, considering another hypothesis about the pathogenesis of mania and its relationship to catecholamines. Their findings showed that during mania, there was an impairment of the ability to process environmental time cues and maintain a normal phase of circadian rhythms. Looking at the pathogenesis of mania at a molecular level, they presented a model in which signal transduction impairment could produce an accumulation of biologically active transducers or second messengers in a cyclic manner. Their findings supported the hypothesis that the ability to process environmental time cues and maintain a normal phase circadian rhythm is impaired in manic-depressive patients.

Lachman and Papolos (1989) also considered the molecular basis of manic-depressive disorder, presenting a model where inherited abnormalities of the transducer and second-messenger system could result in excessive accumulation of these biological mediators and disrupt neurotransmission in neuronal systems that regulate mood and behavior. They considered the evidence presented by other authors relating to subcortical nuclei such as the mesencephalic raphe nucleus.

▶ CONCLUSION

The catecholamine hypothesis of mood disorders (based on elevated DA and NE function in the brain during mania with reductions during depression) has led to extensive hypothesis testing in urine, plasma, CSF, and even postmortem samples. Results have lent significant but not total support to elevations in NE, in particular, but also DA turn-over during mania. Further support for this hypothesis may be found in the association of L-dopa (the precursor of DA), amphetamine (the catecholamine releaser), and piribedil (the DA agonist) with the in-duction of mania in bipolar depressed patients. The fact that lithium's antimanic effects have also been associated with a decrease in the mea-sure of urinary and CSF catecholamines also supports this hypothesis. However, further research is needed regarding the molecular basis of mania and its relationship to catecholamines, as well as a better un-derstanding of catecholamine receptor measures during mania. Finally, more work is needed to clarify the relationship between multiple trans-mitter systems (e.g., serotonin, acetylcholine, and GABA) during the manic state, because alterations in all these systems may be due to another, perhaps second, messenger agent.

▶ REFERENCES

Adler LE, Gerhardt GA, Franks R, et al: Sensory physiology and catecho-lamines in schizophrenia and mania. Psychiatry Res 31:297–309, 1990

Ashcroft GW, Dow RC, Yates CM, et al: Significance of lumbar CSF metabo-lite measurements in affective illness, in CNS and Behavioral Pharma-cology, Vol 3. Edited by Tuomisto J, Paasonen MK. Helsinki, Finland, University of Helsinki, 1976, pp 277–284

Baker NJ, Staunton M, Adler LE, et al: Sensory gating deficits in psychiatric inpatients: relation to catecholamine metabolites in different diagnostic groups. Biol Psychiatry 27:519–528, 1990

Banki CM: Correlation between cerebrospinal fluid amine metabolites and psychomotor activity in affective disorders. J Neurochem 28:255–257, 1977

Beckmann H, St-Laurent J, Goodwin FK: The effect of lithium on urinary MHPG in unipolar and bipolar depressed patients. Psychopharmacol-ogy (Berlin) 42:277–282, 1975

Belmaker RH, Zohar J, Levy A: Unidirectionality of lithium stabilization of adrenergic and cholinergic receptors, in Basic Mechanisms in the Action of Lithium. Amsterdam, Netherlands, Excerpt Medica, 1982, pp 146–153

Berrettini WH, Nurnberger JI Jr, Scheinin M, et al: Cerebrospinal fluid and plasma monoamines and their metabolites in euthymic bipolar patients. Biol Psychiatry 20:257–269, 1985

Bond PA, Jenner FA, Sampson GA: Daily variations of the urine content of 3-methoxy-4-hydroxyphenylglycol in two manic-depressive patients. Psychol Med 2:81–85, 1972

Bowers MB Jr, Henninger GR: Lithium: clinical effects and cerebrospinal fluid acid monoamine metabolites. Communications in Psychopharmacology 1:135–145, 1977

Bunney WE Jr, Garland-Bunney BL: Mechanisms of action of lithium in affective illness: basic and clinical implications, in Psychopharmacology: The Third Generation of Progress. Edited by Meltzer HY. New York, Raven, 1987, pp 553–565

Bunney WE Jr, Goodwin FK, Murphy DL, et al: The "switch process" in manic-depressive illness, II: relationship to catecholamines, REM sleep, and drugs. Arch Gen Psychiatry 27:304–309, 1972

Casper RC, Davis JM, Pandey GN, et al: Neuroendocrine and amine studies in affective illness. Psychoneuroendocrinology 2:105–113, 1977

Corona GL, Cucchi ML, Santagostino G: Blood noradrenaline and 5HT levels in depressed women during amitriptyline or lithium treatment. Psychopharmacology (Berlin) 77:236–241, 1982

De Leon-Jones F, Maas JW, Dekirmenjian H, et al: Urinary catecholamine metabolites during behavioral changes in a patient with manic-depressive cycles. Science 179:300–302, 1973

Ebert MH, Post RM, Goodwin FK: The effect of physical activity on urinary MHPG excretion in depressed patients. Lancet 2:766, 1972

Gerner RH, Post RM, Bunney WE Jr: A dopaminergic mechanism in mania. Am J Psychiatry 133:1177–1180, 1976

Gerner RH, Fairbanks L, Anderson GM, et al: CSF neurochemistry in depressed, manic, and schizophrenic patients compared with that of normal controls. Am J Psychiatry 141:1533–1540, 1984

Goode DJ, Dekirmenjian H, Meltzer HY, et al: Relation of exercise to MHPG excretion in normal subjects. Arch Gen Psychiatry 29:391–396, 1973

Goodnick P: Effects of lithium on indices of 5HT and catecholamines in the clinical context: a review. Lithium 1:65–73, 1990

Goodwin FK, Beckmann H: Urinary MHPG in subtypes of affective illness. Scientific Proceedings in Summary Form, 128th Annual Meeting of the American Psychiatric Association. Washington, DC, American Psychiatric Association, 1975, pp 96–97

Goodwin FK, Murphy DL, Brodie HKH, et al: L-dopa, catecholamines, and behavior: a clinical and biochemical study in depressed patients. Biol Psychiatry 2:341–366, 1970

Goodwin FK, Post RM, Dunner DL, et al: Cerebrospinal fluid amine metabolites in affective illness: the probenecid technique. Am J Psychiatry 130:73–79, 1973

Greenspan K, Schildkraut JJ, Gordon EK et al: Catecholamine metabolism in affective disorders, III: MHPG and other catecholamine metabolites in patients treated with lithium carbonate. J Psychiatr Res 7:171–183, 1970

Halaris AE: Plasma 3-methoxy-4-hydroxyphenylglycol in manic psychosis. Am J Psychiatry 135:493–494, 1978

Jenner FA, Sampson GA: Daily variation of the urine content of 3-methoxy-4-hydroxyphenylglycol in two manic-depressive patients. Psychol Med 2:81–85, 1972

Jimerson DC, Post RM, Reus VI, et al: Predictors of amphetamine response in depression (abstract 170). Scientific Proceedings in Summary Form, 130th Annual Meeting of the American Psychiatric Association. Washington, DC, American Psychiatric Association, 1977, pp100–101

Jimerson DC, Nurnberger JI Jr, Post RM, et al: Plasma MHPG in rapid cyclers and healthy twins. Arch Gen Psychiatry 38:1287–1290, 1981

Kety S, Schildkraut JJ, Bunney WE Jr, et al: Brain amines and affective disorders, in Brain Chemistry and Mental Disease. Edited by Oh BT, McIsaac WM. New York, Plenum, 1971, pp 237–263

Koslow SH, Maas JW, Bowden CL, et al: CSF and urinary biogenic amines and metabolites in depression and mania. Arch Gen Psychiatry 40:999–1010, 1983

Lachman HM, Papolos DF: Abnormal signal transduction: a hypothetical model for bipolar affective disorder. Life Sci 45:1413–1426, 1989

Leckman JF, Maas JW: Plasma MHPG: relationship to brain noradrenergic systems and emerging clinical applications, in Neurobiology of Mood Disorders. Edited by Post RM, Ballenger JC. Baltimore, MD, Williams & Wilkins, 1984, pp 529–538

Linnoila M, Karoum F, Potter WZ: Effects of antidepressant treatments on dopamine turnover in depressed patients. Arch Gen Psychiatry 40:1015–1017, 1983

Maas JW, Koslow SH, Katz MM, et al: Pretreatment neurotransmitter metabolite levels and response to tricyclic anti-depressant drugs. Am J Psychiatry 141:1159–1171, 1984

Martin JB, Reichlin S: Neuropharmacology of anterior pituitary regulation, in Clinical Neuroendocrinology, 2nd Edition. Edited by Martin JB, Reichlin S. Philadelphia, PA, Davis, 1987, pp 45–63

Mason JW, Kosten TR, Giller EL: Multidimensional hormonal discrimination of paranoid schizophrenia from bipolar manic patients. Biol Psychiatry 29:457–466, 1991

Messiha FS, Agileness D, Clower C: Dopamine excretion in affective states and following lithium carbonate therapy. Nature 225:868–869, 1970

Murphy DL, Brodie HKH, Goodwin FK, et al: Regular induction of hypomania by L-dopa in "bipolar" manic-depressive patients. Nature 229:135–136, 1971

Muscettola G, Potter WZ, Pickar D, et al: Urinary 3-methoxy-4-hydroxyphenylglycol and major affective disorders. Arch Gen Psychiatry 41:337–342, 1984

Post RM: Non-lithium treatment for bipolar disorder. J Clin Psychiatry 51 (suppl 8):9–16, 1990

Post RM, Goodwin FK: Approaches to brain amines in psychiatric patients: a re-evaluation of cerebrospinal fluid studies, in Handbook of Psychopharmacology, Vol 13: Biology of Mood and Antianxiety Drugs. Edited by Aversion L, Aversion SD, Snyder SH. New York, Plenum, 1978, pp 147–185

Post RM, Rubinow DR: Dysphoric mania. Arch Gen Psychiatry 46:353–358, 1989

Post RM, Gordon EK, Goodwin FK, et al: Central norepinephrine metabolism in affective illness: MHPG in the cerebrospinal fluid. Science 179:1002–1003, 1973

Post RM, Gerner RH, Carman JS, et al: Effects of low doses of a dopamine-receptor stimulator in mania. Lancet 1:203–204, 1976

Post RM, Stoddard FJ, Gillin JC, et al: Alterations in motor activity, sleep, and biochemistry in a cycling manic-depressive patient. Arch Gen Psychiatry 34:470–477, 1977

Post RM, Lake CR, Jimerson DC, et al: Cerebrospinal fluid norepinephrine in affective illness. Am J Psychiatry 135:907–912, 1978a

Post RM, Gerner RH, Carman JS, et al: Effects of a dopamine agonist piribedil in depressed patients. Arch Gen Psychiatry 35:609–615, 1978b

Post RM, Ballenger JC, Goodwin FK: Cerebrospinal fluid studies of neurotransmitter function in manic and depressive illness, in The Neurobiology of Cerebrospinal Fluid, Vol 1. Edited by Wood JH. New York, Plenum, 1980, pp 685–717

Post RM, Ballenger JC, Uhde TW, et al: Efficacy of carbamazepine in manic-depressive illness: implications for underlying mechanisms, in Neurobiology of Mood Disorders. Edited by Post RM, Ballenger JC. Baltimore, MD, Williams & Wilkins, 1984, pp 777–816

Prange AJ Jr, Sisk JL, Wilson IC, et al: Balance, permission, and discrimination among amines: a theoretical consideration of the actions of L-tryptophan in disorders of movement and affect, in Serotonin in Affective Disorders. Edited by Barchas J, Usdin E. New York, Academic Press, 1973, pp 539–548

Risch SC, Janowsky DS: Cholinergic-adrenergic balance in affective illness, in Neurobiology of Mood Disorders. Edited by Post RM, Ballenger JC. Baltimore, MD, Williams & Wilkins, 1984, pp 652–663

Roos BE, Sjöström R: 5-Hydroxyindoleacetic acid (and homovanillic acid) levels in the cerebrospinal fluid after probenecid application in patients with manic-depressive psychosis. Pharmacologia Clinica 1:153–155, 1969

Schildkraut JJ: The catecholamine hypothesis of affective disorders: a review of supporting evidence. Am J Psychiatry 122:509–522, 1965

Sharma RP, Javaid JI, Faull K, et al: CSF and plasma MHPG, and the CSF MHPG index: pretreatment levels in diagnostic groups and response to somatic treatments. Psychiatry Res 51:51–60, 1994

Shopsin G, Wilk S, Gershon S, et al: Collaborative psychopharmacologic studies exploring catecholamine metabolism in psychiatric disorders, in Frontiers in Catecholamine Research. Edited by Usdin E, Snyder SH. New York, Pergamon, 1973, pp 1173–1179

Silverstone T: Dopamine in manic depressive illness: a pharmacological synthesis. J Affect Disord 8:225–231, 1985

Sjöström R: Cerebrospinal fluid content of 5-hydroxyindoleacetic acid and homovanillic acid in manic-depressive psychosis. Acta Univ Upsaliensis 154:5–35, 1973a

Sjöström R: 5-Hydroxyindoleacetic acid and homovanillic acid in cerebrospinal fluid in manic-depressive psychosis and the effect of probenecid treatment. Eur J Clin Pharmacol 6:75–80, 1973b

Spitzer RL, Endicott J, Robins E: Research Diagnostic Criteria: rationale and reliability. Arch Gen Psychiatry 35:773–782, 1978

Ström-Olsen R, Weil-Malherbe H: Humoral changes in manic-depressive psychosis with particular reference to the excretion of catecholamines in urine. Journal of Mental Science 104:696–704, 1958

Swann AC, Berman N, Frazer A, et al: Lithium distribution in mania: single-dose pharmacokinetics and sympathoadrenal function. Psychiatry Res 32:71–84, 1990a

Swann AC, Secunda SK, Stokes PE, et al: Stress, depression, and mania: relationship between perceived role of stressful events and clinical and biochemical characteristics. Acta Psychiatr Scand 81:389–397, 1990b

Swann AC, Stokes PE, Secunda SK, et al: Depressive mania versus agitated depression: biogenic amine and hypothalamic-pituitary-adrenocortical function. Biol Psychiatry 35:803–813, 1994

Tandon R, Channabasavanna SM, Greden JF: CSF biochemical correlates of mixed affective states. Acta Psychiatr Scand 78:289–297, 1988

Van Praag HM, Korf J: Central monoamine deficiency in depression: causative of secondary phenomenon? Pharmakopsychiatr Neuropsychopharmakol 8:322–326, 1975

Vestergaard P, Sorensen T, Hoppe E, et al: Biogenic amine metabolites in cerebrospinal fluid of patients with affective disorders. Acta Psychiatr Scand 58:88–96, 1978

Wehr TA: Phase and biorhythm studies of affective illness. Ann Intern Med 87:319–335, 1977

Wehr TA, Muscettola G, Goodwin FK: Urinary 3-methoxy-4-hydroxy-phenylglycol circadian rhythm. Arch Gen Psychiatry 37:257–263, 1980

Whybrow PC, Prange AJ Jr: A hypothesis of thyroid-catecholamine-receptor interaction: its relevance to affective illness. Arch Gen Psychiatry 38:106–113, 1981

Wilk S, Shopsin B, Gershon S, et al: Cerebrospinal fluid levels of MHPG in affective disorders. Nature 235:440–441, 1972

Woodward DJ, Moises HC, Waterhouse BD, et al: Modulatory actions of norepinephrine in the central nervous system. Federation Proceedings 38:2109–2116, 1979

Young LT, Warsh JJ, Kish SJ, et al: Reduced brain 5HT and elevated NE turnover and metabolites in bipolar affective disorder. Biol Psychiatry 35:121–127, 1994

CHAPTER 8

ACETYLCHOLINE

David S. Janowsky, M.D., and
David H. Overstreet, Ph.D.

Considerable information has suggested a role for mono-aminergic/cholinergic balance in the pathogenesis of mania. As proposed by Janowsky et al. (1972a), mania may be a manifestation of a relative central cholinergic underactivity and adrenergic overactivity, whereas depression may be due to an opposite relationship. In this chapter, we summarize the research findings from both animal and human studies that suggest that central muscarinic mechanisms are likely to contribute to the psychopathology of mania and bipolarity specifically, as well as to affective disorders in general. The greater part of the chapter focuses on the relationship of acetylcholine and adrenergic-cholinergic balance to manic phenomenology, but evidence of a role for increased cholinergic activity in depression is also reviewed.

The early studies that explored a potential role for acetylcholine in the affective disorders generally utilized bipolar patients, most often those in the manic state. Some of the most dramatic and supportive evidence for a role for adrenergic-cholinergic balance in the affective disorders has been derived from these studies of manic and/or bipolar depressed patients and excited schizoaffective patients; the latter is thought in many cases to be a variant of bipolar disorder. More recently, continuing studies of the role of cholinergic mechanisms in the affective disorders have generally focused on patients with major depressive disorder, with a corresponding de-emphasis on the study of bipolar patients. Because of the more recent relative de-emphasis on bipolar patients, the earlier phenomenologic studies of the 1970s and early 1980s exploring the effects of cholinergic agents in bipolar patients are reviewed in detail in this chapter. This series of studies may lay the groundwork for a new generation of studies considering the role of acetylcholine in manic and bipolar patients as such.

▶ Effects of Cholinomimetics on Manic Symptoms

A number of studies have demonstrated that increasing central cholinergic activity leads to a decrease in manic symptoms. In a seminal study by Rowntree et al. (1950), diisopropyl fluorophosphonate (DFP), a long-acting, irreversible, centrally active cholinesterase inhibitor was given to 9 manic-depressive (i.e., bipolar) patients and to 10 control subjects. Control subjects developed irritability, lassitude, depression, apathy, and slowness or poverty of thoughts, which appeared before the onset of peripheral cholinergic symptoms. Two of the manic-depressive patients, tested while in remission, showed mental changes like those of the control subjects, and two hypomanic patients improved with DFP and continued euthymic after its administration. One hypomanic patient became less manic, and was minimally depressed after each of two courses of DFP, but relapsed on DFP withdrawal. One nearly remitted hypomanic patient became floridly manic on DFP withdrawal, and one depressed bipolar patient showed a considerable increase in depression during DFP administration.

Like Rowntree et al. (1950), Janowsky et al. (1973b) found that the centrally active cholinesterase inhibitor, physostigmine, caused a dramatic yet brief reduction in hypomanic and manic symptoms in eight bipolar patients. Neither placebo nor the noncentrally acting cholinesterase inhibitor, neostigmine, produced such changes, and the changes were reversed by the centrally active antimuscarinic drug, atropine. Thus, it was concluded that physostigmine's antimanic effects were due to a central cholinergic, central muscarinic mechanism. Specific to the earlier study, following physostigmine administration, the Beigel-Murphy manic "elation-grandiosity" scale score was reduced within minutes by 78%, and the "manic intensity" scale score was reduced by 48%. Physostigmine also caused a decrease in specific manic symptoms: is talking reduced by 53%, is active by 62%, jumps from one subject to another by 51%, and looks happy and cheerful by 77%. Grandiosity was significantly decreased in the three patients in whom it was present during the baseline period, and irritability decreased in three patients and increased in five. The effects of physostigmine were of rapid onset and lasted from 20 to 90 minutes. In different patients, the total amount of physostigmine necessary to cause a decrease in manic symptoms varied from 0.25 to 3.0 mg. In addition, the average depression score of the patients, as measured using the Bunney-Hamburg scale, more than doubled, and a statistically significant increase in the patient group's "sadness" score occurred. Five of the eight patients developed a depressed mood, whereas three experienced no increase in depression after receiving physostigmine.

In addition to alleviating manic symptoms and causing an increase in depression in most patients, physostigmine caused a retarded, inhibitory state in the patients, slowing them down in a way similar to that occurring in patients suffering from retarded depression. An "inhibitory scale" was derived from the observed phenomena. This scale consisted of the sum of the scores for each patient on the scales termed lethargic, slow thoughts, wants to say nothing, withdrawn, apathetic, lacks energy, drained, hypoactive, lacks thoughts, motor retarded, and emotionally withdrawn, because these symptoms appeared most consistently to increase in the patients following physostigmine administration (Janowsky et al. 1973b). After physostigmine administration, the average "inhibitory scale" score for the manic patients evaluated quadrupled. Physostigmine did not produce marked sedation, obtunded behavior, slurred speech, or ataxia, nor did it cause the patients to fall asleep, such as might have happened with high doses of sedative drugs. Later studies have consistently demonstrated increased behavioral inhibition across all diagnostic categories (Janowsky and Risch 1987).

The following two cases illustrate the qualitative nature of physostigmine's effects on mania.

Case 1

A 34-year-old white female bipolar manic-depressive patient demonstrated marked flight of ideas, increased talkativeness, and rapid fluctuations from cheerfulness and euphoria to anger and argumentativeness; she also demonstrated manipulative behavior of staff members, consisting of aggressive incisive verbal attacks. Administration of placebo injections caused no change in the patient's clinical state. Administration of physostigmine caused the patient, within several minutes, to become more passive, quiet, and reflective; her anger dissipated. She said that she felt sad and scared but on an "even keel" and that she felt warmth for the ward staff. She showed decreased talkativeness and less flight of ideas. She was neither confused, lethargic, nor disoriented. After receiving a total of 2.0 mg physostigmine, about 20 minutes after the onset of the more subdued behavior, the patient became nauseated and vomited. A dose of 1 mg of atropine administered intravenously partially reversed the "antimanic" state and alleviated the vomiting within 5 minutes of administration.

Case 2

A 40-year-old married white male with a 10-year history of bipolar manic-depressive illness presented during the baseline-placebo phase with moderate anger and irritability, increased interactions, and increased talkativeness. He showed moderate flight of ideas and was very manipulative of staff members. He was moderately euphoric. After receiving a total of 3.0 mg physostigmine intravenously, the patient abruptly showed a complete cessation of his manic symptoms. He became depressed, sad, and dysphoric. He stated that he was "no good" and began to cry. He then ceased to be active and did not wish to communicate. He stopped talking except when spoken to and asked to be left alone. He said he felt moderately drained and sad. He was apathetic, withdrawn, and lethargic and showed psychomotor retardation. Irritability and anger increased as the patient became depressed. A dose of 0.75 mg of atropine caused a partial return of manic symptoms, including talkativeness and increased interactions, and a complete reversal of the patient's dysphoria, lethargy, and drained feelings.

At about the same time that Janowsky et al. (1973b) reported their findings described earlier, Modestin et al. (1973a, 1973b) also reported a lessening of manic symptoms following infusion of physostigmine, but not neostigmine, in two of four manic patients. Davis et al. (1978) likewise reported that physostigmine caused dramatic antimanic effects, particularly in patients with low levels of hostility and/or irritability, and Carroll et al. (1973) reported a decrease in euphoria and in mobility after physostigmine infusion in a manic patient whose symptoms were caused by excessive glucocorticoid administration. More recently, Krieg and Berger (1986) reported pilot data suggesting that RS86, a relatively specific muscarinic (M_1) agonist, had significant antimanic effects in a small group of manic patients.

Although most of the descriptive data offered in the studies mentioned have proven supportive of centrally active cholinomimetic agents exerting an antimanic effect, some authors have suggested that these agents affect only the affective and motoric components of mania and do not affect the cognitive aspects of mania such as grandiose thinking. These investigators questioned whether cholinomimetics actually affect the "core" aspect of mania, manic thinking (Carroll et al. 1973; Shopsin et al. 1975).

▶ Rebounding of Manic Symptoms Following Cholinomimetic Administration

There is evidence that when the central cholinergic system is activated, a late-onset compensatory and antagonistic activation of the adrenergic (i.e., noradrenergic/dopaminergic) system occurs. In an animal model of mania, an increase in cholinergic activity caused by the administration of physostigmine led first to motor inhibition and later to an increase over baseline in locomotion (i.e., hyperactivity), as presumed compensatory increases in adrenergic mechanisms began to exert their effects. This activating effect became apparent as the cholinergic behavioral inhibition induced by physostigmine decreased and was exaggerated if a centrally acting anticholinergic-antimuscarinic agent (i.e., scopolamine) was given at the beginning of the hyperactivity phase (presumably because residual acetylcholine was antagonized). The rebound hyperactivity was prevented if a centrally active anticholinergic drug was given prior to physostigmine administration (Fibiger et al. 1971).

There is also some evidence that a late behavioral rebound into hypermania following physostigmine infusion can also occur in bipolar patients. As noted, Rowntree et al. (1950) observed that one of the manic patients to whom he administered DFP subsequently became hypermanic. Generally, physostigmine, given to hypomanic patients by Janowsky et al. (1973b) and Modestin et al. (1973a, 1973b), did not cause a late-onset rebounding.

However, Shopsin et al. (1975) showed different results, in a study of three highly manic patients given physostigmine. Physostigmine was then given after a varying number of placebo injections and, once started, was given at 5-minute intervals until a behavioral change occurred, or significant side effects appeared, or a total of 6 mg of physostigmine had been given. All three patients, irrespective of different overall dosage of physostigmine, demonstrated a three-phase evolution of physostigmine's effects. Initially, all patients experienced varying degrees of sedation, drowsiness, a desire to sleep but not being able to, some dysthymia and mild slurring of speech (occurring in two patients), confusion, and difficulty concentrating. A reduction in spontaneous speech and activity was apparent during this time. Two patients initially described feelings of comfort and relaxation. This subjective comfort soon dissipated in both cases. During this initial phase, it appeared that flight of ideas, rambling speech, tangentiality, irritability, and cheerfulness were attenuated with diminished verbal aggressiveness and decreased grandiose ideation. The delusional quality of the manic psychopathology, however, was not basically altered, and prompting or provoking the patients resulted in a reappearance of manic ideation. The severity of manic symptoms that reappeared on provocation depended on the observed degree of anergia. All patients spontaneously stated that they were eventually "talked out" and did not want to be bothered. Vomiting did not occur. Apathy and anergia were apparent, and no patient became depressed. Toward the end of physostigmine's administration, and always past the 2-mg mark, all patients showed irritability, sweating, and agitation, with marked restlessness quite apparent in two patients.

The most striking and salient feature emerging from this particular study was the late appearance of "rebounding," a clear-cut change in clinical state taking place 2 hours after the previous physostigmine injection in two patients. A marked exacerbation or intensification of the manic state over baseline levels occurred. In one of the patients, a psychotomimetic or activating effect occurred in the form of primary process behavior, which had not been observed previously, nor since that time. The rebounding phenomenon was transient and lasted 3–4 hours thereafter, with a return to baseline psychopathology at approximately 6 hours following the last physostigmine injection. As did Fibiger et al. (1971), Shopsin et al. (1975) interpreted the rebounding as occurring due to increased central acetylcholine compensatorily activating adrenergic mechanisms, the effects of which were unmasked as acetylcholine levels decreased when the physostigmine was metabolized.

▌ Opposite and Antagonistic Effects of Cholinomimetics and Psychostimulants

A pharmacologic-behavioral model for naturally occurring adrenergic-cholinergic regulation of mood may be found in the interactions and reciprocal effects of psychostimulants (which increase dopaminergic/noradrenergic activity) and cholinomimetics (which increase cholinergic activity). Psychostimulant-induced increases in locomotor activity, self-stimulation, and gnawing behavior are rapidly antagonized by physostigmine, but not by neostigmine (Domino and Olds 1968). Conversely, physostigmine's inhibitory-depressant effects on these variables can be reversed by methylphenidate (Janowsky et al. 1973a).

In humans, methylphenidate, like other stimulant drugs, causes increases in euphoric mood, thinking, talkativeness, and interactions. It usually increases manic symptoms in manic patients, including intensifying flight of ideas, talkativeness, and elation, and, when present, manic grandiosity and paranoia (Janowsky et al. 1972b). In this respect, it is similar to the effects of the dopamine precursor L-dopa's effects in manic and bipolar patients. These effects contrast dramatically with the effects of physostigmine, which induces behavioral inhibition in manic patients, as it does in other patients and in control subjects.

In general, methylphenidate causes a generalized increase in talkativeness and interactions. However, in schizophrenic patients with preexisting psychotic symptoms, methylphenidate also causes significant increases in such symptoms as delusions, hallucinations, and bizarre behavior (Janowsky et al. 1973a).

Because methylphenidate (as well as other stimulants) generally causes behavioral activating effects that in many ways parallel manic symptoms (i.e., increased thoughts, talkativeness, interactions) and specifically causes increases in manic symptoms and euphoria in manic patients, Janowsky et al. (1973a) studied the potential antagonistic effects of methylphenidate and physostigmine in humans as a pharmacologic model of naturally occurring adrenergic-cholinergic balance in bipolar patients.

Specifically, in a series of experiments performed in the early 1970s (Janowsky et al. 1973a), some manic and schizophrenic patients were first given physostigmine and then methylphenidate. Other manic and schizophrenic patients received the reverse sequence, methylphenidate followed by physostigmine. For the patients who were given methylphenidate followed by physostigmine, methylphenidate caused a significant increase in the Janowsky-Davis Behavioral Activation Scale (Janowsky et al. 1973a), consisting of a composite of interaction, talkativeness, cheerfulness, and friendliness ratings. This increase was rapidly reversed following the administration of physostigmine. In schizophrenic patients, psychosis activation also occurred after methylphenidate was given, and this effect was decreased by physostigmine. Conversely, physostigmine-induced behavioral inhibition and anergy were antagonized rapidly by methylphenidate. In contrast, patients who received noncentrally active neostigmine followed by methylphenidate displayed no initial behavioral inhibition, and neostigmine failed to inhibit the activating effects of methylphenidate.

Concerning specific results, Janowsky et al. (1973a) noted that physostigmine decreased the average mania ratings of talkativeness, activity, flight of ideas, happiness, and overall manic intensity scores and elation/grandiosity scores in a group of nine manic patients. Methylphenidate, given on another occasion to six of the same manic patients, significantly increased talkativeness, activity, flight of ideas, and manic intensity scores. Neostigmine exerted no significant effects.

Furthermore, when given sequentially, the increase in the activation scale scores caused by methylphenidate in five manic patients was partially and statistically significantly reversed by physostigmine. Conversely, in six manic patients, physostigmine-induced increases in Behavioral Inhibition Scale scores were partially and statistically significantly reversed by methylphenidate.

Possibly related to the ability of physostigmine to antagonize methylphenidate-induced psychostimulation is the observation that physostigmine caused a rapid, dramatic drop in the norepinephrine metabolite, serum 3-methoxy-4-hydroxphenylglycol (MHPG) in a manic patient, presumably reflecting a drop in central nervous system (CNS) noradrenergic activity. Furthermore, a reciprocal relationship may exist between a subject's response to a psychostimulant and his or her separate response to a cholinomimetic agent. Nurnberger et al. (1983b) noted a negative correlation between amphetamine-induced behavioral excitation and the ability of arecoline, given on another occasion, to decrease rapid eye movement latency, an acetylcholine-sensitive sleep parameter. Similarly, Siever and colleagues (Siever and Uhde 1984; Siever et al. 1981) showed that in a mixed group of affective disorder and control subjects, those with the most dramatic physostigmine and arecoline-induced anergy and negative affect showed a blunted growth hormone response to the noradrenergic agonist clonidine, presumably a reflection of decreased noradrenergic responsiveness.

▶ INDUCTION OF SEVERE DEPRESSION IN
   MARIJUANA-INTOXICATED INDIVIDUALS

In several ways, the acute effects of marijuana, like the psychostimulants, parallel those of hypomania. Thus, marijuana can induce feelings of well-being, euphoria, increased verbalizations, flight of ideas, and sequential thought impairment. El-Yousef et al. (1973) reported on the effects of small doses of physostigmine on the intoxicating effects of marijuana in two volunteer control subjects. Both developed severe depression following very low doses of physostigmine, an unexpected finding. This observation was later replicated by Davis et al. (1978)

in volunteer control subjects, who had, unbeknownst to the investigators, smoked marijuana before receiving physostigmine. In the El-Yousef et al. (1973) study, both subjects were graduate students who were intermittent users of marijuana and had no history of serious emotional disturbance.

The following case report describes one of the cases reported by El-Yousef et al. (1973).

Case 3

The female subject arrived apparently intoxicated on marijuana. She stated "I am 13/15th's as high as I have ever been." She was garrulous, cheerful, full of hilarity, showing flight of ideas, talkativeness, and the inability to remember three two-digit numbers for 30 seconds. She was witty, creative, and able to induce hilarity in those observing her. She described this as her usual response to marijuana. Her pulse rate was elevated to 120 and her conjunctiva were red. Five minutes after receiving a total of 0.25 mg physostigmine, she stated that she was no longer "high," that her thoughts were slowed down, and that she did not feel euphoric. By the time she had received 1.25 mg physostigmine, her clinical state had progressed until she reported and appeared to be lethargic, feeling drained, sad, extremely depressed, and saying she was hopeless, useless, and worthless. She sobbed and cried, manifested extreme psychomotor retardation, and reported having no thoughts. Her pulse rate at this time was 96. She stated that she had never been so depressed in her life, yet could offer no reasons to explain her feelings, and stated that she would have committed suicide had she not known that the syndrome was due to a drug. She appeared to be as depressed as any patient the authors had ever observed. Within 1 minute after atropine administration, she commented that she felt better; improvement progressed over the next ½ hour. However, a feeling of being drained and exhausted physically persisted for several hours after atropine administration.

These results were entirely unexpected. It had been hypothesized that marijuana intoxication would exert anticholinergic properties and antagonize physostigmine's effects. Subsequent studies by Rosenblatt et al. (1972) demonstrated that tetrahydrocannabinol significantly increased physostigmine-induced lethality in rats, an atropine- and methylscopolamine-reversible phenomena. Subsequently, cholinergic behavioral effects were found to be augmented by tetrahydrocannabinol in rats (Duncan and Dagirmanjian 1979).

❯ SELECTIVE DEPRESSIVE EFFECTS IN MANIC, SCHIZOAFFECTIVE, AND DEPRESSED PATIENTS

As can be seen from the earlier review and case examples, a significant proportion of manic patients given centrally acting cholinomimetics develop depressive symptoms. Janowsky et al. (1974) reported that in addition to the six of eight manic patients (described earlier), two depressive patients studied showed increased depressed mood with physostigmine infusion. Likewise, five of six schizoaffective patients (four excited, two depressed) showed depressed mood and sadness after physostigmine infusions. In contrast, of eight schizophrenic patients without an affective component to their illness, only one showed increased mood depression after receiving physostigmine. The affective disorder patients likewise showed statistically significantly increased depression scores when compared with the nonaffective disorder schizophrenic patients. Furthermore, physostigmine caused depression in a large percentage of the manic patients and bipolar patients given physostigmine by Modestin et al. (1973a, 1973b), Davis et al. (1978), and Rowntree et al. (1950). In addition, Oppenheimer et al. (1979) observed that physostigmine caused a depressed mood in a majority of euthymic bipolar patients maintained on lithium. Similarly, Nurnberger (1983a, 1983b) found that euthymic bipolar patients given the direct muscarinic agonist, arecoline, developed depressed mood and other forms of negative affect, including hostility and anxiety.

Conversely, although their control subjects developed behavioral inhibition like the bipolar patients, Oppenheimer et al. (1979) found no increases in depressed mood in their control subject cohort when they were given physostigmine. Similarly, Silva et al. (S. G. Silva, R. A. Stern, R. N. Golden, E. J. Davidson, G. A. Mason, and D. J. Janowsky, "The effects of physostigmine on behavioral inhibition, cognitive processes, mood state and neuroendocrine functioning in healthy males," unpublished manuscript, September 1994) showed no increase in depressed mood in their carefully screened control subjects who were given physostigmine, although the physostigmine-inhibitory syndrome did occur in most of their subjects.

That physostigmine may behaviorally differentiate patients with affective disorder diagnoses from other nonaffective diagnoses has been further supported by the work of Edelstein et al. (1981). These authors reported that schizophrenic patients who responded to physostigmine with a clearing of psychotic symptoms were significantly more likely to respond with symptomatic improvement when given lithium, presumably because they represented a variant of affective disorder. Furthermore, Steinberg et al. (1993) noted that increases in negative affect after physostigmine administration occurred selectively in those personality disorder patients with preexisting affectively unstable personalities (i.e., borderline personalities), when compared with those personality disorder patients who were affectively stable. However, one study of bipolar patients did not affirm that the latter subjects are supersensitive to the mood-depressing effects of cholinomimetics. Nurnberger et al. (1983a) found that changes in affective symptoms in control subjects did not differ from those of euthymic bipolar patients receiving arecoline.

Centrally active cholinomimetic drugs cause a psychomotor retardation-like syndrome, markedly mimicking the psychomotor component of endogenous depression in virtually all subject groups. In addition, there is evidence, in part reviewed earlier, that patients with nonbipolar major depression can develop an intensified depressed mood after central cholinomimetic administration. This was noted by Janowsky et al. (1973a, 1973b), Modestin et al. (1973a, 1973b), and Rowntree et al. (1950). Depressed mood has also been occasionally observed in control subjects receiving intravenous physostigmine or arecoline (Nurnberger et al. 1983a; Risch et al. 1981), but less frequently than in nonaffective disorder patients.

Some Alzheimer patients receiving acetylcholine precursors, including deanol, choline, and lecithin, also have been reported to develop depression. Davis et al. (1979) and Tamminga et al. (1976) found that depressive mood occurred in some schizophrenic patients who were treated with choline. In selective cases, it was furthermore noted that depressed mood was a side effect of choline and lecithin treatments employed to try to reverse the memory deficits of Alzheimer's disease (Bajada 1982; Mohs et al. 1987). Also, Casey (1979) observed that depressed mood occurred in a subset of deanol-treated patients with tardive dyskinesia and other movement disorders. Thus, precursors of acetylcholine, in addition to cholinergic agonists and anticholinesterase agents, have consistently been noted in several studies to induce a depressed mood.

The majority of studies evaluating the effects of cholinomimetic agents on nonbipolar patients with major depressive disorder have demonstrated that these patients are relatively more sensitive to the general behavioral-inhibiting effects of cholinomimetics than are control subjects. Janowsky et al. (1980, 1981) found that rater-evaluated increases in the Behavioral Inhibition Scale score and in the self-rated anxiety, depression, hostility, confusion, and elation subscales of the Profile of Mood States showed significantly greater changes in depressed affective disorder patients than in other nonaffective disorders patient groups or control subjects after physostigmine infusion. However, the actual differences between control subjects, nonaffective psychiatric disorder patients, and the predominantly major depressive disorder patients were not great. Generally, approximately 25% of control subjects and nonaffective disorder patients show exaggerated changes in mood and behavioral inhibition after physostigmine, compared with approximately 75% of affective disorders patients.

The evidence that behavioral supersensitivity to cholinomimetics is a trait rather than a state marker in affective disorder patients is mixed. On the positive side, Oppenheimer et al. (1979) observed, as mentioned earlier, that a significant percentage of euthymic bipolar patients receiving lithium developed a depressed mood after receiving physostigmine, whereas control subjects who received physostigmine alone did not become depressed, but only became anergic. Similarly, Casey (1979) noted that those euthymic tardive dyskinesia patients with a strong past history of affective disorder selectively showed increased affective symptoms while receiving the putative acetylcholine precursor, deanol. However, Nurnberger et al. (1983a) did not observe a differential behavioral sensitivity between a group of euthymic affective disorder patients and control subjects. Thus, presently there are somewhat conflicting data on whether behavioral supersensitivity in affective disorder patients is a state- or trait-linked phenomenon, and the differentiation between bipolar behavioral sensitivity and supersensitivity in patients with major depressed disorder is not clear. Furthermore, no studies published as of this writing have examined the behavioral effects of cholinergic agonists on the unaffected relatives or offspring of affective disorder patients, and thus the state-trait question regarding cholinomimetic behavioral changes remains an open one.

▶ Mood Effects of Centrally Active Anticholinergic Agents

In contrast to the observed effects of centrally acting cholinomimetics, there is evidence that centrally active anticholinergic/antiparkinsonian drugs have mood-elevating properties, although this evidence is generally anecdotal and mostly uncontrolled. As noted by Jellinec et al. (1981) and Smith (1980), antiparkinsonian drugs used to treat drug-induced parkinsonian symptoms have been reported to cause positive feelings and reversal of depressed mood. Pleasurable effects reported by schizophrenic patients who have abused antiparkinsonian drugs include euphoria; being "buzzed or high"; having a reduction in anxiety; having a sense of well-being; and feeling more sociable and more confident, cheerful, and energetic. Anticholinergics are often used as drugs of abuse in conjunction with alcohol and other drugs of abuse. Furthermore, one report by Cold and Strang (1982) suggested that the anticholinergic agent procyclidine caused a switch into mania in a bipolar patient. In addition, several reports have suggested that high doses of atropine and other anticholinergics such as Ditran may alleviate depression; one report has suggested that a tricyclic-antidepressant–induced central anticholinergic syndrome may alleviate depression. Finally, Kasper et al. (1981) observed antidepressant effects with the anticholinergic drug biperiden, especially in patients with endogenous depression who had a nonsuppressing dexamethasone suppression test.

▶ Biological Studies of Cholinergic Mechanisms in Mania and Depression

The preceding paragraphs have discussed in detail the behavioral-phenomenologic effects of increasing both central cholinergic and adrenergic activity in manic symptoms, in patients with major depressive disorder, and in control subjects. In this section, several physiologic and biochemical studies that suggest that acetylcholine may be altered in the affective disorders, especially bipolar disorders, are outlined.

Red Blood Cell Choline in Bipolar Patients

Although there is considerable evidence that centrally acting muscarinic cholinergic drugs can effectually decrease manic symptoms on acute administration, few reliable direct markers of a cholinergic deficit in mania have been noted. One measure of such function may be reflected in the measurement of erythrocyte choline activity. Erythrocyte choline levels have been investigated as a biochemical marker of acetylcholine activity because choline is the major precursor, as well as a major metabolite of acetylcholine. Slight elevations in erythrocyte choline have been noted in patients with bipolar disorders and have also been observed in schizophrenic and depressive patients. Stoll et al. (1991a, 1991b) also noted that relatively increased levels of choline existed in a subgroup of manic patients before lithium treatment. These patients were noted to have a relatively more severe illness at admission and a less desirous outcome at discharge. In addition, and of potential theoretical significance, bipolar patients with relatively low concentrations of red blood cell choline had a history of four times as many previous episodes of mania as they had a history of episodes of depression. This finding contrasted with observations in patients with high erythrocyte choline levels, who had similar numbers of manic and depressive episodes. Thus, those patients with low choline and presumably low central acetylcholine activity had a relatively greater predominance of manic episodes. Interestingly, those patients with low red blood cell choline showed no depressive symptoms in their clinical presentations. If erythrocyte choline in any way reflects central brain choline and acetylcholine activity, these findings may be consistent with depression being caused by high central acetylcholine levels.

Spectroscopic Studies

Clinical in vivo hydrogen magnetic resonance spectroscopy provides another means for more directly assessing human central cholinergic function in vivo. This technique can measure choline-containing substances noninvasively in the brain. Charles et al. (1994) observed that there is a state-dependent increase in choline in the brains of patients with major depression, as compared with the brains of control subjects. This increase in choline reverted to normal after successful drug treatment of the patient's depression. Also, K. R. Krishnan (personal communication, 1994) anecdotally reported lowered brain choline in a small number of manic patients in a collaboration with Charles et al.

Cholinergic Effects of Lithium

There is still considerable speculation about the mechanisms underlying lithium's antimanic and prophylactic effects, and antiadrenergics are often proposed to underlie lithium's efficacy. Given that cholinergic supersensitivity appears associated with bipolar and possibly unipolar affective disorders, it is reasonable to wonder whether cholinergic mechanisms may also contribute to lithium's therapeutic actions.

Depending on the experiment, lithium either increases or decreases cholinergic neurotransmission. As reviewed by Janowsky and Judd (1981), Vizi et al. (1972) studied the effect of lithium on increased acetylcholine output due to nervous system stimulation. These researchers concluded that lithium ultimately contributes to a block of acetylcholine synthesis and a decrease in its release following nerve stimulation. Possibly related, lithium has been reported by Neil et al. (1976) to intensify muscle weakness in myasthenia gravis, an effect thought to be related to its ability to decrease acetylcholine availability.

Lithium also affects acetylcholine activity in CNS preparations. It decreases the affinity of muscarinic receptor ^{3}H-quinuclidinyl benzilate (QNB) binding in the human caudate nucleus and reduces the number of specific QNB binding sites. Also, although exposure to lithium ion caused no effect on the passive release of acetylcholine from cat cerebral cortex, stimulation of a contralateral peripheral nerve did cause acetylcholine release, which was blocked in the presence of lithium ion. Similarly, although lithium initially increased resting acetylcholine release from rat cerebral cortex slices, it later caused blockade of potassium-stimulated acetylcholine release and synthesis (Janowsky and Judd 1981). More recently, Shiromani et al. (1990) noted that oxotremorine-induced hypothermia was decreased following chronic lithium treatment.

Conversely, Jope (1993) observed that chronic administration of lithium to rats resulted in increased synthesis of acetylcholine in vivo in striatum, hippocampus, and cortex, and in vitro in synaptosomes prepared from whole forebrain and from striatum. Samples et al. (1977) found that acute lithium administration led to increased physostigmine-induced lethality/toxicity in rats, an effect thought to be due to increased acetylcholine availability.

In recent years, the possibility that lithium may be exerting its antimanic effects via postsynaptic-postreceptor mechanisms has been proposed. To this end, an in vitro study reported that modest concentrations of lithium (in the therapeutic range) potentiated cholinergic second-messenger responses, but higher neurotoxic doses disrupted the responses (Gao et al. 1993). Furthermore, Avissar and Schreiber (1989) reported that lithium had a selective blocking effect on muscarinic M_1-receptor–mediated increases in guanine nucleotide-binding proteins (G-proteins). Later, Avissar and Schreiber (1992) developed a more general model concerning the interaction of lithium and G-proteins. By blocking the effects of acetylcholine and other transmitters on G-proteins, lithium was proposed to have antimanic, antidepressant, and prophylactic effects on second messengers such as cyclic adenosine monophosphate and the phosphotydalinositol system. Jope (1993) also argued that lithium has selective effects on the cholinergic nervous system and that these effects may contribute to its antimanic properties.

▶ Conclusion

In the previous pages, the potential role of cholinergic muscarinic mechanisms in the pathogenesis of affective disorders has been reviewed, focusing on bipolar disorders. Information suggesting a role for central acetylcholine overactivity in clinical depression as such has only partially been reviewed. However, there are considerable physiologic and phenomenologic data suggesting that cholinergic hypersensitivity occurs in nonbipolar major depressive disorder patients, at least during periods of overt depression (Janowsky and Risch 1987). Furthermore, the effects of centrally active cholinomimetics very closely resemble the phenomenology of retarded depression from a physiologic, neuroendocrine, sleep architectural, and behavioral perspective (Janowsky and Risch 1987). Nevertheless, when the entire literature concerning cholinergic phenomenology as it relates to the affective disorders is reviewed, it is clear that the study of bipolar patients represents a specific avenue of research that is particularly promising. Thus, we believe that exploration of cholinergic mechanisms in mania and in bipolar disorders in general may offer important clues concerning the pathophysiology of the affective disorders, via the discovery of direct cholinergic linkages or via the understanding of downstream phenomena. The specific application of 1990s cutting-edge technologies—including nuclear magnetic resonance and positron-emission tomography (PET) neuroimaging techniques, advances in molecular genetics and CNS neurobiology, and studies of the effects of newer antimanic and antidepressant medications using the pharmacologic bridge strategy—represent especially promising avenues for further research.

▶ References

Avissar S, Schreiber G: Muscarinic receptor subclassification and G-proteins: significance for lithium action in affective disorders and for the treatment of extra-pyramidal side effects of neuroleptics. Biol Psychiatry 26:113–130, 1989

Avissar S, Schreiber G: The involvement of guanine nucleotide binding proteins in the pathogenesis and treatment of affective disorders. Biol Psychiatry 31:435–459, 1992

Bajada S: A trial of choline chloride and physostigmine in Alzheimer's dementia, in Alzheimer's Disease: A Report of Progress. Edited by Corkin S, Davis K, Growden J. New York, Raven, 1982, pp 427–432

Carroll BJ, Frazer A, Schless A, et al: Cholinergic reversal of manic symptoms. Lancet 1:427–428, 1973

Casey DE: Mood alterations during deanol therapy. Psychopharmacology (Berlin) 62:187–191, 1979

Charles HC, Lazeyras F, Krishnan KRR, et al: Brain choline in depression: in vivo detection of potential pharmacodynamic effects of antidepressant therapy using hydrogen localized spectroscopy. Prog Neuropsychopharmacol Biol Psychiatry 118: 1121–1127, 1994

Cold B, Strang M: Mania secondar to procyclidine (Kemadrin) abuse. Br J Psychiatry 141:81–84, 1982

Davis KL, Berger PA, Hollister LE, et al: Physostigmine in man. Arch Gen Psychiatry 35:119–122, 1978

Davis KL, Hollister LE, Berger PA: Choline chloride in schizophrenia. Am J Psychiatry 136:1581–1584, 1979

Domino EF, Olds ME: Cholinergic inhibition of self stimulation behavior. J Pharmacol Exp Ther 164:202–211, 1968

Duncan E, Dagirmanjian R: Tetrahydrocannabinol sensitization of the rat brain to direct cholinergic stimulation. Psychopharmacology (Berlin) 60:237–240, 1979

Edelstein P, Schulz JF, Hirschowitz J, et al: Physostigmine and lithium response in schizophrenia. Am J Psychiatry 138:1078–1081, 1981

El-Yousef M, Janowsky DS, Davis JM, et al: Induction of severe depression in marijuana intoxicated individuals. Br J Addict 68:321–325, 1973

Fibiger HD, Lynch GS, Cooper HP: A biphasic action of central cholinergic stimulation on behavioral arousal in the rat. Psychopharmacologia 20:366–382, 1971

Gao K-M, Fukamauchi F, Chuang D-M: Long-term biphasic effects of lithium treatment on phospholipase C-coupled M3-muscarinic acetylcholine receptors in cultured cerebellar granule cells. Neurochemistry International 22:395–403, 1993

Janowsky D, Judd L: The effects of lithium on cholinergic mechanisms, in Biological Psychiatry. Edited by Perris C, Struwe G, Janson B. Amsterdam, Netherlands, Elsevier/North-Holland Biomedical Press, 1981, pp 653–656

Janowsky DS, Risch SC: Role of acetylcholine mechanisms in the affective disorders, in Psychopharmacology: The Third Generation of Progress. Edited by Meltzer HY. New York, Raven, 1987, pp 527–534

Janowsky DS, El-Yousef MK, Davis JM, et al: A cholinergic-adrenergic hypothesis of mania and depression. Lancet 2:632–635, 1972a

Janowsky DS, El-Yousef MK, Davis JM, et al: Cholinergic antagonism of methylphenidate-induced stereotyped behavior. Psychopharmacologia 27:295–303, 1972b

Janowsky DS, El-Yousef MK, Davis JM: Antagonistic effects of physostigmine and methylphenidate in man. Am J Psychiatry 130:1370–1376, 1973a

Janowsky DS, El-Yousef MK, Davis JM, et al: Parasympathetic suppression of manic symptoms by physostigmine. Arch Gen Psychiatry 28:542–547, 1973b

Janowsky DS, El-Yousef MK, Davis JM: Acetylcholine and depression. Psychosom Med 36:248–257, 1974

Janowsky DS, Risch SC, Parker D, et al: Increased vulnerability to cholinergic stimulation in affect disorder patients. Psychopharmacol Bull 16:29–31, 1980

Janowsky DS, Risch SC, Judd LL, et al: Cholinergic supersensitivity in affect disorder patients: Behavioral and neuroendocrine observations. Psychopharmacol Bull 17:129–132, 1981

Jellinec T, Gardos G, Cole J: Adverse effects of antiparkinsonian agents. Psychiatry 138:1567–1571, 1981

Jope RS: Lithium selectively potentiates cholinergic activity in rat brain. Prog Brain Res 98:317–322, 1993

Kasper S, Moises HW, Beckmann H: The anticholinergic biperiden in depressive disorders. Pharmacopsychiatry 14:195–198, 1981

Krieg JC, Berger M: Treatment of mania with the cholinomimetic agent RS-86. Br J Psychiatry 148:613–615, 1986

Modestin JJ, Hunger J, Schwartz RB: Uber die depressogene Wirkung von Physostigmine. Archiv für Psychiatrie und Nervenkrankheiten 218:67–77, 1973a

Modestin JJ, Schwartz RB, Hunger J: Zur Frage der Beeinflussung Schizophrener Symptome Physostigmine. Pharmacopsychiatria 3:300–304, 1973b

Mohs R, Hollander E, Haroutunian V, et al: Cholinomimetics in Alzheimer's disease. Int J Neurosci 32:775–776, 1987

Neil FJ, Himmelhoch JJ, Licata SM: Emergence of myasthenia gravis during treatment with lithium carbonate. Arch Gen Psychiatry 33:1090–1092, 1976

Nurnberger JL Jr, Jimerson DC, Simmons-Alling S: Behavioral, physiological and neuroendocrine response to arecoline in normal twins and well state bipolar patients. Psychiatry Res 9:191–200, 1983a

Nurnberger JL Jr, Sitaram N, Gershon ES, et al: A twin study of cholinergic REM induction. Biol Psychiatry 18:1161–1173, 1983b

Oppenheimer G, Ebstein R, Belmaker R: Effects of lithium on the physostigmine-induced behavioral syndrome and plasma cyclic GMP. J Psychiatr Res 14:133–138, 1979

Risch SC, Cohen PM, Janowsky DS, et al: Physostigmine induction of depressive symptomatology in normal human subjects. Psychiatry Res 4:89–94, 1981

Rosenblatt JC, Janowsky DS, Davis JM, et al: The augmentation of physostigmine toxicity in the rat by Δ^9 tetrahydrocannibinol. Research Communications in Chemical Pathology and Pharmacology 3:479–482, 1972

Rowntree DW, Neven S, Wilson A: The effect of di-isopropylfluorophosphonate in schizophrenia and manic depressive psychosis. J Neurol Neurosurg Psychiatry 13:47–62, 1950

Samples JR, Janowsky DS, Pechnick R, et al: Lethal effects of physostigmine plus lithium in rats. Psychopharmacology (Berlin) 52:307–309, 1977

Shiromani PJ, Overstreet DH, Lucero S, et al: Dietary lithium blunts oxotremorine-induced hypothermia in a genetic animal model of depression. Lithium 1:186–190, 1990

Shopsin B, Janowsky DS, Davis JM, et al: Rebound phenomena in mania patients following physostigmine. Neuropsychobiology 1:180–187, 1975

Siever LJ, Risch SC, Murphy DL: Central cholinergic-adrenergic balance in the regulation of affective state. Psychiatry Res 5:108–109, 1981

Siever LJ, Uhde TW: New studies and perspectives on the noradrenergic receptor system in depression: effects of the alpha-2 adrenergic agonist clonidine. Biol Psychiatry 19:131–156, 1984

Smith JA: Abuse of antiparkinsonian drugs: a review of the literature. J Clin Psychiatry 41:351–354, 1980

Steinberg B, Weston S, Trestman RL, et al: Affective instability in personality disordered patients correlates with mood response to physostigmine challenge. Biol Psychiatry 33:86A, 1993a

Stoll A, Cohen BM, Hanin I: Erythrocyte choline concentration in psychiatric disorders. Biol Psychiatry 29:309–321, 1991a

Stoll AL, Cohen BM, Snyder MB, et al: Erythrocyte choline concentration in bipolar disorder: a predictor of clinical course and medication response. Biol Psychiatry 29:1171–1180, 1991b

Tamminga C, Smith RC, Change S, et al: Depression associated with oral choline. Lancet 2:905, 1976

Vizi ES, Illes A, Ronia A, et al: Effect of lithium ions on the release of acetylcholine from the cerebral cortex. Neuropharmacology 2:521–530, 1972

CHAPTER 9

GAMMA-AMINOBUTYRIC ACID

Frederick Petty, M.D., Ph.D.,
Gerald L. Kramer, B.A., and
Lori L. Davis, M.D.

H istorically and traditionally, the biogenic amines are considered key agents in the neurochemical theories of bipolar
disorder.

▶ NEUROCHEMICAL THEORIES OF BIPOLAR ILLNESS

These hypotheses were first formulated in the mid-1960s (Bunney and
Davis 1965; Schildkraut 1965). The essential features of this theory
were that catecholamine excess is associated with the manic state,
whereas a deficiency of catecholamines is correlated with depression.
Interestingly enough, a permissive theory postulated that serotonin
was low in both mania and depression (Goodwin and Jamison 1990).
The authors' data suggested that γ-aminobutyric acid (GABA) is also
deficient in a subset of patients, while both manic and depressed (Petty
et al. 1993b). The primary evidence supporting the biogenic amine
hypothesis is derived from the observation that the catecholamine de-
pletor reserpine could precipitate depressive symptoms, and the catecholamine precursor L-dopa increased ratings of psychosis and anger
as well as hypomania in some patients (Goodwin et al. 1970; Murphy
et al. 1971). In the last 20–30 years, a large body of research has
focused on studies of the biogenic amines and also of acetylcholine in

157

bipolar disorder. Current thinking on the biochemical etiology of mood disorders reflects increased sophistication regarding neurotransmitter interactions, and a simplistic monotransmitter model is no longer tenable (Goodwin and Jamison 1990).

Emrich et al. (1980) first proposed a GABA theory of mood disorders that was based on their observation of a therapeutic moodstabilizing effect of valproate in patients with bipolar disorder. In the ensuing years, a variety of empirical evidence has developed to support a role for GABA. However, most studies have been done in unipolar major depressive disorders; this evidence has been reviewed (Petty et al. 1993a). Briefly, brain levels, cerebrospinal fluid (CSF) levels, and plasma levels of GABA are low in unipolar major depression. Because there is no correlation between the severity of depressive symptoms and levels of plasma GABA (Petty et al. 1992), and because low plasma GABA levels do not appear to normalize with clinical improvement (Petty 1994; Petty et al. 1993a), we have proposed that low plasma GABA may represent a trait-like marker for major depressive illness in a subset of patients. Data from pharmacologic studies and animal models of depression also strongly support a GABA deficit model in depressed states (Petty and Sherman 1981). We have also proposed a unifying neurochemical theory for depression in which norepinephrine plays a central role, and in which the modulating effects of serotonin and GABA are considered (Petty et al. 1993a). Briefly, depression is conceptualized as correlating with decreased limbic noradrenergic function. GABA facilitates noradrenergic release in limbic terminals; an intact serotonergic system is required for antidepressant treatment to work. Therefore, depression may be accompanied by low norepinephrine, low serotonin, and/or low GABA, and the reversal of depressive symptoms may be mediated by drugs that have primary action on any of these three neurotransmitter systems. There are considerably less data regarding the role of GABA in bipolar illness; however, the data are carefully addressed in this chapter. Low plasma GABA represents a potential trait vulnerability marker for a subset of patients with bipolar illness.

The criteria for a biological trait vulnerability marker emphasize that the putative marker should differentiate well from ill subjects in the symptomatic state and that the abnormality should continue into the clinically remitted state. Additionally, a marker should be state independent and should be seen in a proportion of vulnerable subjects, (i.e., those with family history) who have not yet reached the age at risk. Low plasma GABA differentiates well from ill subjects in about one-third of bipolar subjects (Petty et al. 1993b) and is also seen in euthymic unmedicated bipolar patients (Berrettini et al. 1982). Plasma GABA levels do not correlate with severity of symptoms for either depression or mania (i.e., state independent); however, the key research in identifying whether the marker is familial and segregates with illness in families with affective disorders has not yet been done. Additionally, a formal state-trait analysis (Kraemer et al. 1994) has not yet been performed to determine what proportion of the variance in plasma GABA is attributable to the trait of bipolar illness. Although the findings of state-independent low plasma GABA must be considered preliminary, they are certainly promising and deserve further research.

▶ Valproate in the Treatment of Bipolar Disorder

Since the introduction of lithium into psychiatric practice, it has been evident that this agent is reasonably specific as a treatment for bipolar disorder. Although lithium has some antidepressant characteristics in patients with nonbipolar depression as well as utility in the treatment of aggressive and impulsive behavior, schizophrenia, and schizoaffective disorder, it certainly does not have the broad spectrum of utility that other psychotropic agents, such as the neuroleptics, antidepressants, or benzodiazepines, have. Because patients with epilepsy often exhibit psychopathology reminiscent of some aspects of manic-depressive illness, it is natural that anticonvulsants have been tested in therapeutic trials for patients with mood disorders. Phenytoin or barbiturates do not appear to have any particular efficacy in the treatment of mood disorders; however, carbamazepine and valproic acid are efficacious, as demonstrated simultaneously and independently by research groups in Japan and Germany (Emrich et al. 1980; Okuma et al. 1979).

Valproic acid is a small branch chain carboxylic acid originally developed as an industrial solvent in Germany in the late 1800s. The anticonvulsant property of valproic acid was discovered serendipitously when it was used as a solvent (vehicle) to dissolve an experimental antiepileptic drug for preclinical testing. Although the drug was later found not to have anticonvulsant efficacy in animal models, the vehicle, valproic acid, was found to be anticonvulsive effective. Valproic acid is considered to have a primary action as a facilitator of GABA. In open-label trials in France in the mid-1960s, Lambert (1984) found that valproic acid was helpful in treating patients with mood disorders. Subsequently, Emrich et al. (1980) demonstrated in open trials that valproic acid had mood-stabilizing characteristics in bipolar patients. In open trials, sodium valproate demonstrated antimanic efficacy (Calabrese and Delucchi 1989), particularly for patients with rapid-cycling bipolar disorder. Controlled trials of valproic acid in mania have also suggested that valproate is a potentially useful antimanic agent (McElroy et al. 1992; Pope et al. 1991). Divalproex sodium (a stable coordination compound of valproic acid and sodium valproate) was found effective in a randomized double-blind, parallel-group, multicenter study of patients with acute mania (Bowden et al. 1994).

For the sake of discussion, it is assumed that valproic acid will eventually be demonstrated to a specific agent with broad-spectrum efficacy in bipolar illness in both the manic and depressed phases as well as in prophylaxis, much like lithium. Regarding a GABA theory of bipolar illness, because only 50% of bipolar patients demonstrate a robust response to valproic acid, one would conclude that such a theory could account for only a proportion of patients with this illness. Furthermore, valproic acid has effects on neurotransmitter systems other than GABA, particularly the biogenic amines.

The acute neurochemical effects of valproate on the GABA system are complex (Loscher 1993a). Although acute administration of valproate leads to increased brain tissue levels of GABA, these changes are not striking at clinically relevant doses (Loscher and Horstermann 1994). At lower doses, GABA concentrations in synaptosomes and nerve terminals are increased significantly by acute administration of valproate (Loscher and Vetter 1985), and the activity of GABA transaminase (GABA-T, the GABA metabolizing enzyme), is decreased

(Loscher 1993b). Valproate enhances the function of the GABA-A (GABA type A) receptor at the level of the chloride channel similar to benzodiazepine (Concas et al. 1991). In vivo release of GABA in the ventral hippocampus studied with microdialysis has shown a biphasic response to interperitoneal valproate, with low doses reducing and high doses increasing GABA levels in extracellular fluid (Biggs et al. 1992). However, when perfused directly into the brain, valproate inhibited GABA release in the substantia nigra (Wolf and Tscherne 1994), which appears to contradict other reports that valproate enhanced GABA turnover in this brain region (Loscher 1989); therefore, the simplistic notion that valproate is a specific "GABA mimetic" is probably incorrect, particularly because valproate has well-documented effects on neurotransmitter systems other than GABA, including biogenic amines (Loscher 1993a).

In both seizure disorders and bipolar illness, the therapeutic effects of valproate are achieved only with chronic drug administration. It is therefore somewhat surprising that virtually no basic neurochemistry research has been done on the chronic neurochemical effects of valproate administration. One study has shown that chronic valproate administration increased the density of GABA-B (GABA type B) receptors in the hippocampus, but not the frontal cortex, similar to the action of chronic lithium and carbamazepine (Motohashi 1992). In humans, subchronic (4 days) administration of valproate increased plasma GABA in healthy control subjects (Loscher and Schmidt 1980) and increased CSF and plasma GABA in patients with epilepsy (Loscher and Schmidt 1981; Loscher and Siemes 1985).

In summary, although valproic acid is known to have a number of primary effects on the GABA system with acute administration, it is not known whether these neurochemical effects are indeed responsible for its clinical efficacy in bipolar disorder. The chronic neurochemical effects of valproate are also not yet known.

▶ Low Plasma GABA in Bipolar Disorder

Plasma levels of GABA are significantly lower in control subjects than in patients with bipolar disorder (whether bipolar mania or bipolar depression) and in euthymic bipolar patients currently not on medication (Berrettini et al. 1982; Petty et al. 1993b). These data are best interpreted as demonstrating a different distribution for plasma GABA levels in mood disorder patients than in control subjects, with about 30% of bipolar manic and 40% of bipolar depressed patients having plasma GABA levels lower than 95% of control subjects. In other words, the majority of bipolar patients have plasma GABA levels in the normal control range. Therefore, low plasma GABA identifies a subset of approximately one-third of bipolar patients.

This finding must be interpreted with some caution. First, low plasma GABA is not specific to bipolar disorder, because it has also been shown in patients with primary unipolar major depression and in patients with alcoholism (Petty et al. 1992, 1993c). However, it may be specific for these two conditions (i.e., mood disorders and alcoholism) because plasma GABA levels in patients are normal with anxiety disorders, with eating disorders, and with schizophrenia. Other psychiatric syndromes closely associated with the mood disorders, such as obsessive-compulsive disorder and severe personality disorders, have not yet been studied with regard to plasma GABA measures. Thus, finding low plasma GABA in mood disorders and alcoholism may be taken as corroborative evidence of the close relationship between these two psychiatric syndromes (Coryell et al. 1992).

In addition to specificity, another major difficulty in interpreting plasma GABA levels is related to their origin. Studies of CSF GABA in major depression have consistently demonstrated a lower level of GABA in CSF in patients with major depressive disorders than in control subjects (for a review, see Petty et al. 1993a). Studies of CSF GABA in patients with bipolar disorder have been limited and generally inconclusive (Berrettini et al. 1986). The precise origin of plasma GABA in humans is difficult to prove; however, a variety of indirect evidence has suggested that plasma GABA is an accurate reflection of brain GABA activity or function (for a review, see Petty et al. 1993b).

▶ CAN PLASMA GABA PREDICT TREATMENT RESPONSE?

As part of a multicenter, double-blind, randomized, acute-phase, placebo-controlled trial of divalproex in mania (Bowden et al. 1994), plasma concentrations of GABA were measured before and after treatment in a subset of 63 patients. A preliminary analysis of these data (Petty et al. 1995) has revealed three interesting findings. First, there was no correlation demonstrated between baseline levels of plasma GABA after a minimum 3-day washout and severity of manic symptomatology as determined by a mania rating scale. This finding is compatible with plasma GABA being a state-independent marker of bipolar illness in the manic phase.

The second significant finding of this research was that pretreatment levels of plasma GABA predicted response to divalproex ($n = 19$) but not to lithium ($n = 13$) or placebo ($n = 31$). However, the correlation was such that patients with the higher levels of plasma GABA were more likely to respond to divalproex with improvement in their acute manic symptoms than patients with lower plasma GABA levels. This particular finding was opposite to that which the researchers predicted and seemed counterintuitive. However, with a GABA disequilibrium hypothesis of bipolar illness, this finding can be explained. Additionally, it is consistent with a report (Arteaga et al. 1993) that chronic administration of valproic acid induces platelet GABA-T (the GABA metabolizing enzyme). If similar effects are found in patients with mania, induction of the brain enzyme that shares the characteristics of the platelet enzyme would also be expected. Increased activity of GABA-T would result in lower GABA levels.

The third major finding of this work was that plasma levels of GABA decreased during treatment with divalproex and with lithium, although the small sample size precludes significance in the lithium-treated patients. Again, if low plasma GABA is a correlate of the manic state, it would be expected that levels would normalize with clinical improvement, which they clearly do not. This result is additional evidence that low plasma GABA is a state-independent biological marker of bipolar illness.

Preliminary data have also been obtained for plasma GABA as a predictor of treatment response or outcome in two other clinical situations. First, in a series of patients with severe depression, baseline levels of plasma GABA predicted response to electroconvulsive therapy (ECT) (Devanand et al. 1991). In this case, as for the previously described prediction of treatment response to divalproex in acute mania, when the patients were arbitrarily divided into two groups (one with plasma GABA levels above the median and one below), patients with higher levels of plasma GABA before ECT had a greater tendency to respond than patients with lower levels of plasma GABA.

The second clinical situation in which baseline plasma GABA levels predicted treatment response was in patients with schizophrenia treated with neuroleptics who received alprazolam as supplemental therapy in an attempt to determine whether alprazolam potentiated the antipsychotic effects of the neuroleptic (Wolkowitz et al. 1993). Again, in this clinical situation, there was a tendency for patients with the higher levels of baseline pretreatment plasma GABA to demonstrate a more robust response to the addition of alprazolam.

In summary, in three clinical conditions in which the patients were symptomatic with a severe mental illness (mania, schizophrenia, or major depressive disorder), higher levels of plasma GABA predicted a treatment response to a therapeutic agent considered to have a primary action on the GABA system (divalproex, alprazolam, or ECT). Additionally, in all three cases, the treatment led to a lowering of plasma GABA levels.

▶ GABA THEORY OF BIPOLAR ILLNESS: SPECULATIONS AND DIRECTIONS OF FUTURE RESEARCH

A GABA theory of bipolar illness is best formulated in the context of considering low plasma GABA to characterize a subset of patients with mood disorders as well as alcohol dependence. There is a close clinical and perhaps genetic relationship between alcohol dependence and mood disorders (Coryell et al. 1992; Petty et al. 1992). Therefore, the authors' theory is not exclusively applicable to bipolar disorder but considers a subset of patients with bipolar disorder, unipolar major depressive disorder, or alcoholism to have "low GABA disease." It is hypothesized that these individuals inherit a genetic defect that leads to their having a trait-like characteristic of low extracellular GABA, the phenotype of which can be measured as low plasma GABA. When these individuals are subjected to environmental circumstances that

cause them to become symptomatic, it is hypothesized that their extracellular levels of GABA are increased above the individual asymptomatic baseline. Because the baseline is lower than in healthy control
subjects, the mood-disordered person might have GABA in the normal
range while ill. It is hypothesized that the increased GABA over baseline leads to the development of psychiatric symptomatology. Depending on other neurotransmitters, presumably norepinephrine and/or
serotonin, the precise manifestation of psychiatric symptoms may be
seen as a clinical syndrome that is classically described as either depression or mania. With treatment, or with the passage of time and clinical
remission, the elevated extracellular levels, seen during symptomatic
worsening, return to the euthymic presymptomatic baseline, along
with clinical improvement and remission. When persons with "low
GABA disease" are euthymic, stable, and not severely craving alcohol,
their GABA levels have reverted to the premorbid low GABA condition (see Figure 9–1).

In other words, this theory postulates that a subset of patients with
mood disorders has a genetically determined low plasma GABA baseline that is a trait marker. An elevation of plasma GABA over the low

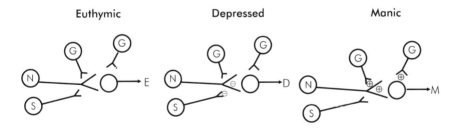

Figure 9–1. Hypothetical neuronal map of the γ-aminobutyric acid
(GABA) (G) theory of mood disorders. Map accounts for theorized
neurotransmitter interactions in patients with bipolar illness while
euthymic (E), depressed (D), or manic (M). Note that in the euthymic
or depressed state, the baseline GABA for some bipolar patients will be
lower than that for healthy control subjects. N = norepinephrine.
S = serotonin.

trait levels is a state characteristic during symptomatic worsening. Low GABA may be seen either during illness or when a person is asymptomatic and well. This concept is difficult, because it implies that plasma GABA has both state and trait characteristics. It is hypothesized that fluctuations in GABA levels above the euthymic baseline are state related. For the subset of patients with "low GABA disease," the baseline euthymic state is also the trait level. In some cases while symptomatic, plasma GABA levels might be elevated above the euthymic trait level and might be measured in the healthy control range. One implication of this theory is that the proportion of patients with mood disorders and a low GABA trait may be higher than the 40% seen in symptomatic cases.

Several predictions of this theory can be tested clinically. First of all, the characteristic of low plasma GABA should cosegregate with illness and should be found in a greater proportion of offspring of ill parents who have not yet reached the age at risk for illness. In other words, manic-depressive parents with low plasma GABA would be expected to have a greater proportion of their offspring also characterized by low plasma GABA than control subjects with no family history of mental illness.

Finally, nuclear magnetic resonance (NMR) spectroscopy has the capability of measuring GABA levels in vivo in the human brain (Rothman et al. 1993). Future studies with NMR scanning should be undertaken in patients with mood disorders and alcoholism to ascertain whether their brain levels of GABA are indeed different from levels in control subjects. However, NMR scanning cannot discriminate between intracellular and extracellular GABA levels in the brain. Although, because most GABA is intracellular (millimolar versus nanomolar concentrations), we predict that no significant differences will be found in individuals with low plasma GABA compared with control subjects using NMR.

In summary, the data implicating a role for GABA in the biochemical pathology of mood disorders are as compelling as that implicating any other neurotransmitter. Several testable hypotheses of a GABA theory of bipolar illness should be the subject of future research. Particularly, studies of individuals at risk may lead to strategies for prophylactic intervention in children of parents with bipolar disorder.

▶ REFERENCES

Arteaga R, Herranz JL, Armijo JA: Platelet GABA-transaminase in epileptic children: influence of epilepsy and anticonvulsants. Epilepsy Res 14:73–85, 1993

Berrettini WH, Nurnberger JI, Hare T, et al: Plasma and CSF GABA in affective illness. Br J Psychiatry 141:483–487, 1982

Berrettini WH, Nurnberger JI, Hare TA, et al: CSF GABA in euthymic manic-depressive patients and controls. Biol Psychiatry 21:842–844, 1986

Biggs CS, Pearce BR, Fowler LJ, et al: The effect of sodium valproate on extracellular GABA and other amino acids in the rat ventral hippocampus: an in vivo microdialysis study. Brain Res 594:138–142, 1992

Bowden CL, Brugger AM, Swann AC, et al: Efficacy of divalproex vs lithium and placebo in the treatment of mania. JAMA 271:918–924, 1994

Bunney WE Jr, Davis J: Norepinephrine in depressive reactions. Arch Gen Psychiatry 13:483–494, 1965

Calabrese JR, Delucchi GA: Phenomenology of rapid cycling manic depression and its treatment with valproate. J Clin Psychiatry 50 (suppl):30–34, 1989

Concas A, Mascia MP, Sanna E, et al: *In vivo* administration of valproate decreases t-[35S] butylbicyclophosphorthionate binding in rat brain. Naunyn Schmiedebergs Arch Pharmacol 343:296–300, 1991

Coryell W, Winokur G, Keller M, et al: Alcoholism and primary major depression: a family study approach to co-existing disorders. J Affect Disord 24:93–99, 1992

Devanand D, Sackeim H, Kramer G, et al: ECT and plasma GABA. Paper presented at the annual meeting of the Society for Biological Psychiatry, New Orleans, LA, May 1991

Emrich HM, Zerssen DV, Kissling W, et al: Effect of sodium valproate on mania: the GABA-hypothesis of affective disorders. Archiv für Psychiatrie und Nervenkrankheiten 229:1–16, 1980

Goodwin FK, Jamison KR: Manic-Depressive Illness. New York, Oxford University Press, 1990

Goodwin FK, Murphy DL, Brodie HK, et al: L-dopa, catecholamines, and behavior: a clinical and biochemical study in depressed patients. Biol Psychiatry 2:341–366, 1970

Kraemer HC, Gullion CM, Rush AJ, et al: Can state and trait variables be disentangled?: a methodological framework for psychiatric disorders. Psychiatry Res 52:53–69, 1994

Lambert PA: Acute and prophylactic therapies of patients with affective disorders using valpromide (dipropylacetamide), in Anticonvulsants in Affective Disorders. Edited by Emrich HM, Okuma T, Muller AA. Amsterdam, Netherlands, Excerpta Medica, 1984, pp 33–44

Loscher W: Valproate enhances GABA turnover in the substantia nigra. Brain Res 501:198–203, 1989

Loscher W: Effects of the antiepileptic drug valproate on metabolism and function of inhibitory and excitatory amino acids in the brain. Neurochem Res 18:485–502, 1993a

Loscher W: In vivo administration of valproate reduces the nerve terminal (synaptosomal) activity of GABA aminotransferase in discrete brain areas of rats. Neurosci Lett 160:177–180, 1993b

Loscher W, Horstermann D: Differential effects of vigabatrin, gamma-acetylenic GABA, aminooxyacetic acid, and valproate on levels of various amino acids in rat brain regions and plasma. Naunyn Schmiedebergs Arch Pharmacol 349:270–278, 1994

Loscher W, Schmidt D: Increase of human plasma GABA by sodium valproate. Epilepsia 21:611–615, 1980

Loscher W, Schmidt D: Plasma GABA levels in neurological patients under treatment with valproic acid. Life Sci 28:2383–2388, 1981

Loscher W, Siemes H: Cerebrospinal fluid-aminobutyric acid levels in children with different types of epilepsy: effect of anticonvulsant treatment. Epilepsia 26:314–319, 1985

Loscher W, Vetter M: In vivo effects of aminooxyacetic acid and valproic acid on nerve terminal (synaptosomal) GABA levels in discrete brain areas of the rat. Biochem Pharmacol 34:1747–1756, 1985

McElroy SL, Keck PE, Pope HG, et al: Valproate in the treatment of bipolar disorder: literature review and clinical guidelines. J Clin Psychopharmacol 12:42S–52S, 1992

Motohashi N: GABA receptor alterations after chronic lithium administration: comparison with carbamazepine and sodium valproate. Prog Neuropsychopharmacol Biol Psychiatry 16:571–579, 1992

Murphy DL, Brodie HK, Goodwin FK, et al: Regular induction of hypomania by L-dopa in "bipolar" manic-depressive patients. Nature 229:135–136, 1971

Okuma T, Inanaga K, Otsuki S, et al: Comparison of the antimanic efficacy of carbamazepine and chlorpromazine: a double-blind controlled study. Psychopharmacology (Berlin) 66:211–217, 1979

Petty F: Plasma concentrations of gamma-aminobutyric acid (GABA) and mood disorders: a blood test for manic depressive disease. Clin Chem 40:296–302, 1994

Petty F, Sherman AD: GABAergic modulation of learned helplessness. Pharmacol Biochem Behav 156:567–570, 1981

Petty F, Kramer GL, Gullion CM, et al: Low plasma gamma-aminobutyric acid levels in male patients with depression. Biol Psychiatry 32:354–363, 1992

Petty F, Kramer GL, Hendrickse W: GABA and depression, in Biology of Depressive Disorders, Part A: A Systems Perspective. Edited by Mann JJ, Kupfer DJ. New York, Plenum, 1993a, pp 79–108

Petty F, Kramer GL, Fulton M, et al: Low plasma GABA is a trait-like marker for bipolar illness. Neuropsychopharmacology 9:125–132, 1993b

Petty F, Fulton M, Moeller FG, et al: Plasma gamma-aminobutyric acid (GABA) is low in alcoholics. Psychopharmacol Bull 29:277–281, 1993c

Petty F, Rush AJ, Davis JM, et al: Plasma GABA predicts acute response to divalproex in mania. Biol Psychiatry 39:278–284, 1996

Pope HG, McElroy SL, Keck PE, et al: Valproate in the treatment of acute mania. Arch Gen Psychiatry 48:62–68, 1991

Rothman DL, Petroff OAC, Behar KL, et al: Localized H-1 NMR measurements of gamma-aminobutyric acid in human brain in vivo. Proc Natl Acad Sci U S A 90:5662–5666, 1993

Schildkraut JJ: The catecholamine hypothesis of affective disorders: a review of supporting evidence. Am J Psychiatry 122:509–522, 1965

Wolf R, Tscherne U: Valproate effect on gamma-aminobutyric acid release in pars reticulata of substantia nigra: combination of push-pull perfusion and fluorescence histochemistry. Epilepsia 35:226–233, 1994

Wolkowitz OM, Harris D, Turetsky NG, et al: Alprazolam-neuroleptic treatment of schizophrenia. Paper presented at the 146th annual meeting of the American Psychiatric Association, San Francisco, CA, May 22–27, 1993

CHAPTER 10

ELECTROPHYSIOLOGY

Richard C. Josiassen, Ph.D.,
Chand Nair, M.D., and
Rita A. Shaughnessy, Ph.D., M.D.

F or more than half a century, it has been expected that the recording of human cerebral electrical activity would play a role in the identification of neurophysiological mechanisms underlying psychopathology. To put this expectation into some context, it is important to go back to the work of the British physiologist Richard Caton (1875), who is credited with the demonstration that as nerve impulses flow in and out of the brain, the "feeble currents" are detectable from the exposed cortex, based on work on the exposed brains of cats, rabbits, and monkeys. His experiments were aimed at demonstrating brain electrical changes in response to visual stimulation. Simultaneously, he performed the pioneering study of cerebral event-related potentials (ERPs), providing a method for mapping the localization of cerebral electrical potentials evoked by sensory stimulation. These have become the two general categories of electrical activity available from the intact human scalp: the electroencephalogram (EEG) and the ERP.

At first there was little interest in these observations, and several decades passed before Hans Berger (1929) demonstrated that the EEG could be recorded from the surface of the human head. He placed scalp electrodes on the front and back of the head and viewed much of what he saw as a measure of global cortical activity. It has been suggested that the fact that Berger was a psychiatrist and a "bit of a crank" may

171

have contributed to the general skepticism that attended his early reports of the EEG (Walter 1963). Within a few years, however, the EEG achieved acceptance as a genuine phenomenon when Adrian and Matthews demonstrated it before a meeting of the Physiological Society in London (Walter 1963). This recognition led to the rapid development of electroencephalography, and almost immediately, the EEG became a clinical tool for measurement of brain activity, with obvious applications in cases of brain tumors, epileptic conditions, head injury, drug overdose, and even brain death. Thus, the EEG quickly found a place in the armamentarium of neurological diagnosis.

The advent of EEG also raised optimistic expectations among the psychiatric community. Based on the pioneering efforts of Hans Berger in Germany; the early work of Lee Edward Travis at the University of Iowa (Travis and Dorsey 1931), who introduced EEG into the United States; and the early systematic studies of Donald Lindsley (1933), Herbert Jasper (Jasper et al. 1939), John Knott (1938), and countless others, it was hoped that the underlying brain electrical events critical to psychopathologic behavior would be signaled by specific and identifiable changes in electrical patterns recorded from the human scalp. It was hoped that the technique of EEG, and later the ERPs, would yield patterns characteristic for schizophrenia, mania, and other "functional" psychiatric disorders. Although this hope was intuitively appealing, and bolstered by the truism that all behavior is constrained within the structural and functional capacity of the central nervous system, the electrophysiological signals from patients with classical forms of psychiatric disorders did not contain distinctive "signature" patterns. Mounting evidence supports the conclusion that "higher-level" processing of sensory input and cerebral activity involved in preparing for and carrying out action may influence brain electrical patterns (for a comprehensive review, see Coles et al. 1985). For the most part, however, the hope that differences in brain electrical patterns could reliably distinguish among diagnostic groups has gone unfulfilled.

▶ ELECTROPHYSIOLOGICAL STUDIES OF MANIA

Mania, widely considered one of the major psychotic disorders, has stimulated a broad range of electrophysiological research, although the effort has not been as systematic or comprehensive as that in other areas of psychopathology, such as schizophrenia or major depressive disorders. For obvious practical reasons, investigators have seldom been able to deal with unmedicated patients during a manic phase. The illness, with its characteristic symptoms of irritability, distractibility, psychomotor agitation, and pressured speech, often renders manic patients unable to cooperate with the demands of testing. Added to the problem of patient cooperation is the historical lack of reliable and valid diagnoses. Much of the clinical description in the early literature is fuzzy and difficult to interpret within contemporary nomenclature.

In this review chapter, the electrophysiological variables discussed are limited to signals that can be recorded from the intact human scalp—the EEG and the ERP. In addition to reviewing the published literature, multisensory ERP data recently found from a small sample ($N = 11$) of unmedicated manic patients (R. C. Josiassen, R. E. Antelo, and C. Nair, unpublished data, 1994) is also briefly described. Because this chapter is intended as a brief review, it was often not possible to indulge in the luxury of many qualifying statements or details. Any brief review of electrophysiological studies must make some arbitrary choices of what to include as both independent and dependent variables. In this review, the literature on autonomic and somatic activity in mania is not discussed. The older literature in these areas has been reviewed by Christie et al. (1980) and Lader (1975). Literature on electrodermal variables has been reviewed by Stern and Janes (1973) and by Zahn (1985). The eye tracking literature in mania has been reviewed by Levy et al. (1994).

▶ EEG Studies of Mania

Qualitative Studies

The earliest qualitative studies showed that scalp-recorded EEG contained a wide range of frequencies (oscillations per second) that could be visually detected. The continuous "roar" or "noise" of brain electricity is not simply a hodgepodge of frequencies, but seems to be organized according to some law and order among various frequencies and amplitudes. The frequencies are traditionally broken down into the following bands or ranges: delta—below 3.5 cycles per second (cps), theta—4–7.5 cps, alpha—8–13 cps, and beta—above 13 cps (usually 14–40 cps). In the healthy adult, the slow ranges (0.3–7 cps) and the very fast range (above 30 cps) are sparsely represented; medium (8–13 cps) and fast (14–30 cps) ranges predominate. The synchronous rhythm of these frequencies as well as the actual voltage, wave morphology, and spatial distribution across the scalp are all important visual guides for evaluating these brain signals.

For the most part, the original EEG literature in mania consisted of simple case reports of findings based on visual interpretation of individual records by a trained electroencephalographer. Using this approach, investigators often failed to find clear-cut EEG abnormalities associated with mania. On the contrary, the discovery of gross abnormalities in manic patients usually led to a revision of the original psychiatric diagnosis. For example, Strauss (1955) reported four cases that had been diagnosed and treated as affective illness in which the EEG aided correct neurologic diagnosis of intracranial neoplasm.

The absence of a convincing association between specific EEG abnormalities and clinical manifestations of mania led some investigators to look at the distributions of specific EEG characteristics in manic as compared with healthy control populations. In one of the first such studies, Davis and Davis (H. Davis and Davis 1937; P. A. Davis and Davis 1939) compared EEG findings in 100 healthy adult control subjects and 70 psychiatric patients, followed by a further study of 232 psychiatric patients, of which 64 were manic. They concluded that manic patients tend to have alpha activity mixed with fast activity, whereas the depressed patients tend to have alpha activity mixed with slow activity. P. A. Davis (1941a, 1941b, 1942) then visually rated EEG tracings from manic patients on a five-point scale and found that manic patients had a higher incidence of irregular and abnormal records than the earlier literature had suggested. In addition, among 111 manic-depressive patients (82 depressed, 22 manic, and 7 mixed), she found very little change in EEG when patients switched from one phase of the illness to another.

Following the lead of Davis and Davis, other investigators carried out more exhaustive studies of EEG characteristics in mania. The reports of Greenblatt et al. (1944) and Hurst et al. (1954) deserve special comment. Greenblatt et al. reviewed EEG findings in 1,593 psychiatric patients, including 145 manic-depressive depressed type and 82 manic-depressive manic type. Derived from simple compilations of abnormal findings, Greenblatt et al. reported a 31% and 42% incidence of EEG abnormality among manic-depressive depressed and manic-depressive manic patients, respectively. Hurst et al. carried out one of the most exhaustive studies of the EEG in mania using frequency analysis in addition to the standard visual inspection of EEG recording. They verified the earlier finding of Davis and Davis that mean alpha frequency was higher in patients with predominantly manic symptoms than in those with predominantly depressive symptoms.

Within this early EEG literature on mania, there was a wide scattering of reported EEG abnormalities. It was suggested that samples with the highest incidence of abnormalities may have been biased by overrepresentation of patients referred for a clinical EEG examination due to signs of brain disease, such as convulsive disorder or infection. Despite consistent findings that mean alpha frequency was higher in patients with manic symptoms than in those with depressive symptoms, and that the "mitten pattern," a slow wave-and-spike pattern that occurs only in sleep, was found in 20% of manic patients, most early researchers concluded that there were no clear and convincing EEG abnormalities specific to manic disorder (for a review of the early EEG findings, see Shagass and Schwartz 1961).

Early Activated EEG Studies

The lack of resting EEG abnormalities did not preclude the possibility that "activating" the EEG might reveal differential responsiveness in mania. Liberson (1944) used the term *functional electroencephalography* to designate this approach, and various procedures for activating the EEG were utilized by the early investigators. Greenblatt et al. (1944) interpreted an excessive response to hyperventilation as one of their criteria for "abnormality." Unfortunately, they did not indicate to what extent this interpretation contributed to their classification of abnormal EEG findings in their manic population. Liberson (1944) reported the results obtained in 945 psychiatric patients under conditions of early-morning fasting with undisturbed recording to produce a drowsy state, and visual stimulation with flashes of light at two per second. His population included 51 manic-depressive depressed patients, 49 manic patients, 111 patients with involutional melancholia, and 38 reactive depressive patients. He found drowsy EEG patterns in 70% of manic patients, 55% of the manic-depressive depressed patients, and 50% of the involutional melancholia patients. The drowsy patterns varied from one group to another with respect to locus, speed, and pattern of onset. Diaz-Guerrero et al. (1946) compared six manic-depressive patients and healthy control subjects with respect to all-night sleep EEGs. They found not only that the patients had greater difficulty in falling asleep and staying asleep, but also that the EEGs showed a greater proportion of their sleep to be light and oscillating more frequently from one level of sleep to another than the sleep of the control subjects. Hurst et al. (1954) found a more pronounced photic driving from repetitive light flashes in manic patients than in control subjects.

Quantitative EEG Studies

Although the limitations of visual EEG inspection were well recognized by early investigators (Adrian 1944), further developments in EEG measurement required the introduction of analog circuitry and digital computer analysis (Clynes and Kohn 1961; Goldstein et al. 1963; Marjerrison et al. 1968). These technological developments in signal processing raised the possibility that EEG signals may contain useful information that is not evident to the naked eye. Computer-assisted quantitative EEG studies revealed a number of interesting findings. For example, Dalen (1965) studied patients with recurrent manic conditions that probably met DSM-III (American Psychiatric Association 1980) criteria for bipolar disorder. Some patients were found to have a positive family history of affective disorder and a normal EEG, whereas others had EEG abnormalities, a negative history of affective disorder, and a history of perinatal complications. This finding suggested an association of perinatal hazard, abnormal or borderline EEGs, and absence of familial affective disease. Cook et al. (1986) reported comparable findings in patients with bipolar illness.

Shagass et al. (1982) considered several indices of amplitude, frequency, and variability as measures of activation in several diagnostic groups. They concluded that under eyes-closed conditions, manic patients, like schizophrenic patients, are higher in activation than control subjects, whereas depressive patients are lower than control subjects. The effect of eye opening, however, was large for depressive patients, normal for manic patients, and small for schizophrenic patients. Thus, these authors suggested some diagnostic specificity was achieved by combining markers. Flor-Henry and Koles (1984) found that alpha was low (indicating activation) in manic patients, but not in depressive patients. Flor-Henry and Koles (1980) compared EEG characteristics of control subjects and depressive, manic, and schizophrenic patients during rest (eyes open) and during verbal and spatial processing. At rest, manic and depressive patients had lower right-hemisphere (especially right parietal alpha) activity than did healthy control subjects. During the activation tasks, control subjects showed greater left-hemisphere than right-hemisphere activation during verbal versus spatial tasks, whereas the manic patients showed a trend toward reversed laterality.

Polysomnographic Studies of Mania

As is well known, sleep disturbance is one of the more striking and clinically important features of major mood disorders. Extensive investigation using all-night polysomnography has demonstrated that sleep in major depression is characterized by more frequent awakenings and lighter sleep (stage 1) and less deep stages of sleep (stages 3 and 4), resulting in shallow and fragmented sleep (Reynolds and Kupfer 1987). There have been few comparable studies in mania. The previously noted results of the earlier qualitative EEG studies (Diaz-Guerrero et al. 1946; Liberson 1944) generally found disturbed sleep continuity. Akiskal (1984) reported that 12 patients with chronic hypomania had polysomnography features similar to patients with chronic depression and an increased number of awakenings. Linkowski et al. (1986) found shortened total sleep time and decreased sleep efficiency in six manic patients. The report of Hudson et al. (1992) merits special comment. Hudson et al. reported polysomnography features obtained in 2–4 consecutive nights in 19 young manic patients, 19 age-matched patients with major depression, and 19 age-matched healthy control subjects. Manic and depressed patients displayed nearly identical polysomnography abnormalities compared with the healthy control subjects, including disturbed sleep continuity, increased percentage of stage 1 sleep, shortened rapid eye movement (REM) latency, and increased REM density. They concluded that the polysomnography features were consistent with the possibility that the sleep disturbances in mania and major depression are caused by the same neural mechanism.

▶ ERP Studies of Mania

EEG studies proceeded for some time without seriously raising the question of the other category of electrical activity, namely the ERPs. In 1875, Caton had demonstrated that electrical potentials can be stimulated in the brain by a sensory stimulus and that there is a degree of cortical localization of the sensory area activated. ERPs should not be confused with the spontaneous EEG or with action potentials occurring in single axons. When a sensory stimulus is presented, a series of electrical events is initiated at the receptor organ, conducted into the brain, and propagated through the various sensory pathways. However, ERP signals recorded from the intact scalp are so much smaller in amplitude than the continuously changing EEG background ($0.1–30~\mu V$ versus $10–100~\mu V$) that they are essentially buried within the ongoing spontaneous EEG "noise." Thus, scalp-recorded ERPs require computer-assisted "signal averaging," in which EEG epochs that are time locked to repeated presentations of specific stimuli are algebraically averaged together. In this way, the random EEG activity is averaged out, and the ERP signal emerges as a composite waveform made up of distinct components that offer the opportunity to map the temporal features and spatial distribution of the underlying neural mechanisms involved in sensory and cognitive processing.

Sensory ERPs

The pioneering sensory ERP work of Shagass and Schwartz (1961) focused on the possibility that reduction in neural excitability underlies psychopathology. Pairs of weak sensory stimuli were administered to patients, with the paired stimuli separated by varying time intervals (interstimulus intervals). Amplitude and latency of ERPs to the first and second stimuli of the pair were measured. When the second stimulus of the pair yielded the same ERP response as the first stimulus, neural recovery was assumed to be complete. Relative recovery functions were assessed by comparing diagnostic groups and healthy control subjects. Results suggested that psychopathology is accompanied by a reduction in brain excitability and that patterns of reduction may differ among various diagnostic groups. Sensory ERPs evoked with the presentation of distinct sensory stimuli have been described in various psychopathologic groups. Abnormalities of these sensory ERPs are thought to be a sign of physiological deviance reflecting impaired neural processing of sensory and perceptual input.

The early ERP reports were encouraging. Shagass and Schwartz (1961) confined their measurements to the recovery function of the primary complex of the somatosensory response (somatosensory ERPs occurring within the first 45 milliseconds [msec] poststimulus). They demonstrated that in healthy control subjects, the first 200 msec of the recovery function is biphasic, with an early peak of recovery occurring by 20 msec and a later one at about 100 msec. There is a period of subnormal responsiveness between these peaks. Shagass and Schwartz reported mean recovery curves for 13 healthy control subjects and a group of 21 "psychotic depressive" patients (which included manic patients). The results indicated a marked reduction of early somatosensory recovery in the psychotic-depressed patients. Moreover, effective treatment with electroconvulsive therapy or antidepressant drugs returned the recovery curves to the normal pattern, except in those patients diagnosed as manic (Shagass and Schwartz 1961). Almost a quarter century later, Freedman et al. (1983) reported recovery function findings in mania using an auditory ERP technique. Auditory stimuli are paired at intervals separated by 0.5 seconds, and the P50 amplitude to the second stimulus is compared with the P50 amplitude to the first stimulus. In healthy control subjects, an amplitude reduction (inhibition) to the second stimulus is commonly observed; however, in acute manic patients, Freedman et al. noted a lack of inhibition in the auditory P50 to the second stimulus. This finding is similar to the fixed P50 deficit seen in schizophrenic patients, which is unchanged by neuroleptic treatment. The P50 deficit in manic patients, however, appears to be transient and seems to be mediated by norepinephrine (Adler et al. 1990). Thus, similar auditory P50 deficits in mania and schizophrenia are possibly associated with different biochemical abnormalities.

Following the early results of Shagass, Buchsbaum launched a research program using visual ERP in the study of affective disorder. Buchsbaum et al. (1973) found that patients with bipolar affective disorder, whether manic or depressed, had larger amplitude visual ERP components in the mid-latency range (P100–N140 components) as compared with healthy control subjects. Unipolar depressed patients had smaller amplitudes compared with control subjects. Buchsbaum et al. (1971) had previously reported that lithium efficacy may be predicted with auditory ERPs. In an unusual case study, Buchsbaum et al. (1977) reported that amplitude characteristics of middle and late auditory ERPs (P200 and P100) tended to covary with changes in clinical state in a 39-year-old woman with regular and rapid switches from mania to depression. The patient was studied for 113 consecutive days through five switches in clinical state. Shagass et al. (1980) found a number of differences between unmedicated patients with psychotic depression (85% were diagnosed as manic-depressive depressed) and healthy control subjects. Patients showed larger amplitude early ERP components (> 100 msec poststimulus) in the somatosensory and auditory modalities, and reduced amplitude in later ERP components compared with control subjects. Unfortunately, none of the patients in the Shagass et al. (1980) report were recorded during a manic phase.

Recent ERP Study in Mania

In the unpublished investigation by Josiassen et al. cited earlier, multisensory ERP findings were obtained from 11 healthy control subjects and 11 actively manic patients who had been unmedicated for at least 2 weeks. Patients and control subjects were matched for gender and age (within 2 years). The statistical analysis of these signals was performed on computer-generated amplitude measures using arbitrarily defined, overlapping time segments (epochs) of the ERPs. The group mean average deviations along with results of the two-way analyses of variance comparing manic patients and healthy control subjects are briefly summarized in Table 10–1 and Table 10–2.

The one statistically significant main effect ($P < .01$) for group was in the auditory evoked potential (AEP) 100–239 msec epoch where the mean average deviation value (across all leads) was smaller for manic patients than control subjects (1.71 μV versus 2.64 μV). There were no statistically significant group effects in either the somatosensory evoked potential (SEP) or visual evoked potential (VEP) comparisons. Because the relatively small sample size ($N = 11$ each) limited the statistical power to detect significant effects, two trends toward significant group effects are noted in Table 10–1 and Table 10–2: the left SEP 15–49 msec epoch (1.39 μV versus 1.07 μV) and the AEP 140–239 msec epoch (1.21 μV versus 1.58 μV). Significant group × lead interactions were found in 6 of 12 somatosensory ERP epochs and in 2 of 6 auditory ERP epochs. The interaction from the left SEP and right SEP 15–49 msec epoch resulted from the manic group having primary somatosensory responses (N20, P30, P45 peaks) of nearly twice the amplitude of the healthy control subjects for both right and left median nerve stimulation. All the other interactions in the somatosensory and auditory modalities resulted from the manic group having lower mean amplitude values from central recordings. In general, the early ERP amplitudes (< 100 msec poststimulus) were larger in the manic patients than in the healthy control subjects, whereas in the later epochs the mean amplitudes were larger in the control subjects than in the manic patients.

Cognitive ERPs

ERP signals have also been recorded in conjunction with performance of complex cognitive tasks (e.g., selective attention, short-term memory). Systematic changes in ERP activity are considered representative of the engagement of different neural processes mediating the cognitive task. Sutton et al. (1965) were the first to show that a portion of the auditory ERP was sensitive to how a subject perceived the probability of an event. When a rare event was presented, the auditory ERP showed a prominent positive deflection, "the P300 wave," having a

Table 10–1. Mean somatosensory evoked potential (SEP) amplitudes (average deviations, μV) of 11 manic patients and 11 healthy control subjects matched for age and gender (main effect for leads was $P < .0001$ in all epochs)

Epoch (msec)	Left SEP		Right SEP	
	Manic patients	Control subjects	Manic patients	Control subjects
15–30	1.07	0.94	1.05	0.95
15–49	1.39	1.07[a,b]	1.34	1.23[b]
31–99	1.67	1.62	1.73	1.87
50–199	2.05	2.58[a]	2.22	2.77[c]
100–299	2.06	2.34	2.19	2.59[c]
200–450	1.69	1.80[d]	1.76	1.99[d]

[a]Diagnosis × lead interaction ($P < .05$).
[b]Trend toward significant group effect ($P < .09 > .05$).
[c]Diagnosis × lead interaction ($P < .0001$).
[d]Diagnosis × lead interaction ($P < .01$).

Table 10–2. Mean visual evoked potential (VEP) and auditory evoked potential (AEP) amplitudes (average deviations, μV) of 11 manic patients and 11 healthy control subjects matched for age and gender (main effect for leads was $P < .0001$ in all epochs)

VEP epoch (msec)	Manic patients	Control subjects	AEP epoch (msec)	Manic patients	Control subjects
15–30	1.93	1.83	15–49	1.01	0.87
15–49	1.94	1.90	40–99	1.44	1.51
31–99	2.50	2.74	40–139	1.68	1.83
50–199	2.90	2.86	100–239	1.71	2.58[a,b]
100–299	2.39	2.66	140–239	1.21	1.58[c]
200–450	2.59	2.31	40–450	1.76	2.03[d]

[a]Main effect of group ($P < .01$).
[b]Diagnosis × lead interaction ($P < .0001$).
[c]Trend toward significant group effect ($P < .09 > .05$).
[d]Diagnosis × lead interaction ($P < .02$).

latency of approximately 300 msec poststimulus. Another robust cognitive ERP is the contingent negative variation (CNV). This slow negative shift of potential occurs approximately 400 msec after the presentation of a warning stimulus and normally terminates after the presentation of an "imperative stimulus" (i.e., a stimulus demanding a behavioral response or decision by the subject).

There have been relatively few cognitive ERP studies in manic patients. Only Kaskey et al. (1980) have reported the P300 in mania, and their study assessed the effects of lithium in 15 manic patients (pretreatment and posttreatment) rather than a between-group comparison. Lithium did not appear to increase P300 amplitude to all stimuli, but it did increase the difference in P300 to critical and noncritical stimuli. This finding, along with a decrease in commission errors, was interpreted to indicate that lithium enhances selective attention—a conclusion supported by a possible enhancement of the CNV by lithium (Tecce 1972). Visual inspection of Tecce's records suggests that the P300 component can be recorded in manic patients, and Tecce commented that the P300 component in the sample had a normal scalp distribution. Another cognitive ERP finding in mania was a reduction in CNV amplitude, an abnormality seen in other psychoses (Small and Small 1971).

▶ EFFECTS OF LITHIUM ON EEG AND ERPS

Lithium carbonate is the most extensively studied treatment for mania, and several electrophysiological findings regarding the effects of lithium of EEG and ERP characteristics have been replicated. At therapeutic doses, lithium carbonate has been found to increase density at delta and theta wave bands and to slow the peak alpha frequency (Heninger 1978). The latter finding, slowing of the alpha frequency, is interesting in relation to the faster alpha frequency observed in untreated manic patients as compared with depressive patients (P. A. Davis 1941b, 1942; Greenblatt et al. 1944; Hurst et al. 1954). These EEG changes correlated with clinically reduced symptoms of mania. The most consistent effects of lithium on ERPs is to increase the amplitude of positive components of both somatosensory and auditory modalities, as reported by Heninger (1978). Heninger also described increased mid-latency components in the somatosensory and auditory modalities; however, these findings were not replicated (Shagass and Straumanis 1978). A more extensive study by Straumanis et al. (1981)

found that lithium increased the amplitude of positive ERP components at both early and late latency ranges, with a tendency to reduce the amplitude of negative ERP components. Topography of the ERP peaks in the Straumanis et al. report was not altered by lithium, and there were no convincing associations between ERP changes and clinical changes in the patients.

▶ DIAGNOSTIC DIFFERENTIATION

Although an enormous literature has developed in the field of neuroelectrical signals from clinically defined psychopathologic groups, within this literature there are only a modest number of positive findings showing altered patterns of neural activity in mania. Using data from 242 unmedicated patients and 94 healthy control subjects, Shagass et al. (1984) used statistically derived factor scores to determine the extent to which single nonredundant measures (discriminant scores) of brain electrical events could differentiate between various groups of psychiatric patients and healthy control subjects. The diagnostic groups included 37 neurotic patients, 25 patients with personality disorders, 78 overt schizophrenic patients, 20 latent schizophrenic patients, 39 major-depression patients, 13 manic patients, and 94 healthy control subjects. Using equalized sample sizes, the sensitivity, specificity, and diagnostic confidence were computed between the manic group and the other groups. Diagnostic confidence rates greater than 75% were obtained between the manic patients and the major-depression patients (75%), patients with personality disorders (87.6%), neurotic patients (81%), and healthy control subjects (91.6%). It should be pointed out that a statistically meaningful discrimination was not obtained between manic and schizophrenic patients. The overall positive nature of these EEG results is encouraging and demonstrates statistically derived EEG differences between manic patients and other diagnostic groups. However, discriminant analysis capitalizes on chance, and it is difficult to specify clearly the degree to which these results are possible chance effects. Moreover, the manic group was very small, precluding any attempts to replicated the discrimination with other manic groups.

Using ERPs, a similar approach to diagnostic discrimination has also been reported. Josiassen et al. (1988) showed highly significant between-group differences on ERP measures (population $N = 836$). In this report, significant discriminant functions were found between manic patients and the following groups: healthy control subjects ($P < .001$), patients with personality disorders ($P < .01$), schizophrenic patients ($P < .002$), schizotypal/borderline patients ($P < .007$), and major depressive patients ($P < .002$). Again, these findings suggested many differences in brain electrical activity between manic patients and other psychiatric groups; however, the "brute force" nature of the statistical approach in the analysis makes it difficult to evaluate the details of specific ERP differences.

▶ CONCLUSION

Two contrasting impressions are gained from surveying the EEG and ERP literature on mania. On the one hand, it is difficult not to be disappointed by the relatively small yield of results after more than 50 years of EEG research and 25 years of ERP investigation. What has been learned with EEG and ERP measurements has centered around the demonstration of statistical group differences using relatively small groups with considerable overlap of measurements. There has been considerable difficulty moving beyond the relatively simple group differences approach. On the other hand, the few positive findings that have emerged using relatively small samples of patients do support an optimistic outlook for the future.

It seems reasonably clear that the increasing yield of encouraging results in this field will depend on continuing technical and methodological improvement. Neuroelectric activity and accompanying cerebral metabolism are both exquisitely sensitive to transient fluctuations in psychopathological symptoms, drug treatment, and secondary consequences of the illness, and to a large extent, experimental methods have yet to be devised that adequately control for these sources of artifact. Computer technology has provided the means for quantifying and reducing large amounts of data, for examining the relationships among many kinds of variables, and for testing concepts about the mathematical properties of brain potentials with relative ease. More and more factors requiring experimental control subjects have been identified, leading to improved methodology. Also, concurrent advances in classification and quantification of clinical variables have improved diagnostic criteria. Thus, although electrophysiological methods have been available for quite some time, the specific techniques currently in use have advanced greatly from those techniques employed in the past and will undoubtedly become much more sophisticated in the future. In essence, psychiatric electrophysiology has only just begun to harness its technology. From this perspective, there should be little discouragement about the paucity of its important contributions to research in mania and considerable optimism about its future productivity.

▶ REFERENCES

Adler LE, Gerhardt GA, Franks R, et al: Sensory physiology and catecholamines in schizophrenia and mania. Psychiatry Res 31:297–309, 1990
Adrian ED: Brain rhythms. Nature 153:360, 1944
Akiskal HS: Characterologic manifestations of affective disorders: toward a new conceptualization. Integrative Psychiatry 2:83–88, 1984
American Psychiatric Association: Diagnostic and Statistical Manual of Mental Disorders, 3rd Edition. Washington, DC, American Psychiatric Association, 1980
Berger H: Uber das elektrenkephalogram des menschen. Archiv für Psychiatrie und Nervenkrankheiten 87:527–570, 1929
Buchsbaum MS, Goodwin FK, Murphy DL, et al: AERs in affective disorders. Am J Psychiatry 128:19–25, 1971
Buchsbaum MS, Landau S, Murphy DL, et al: Average evoked response in bipolar and unipolar affective disorders: relationship to sex, age of onset and monoamine oxidase. Biol Psychiatry 7:199–212, 1973
Buchsbaum MS, Post RM, Bunney WE: Average evoked response in a rapidly cycling manic-depressive patient. Biol Psychiatry 12:83–99, 1977
Caton R: The electric currents of the brain. BMJ 2:278, 1875
Christie MJ, Little BC, Gordon AM: Peripheral indices of depressive states, in Handbook of Biological Psychiatry, Part II: Brain Mechanisms and Abnormal Behavior—Psychophysiology. Edited by Van Praag HM, Lader MH, Rafaelson OJ, et al. New York, Marcel Dekker, 1980
Clynes M, Kohn M: Portable four channel on-line digital average response computer CAT II, in Digest of IVth International Conference on Medical Electronics. New York, 1961, pp 92–102
Coles M, Donchin E, Porges SW (eds): Psychophysiology. New York, Guilford, 1985

Cook BL, Shukla S, Hoff AL: EEG abnormalities in bipolar affective disorder. J Affect Disord 11:147–149, 1986

Dalen P: Family history, the electroencephalogram and perinatal factors in manic conditions. Acta Psychiatr Scand 41:527–563, 1965

Davis H, Davis PA: The human electroencephalogram in health and in certain mental disorders. Archives of Neurology and Psychiatry 37:1461–1462, 1937

Davis PA: Electroencephalograms of manic-depressive patients. Am J Psychiatry 98:430–433, 1941a

Davis PA: Technique and evaluation of the electroencephalogram. Journal of Neurophysiology 4:92–114, 1941b

Davis PA: Comparative study of the EEGs of schizophrenic and manic-depressive patients. Am J Psychiatry 99:210–217, 1942

Davis PA, Davis H: The electroencephalograms of psychotic patients. Am J Psychiatry 95:1007–1025, 1939

Diaz-Guerrero R, Gottlieb JS, Knott JR: The sleep of patients with manic-depressive psychosis, depressive type: an electroencephalographic study. Psychosom Med 8:399–404, 1946

Flor-Henry P, Koles ZJ: EEG studies in depression, mania and normals: evidence for partial shifts of laterality in the affective psychoses. Advances in Biological Psychiatry 4:21–43, 1980

Flor-Henry P, Koles ZJ: Statistical quantitative EEG studies of depression, mania, schizophrenia and normals. Biol Psychiatry 19:257–279, 1984

Freedman R, Adler LE, Waldo MC, et al: Neurophysiological evidence for a defect in inhibitory pathways in schizophrenia: comparison of medicated and drug-free patients. Biol Psychiatry 18:537–551, 1983

Goldstein L, Murphree HB, Sugerman AA, et al: Quantitative electroencephalographic analysis of naturally occurring (schizophrenic) and drug-induced psychotic states in human males. Clin Pharmacol Ther 4:10–17, 1963

Greenblatt M, Healey MM, Jones GA: Age and electroencephalographic abnormality in neuropsychiatric patients: a study of 1593 cases. Am J Psychiatry 101:82–90, 1944

Henninger GR: Lithium carbonate and brain function. Arch Gen Psychiatry 35:228–233, 1978

Hudson JI, Lipinski JF, Keck PE, et al: Polysomnographic characteristics of young manic patients: comparison with unipolar depressed patients and normal control subjects. Arch Gen Psychiatry 49:378–383, 1992

Hurst LA, Mundy-Castle AC, Beerstecher DM: The electroencephalogram in manic-depressive psychosis. Journal of Mental Science 100:220–240, 1954

Jasper HH, Fitzpatrick CP, Solomon P: Analogies and opposites in schizophrenia and epilepsy. Am J Psychiatry 95:835–851, 1939

Josiassen RC, Shagass C, Roemer RA: Dealing with differential gender and age effects in evoked potential studies of psychopathology. Biol Psychiatry 23:612–627, 1988

Kaskey GB, Salzman LF, Ciccone JR, et al: Effects of lithium on evoked potentials and performance during sustained attention. Psychiatry Res 3:281–289, 1980

Knott JR: Reduced latent time of blocking of the berger rhythm to light stimuli. Proceedings of the Society for Experimental Biology and Medicine 38:216–217, 1938

Lader MH: The Psychophysiology of Mental Illness. London, England, Routledge & Kegan Paul, 1975

Levy DL, Holzman PS, Matthysse S, et al: Eye tracking and schizophrenia: a selective review. Schizophr Bull 201:47–62, 1994

Liberson WT: Functional electroencephalography in mental disorders. Diseases of the Nervous System 5:357–364, 1944

Lindsley DB: Some neurophysiological sources of action current frequencies. Psychol Med 44 (suppl):33–60, 1933

Linkowski P, Kerkhofs M, Rielaert C, et al: Sleep during mania in manic-depressive males. Eur Arch Psychiatry Neurol Sci 235:339–341, 1986

Marjerrison G, Krause AE, Keogh RP: Variability of the EEG in schizophrenia: quantitative analysis with a modulus voltage integrator. Electroencephalogr Clin Neurophysiol 24:35, 1968

Reynolds CF, Kupfer DJ: Sleep research in affective illness: State of the art circa 1987. Sleep 10:199–215, 1987

Shagass C, Schwartz M: Reactivity cycle of somatosensory cortex in humans with and without psychiatric disorder. Science 134:1757–1759, 1961

Shagass C, Straumanis JJ: Drugs and human sensory evoked potentials, in Psychopharmacology: A Generation of Progress. Edited by Lipton MA, DiMascio A, Killam KF. New York, Raven, 1978, pp 112–127

Shagass C, Roemer RA, Straumanis JJ, et al: Topography of sensory evoked potentials in depressive disorders. Biol Psychiatry 15:183–207, 1980

Shagass C, Roemer RA, Straumanis JJ: Relationships between psychiatric diagnosis and some quantitative EEG variables. Arch Gen Psychiatry 39:1423–1435, 1982

Shagass C, Roemer RA, Straumanis JJ, et al: Psychiatric diagnostic discriminations with combinations of quantitative EEG variables. Br J Psychiatry 144:581–592, 1984

Small JG, Small IF: Contingent negative variation (CNV) correlations with psychiatric diagnosis. Arch Gen Psychiatry 25:550–554, 1971

Stern JA, Janes CL: Personality and psychopathology, in Electrodermal Activity in Psychological Research. Edited by Prokasy WF, Raskin DC. New York, Academic Press, 1973, pp 76–85

Straumanis JJ, Shagass C, Roemer RA, et al: Cerebral evoked potential changes produced by treatment with lithium carbonate. Biol Psychiatry 16:113–129, 1981

Strauss H: Intracranial neoplasms masked as depressions and diagnosed with the aid of electroencephalography. J Nerv Ment Dis 122:185–189, 1955

Sutton S, Braren M, Zubin J, et al: Evoked potential correlates of stimulus uncertainty. Science 150:1187–1188, 1965

Tecce JJ: Contingent negative variation (CNV) and psychological processes in man. Psychol Bull 77:73–108, 1972

Travis LE, Dorsey JM: Mass responsiveness in the central nervous system. Archives of Neurology and Psychiatry 26:141–145, 1931

Walter WG: Technique-interpretation, in Electroencephalography. Edited by Hill D, Parr G. New York, Macmillan, 1963, pp23–29

Zahn TP: Psychophysiological approaches to psychopathology, in Psychophysiology. Edited by Coles R, Donchin E, Porges SW. New York, Guilford, 1985, pp 89–102

Chapter 11

BRAIN IMAGING

Mark S. George, M.D.,
Terence A. Ketter, M.D., F.R.C.P.C.,
Tim A. Kimbrell, M.D., and
Robert M. Post, M.D.

Seeing. We might say that the whole of life lies in that verb.

Teilhard De Chardin

Once we have seen or encountered something, we know it in a different, more comprehensive manner than if we were merely intellectually acquainted with it. That is, academic or general knowledge is quite different from the personal, acquainted knowledge that comes with actually visiting and seeing something. In French, this distinction is formalized by the use of different verbs depending on whether one has visited or seen something (*connaitre*) or is merely informed about it (*savoir*). With new imaging technologies, clinicians and researchers are now able actually to see the brain in illness and health and acquire a new level and type of knowledge and understanding (e.g., *connaitre* rather than *savoir* the brain in mania).

Imaging studies limited to mania, as opposed to mood disorders in general, have been hampered by several factors, including the difficulty of scanning actively manic patients. Despite these obstacles, imaging studies are beginning to implicate specific brain regions that are abnormal in manic patients. Structural studies using computed tomography (CT) and magnetic resonance imaging (MRI) have found

191

differences in the frontal and temporal lobes in bipolar disorder patients. Additionally, resting functional studies with positron-emission tomography (PET) and single photon emission computed tomography (SPECT) have revealed that some subjects with mood disorders have decreased activity in the prefrontal lobes and basal ganglia, compared with healthy control subjects. Preliminary new PET findings have hinted at increased temporal lobe activity in bipolar patients compared with unipolar subjects. Lastly, pharmacological and neuropsychological activation studies that image transient happiness or euphoria have provided further information about brain regions likely to be involved in the pathogenesis of mania.

In this chapter, the new imaging tools available to the psychiatric researcher are briefly described. The results from studies using these technologies to investigate the brain in mania are then critically reviewed. Finally, these diverse imaging modality results are synthesized into a preliminary neuroanatomy of mania.

▶ REVIEW OF NEW IMAGING TECHNOLOGIES

Repeatedly in the field of medicine, new technologies that are used to redefine the study of a disease have emerged (McHenry 1969). In cardiology, this first occurred with the development of the electrocardiogram (ECG), and later with more advanced techniques of catheterization. In the field of epilepsy, a technologically driven revolution occurred with the development of the electroencephalogram (EEG) (Temkin 1945). Prior to the EEG, there was at best a partial consensus about the pathophysiology of epilepsy. Controversies existed about whether epilepsy was a brain-generated or peripherally generated illness, about appropriate treatments, and so on. It was largely after the use of EEG became widespread, with its ability to "image" the abnormal electrical discharges, that epilepsy evolved from an illness whose treatment was mostly long-term support, to a group of well-defined illnesses with distinct pathophysiologies and treatments (focal versus primarily generalized, myoclonic, or petit mal) (Engel 1989; Penfield and Jasper 1954).

The new imaging technologies available today offer the promise of doing the same for several umbrella classifications of diseases in current psychiatry, most notably the schizophrenias and the mood disorders. In the area of mood dysregulation, it is already apparent that "clinical depression" encompasses several diseases with distinct pathophysiologies, ranging from depressions that stem from known biological abnormalities such as hypothyroidism or poststroke (referred to as secondary depressions) to the more idiopathic and genetic syndromes of recurrent brief, unipolar and bipolar depression (primary mood disorders). The new imaging tools have already advanced our knowledge and understanding of these diseases. The focus of this chapter is the review of brain-imaging studies in mania. However, the findings in mania are necessarily discussed in the context of findings in other depressions as well.

Structural Scans: CT and MRI

The current revolution in neuroimaging began with the development of the ability to sample gamma ray emissions in a circular or tomographic way, using the newfound power of computers. This key advance, sampling radioactivity in a circular way and then reconstructing it with computers to provide an image of the head, is the basis for SPECT and PET. CT scan involves radiation and is poor at resolving structures in the brain stem or posterior fossa. MRI typically involves sampling the degree to which hydrogen ions return to their normal configuration following a transient but powerful magnetic pulse (M. S. Cohen and Bookheimer 1994). Thus, MRI involves no radiation and has remarkable resolving power (on the order of 1–2 mm). It is also very good at imaging structures surrounded by bone, such as the brain stem and cerebellum.

Functional Neuroimaging:
SPECT, PET, and function MRI (fMRI)

In contrast to CT and traditional MRI, which image the structure of the brain, several new technologies have been developed with the power to look at brain function. These technologies have proved a point first formulated by the English neurologist J. Hughlings Jackson, namely, that brain structure does not equal function and vice versa

(Jackson 1873; Taylor 1958). That is, structural brain damage, such as a tumor or scar producing an epileptic focus, can either obliterate the function normally subserved by that portion of the brain or it can heighten its functions (Jackson 1874). Additionally, one can have normal brain structure (at least to the limit of measurement available with current technology) and have markedly abnormal function (areas of the brain that are normal structurally, but that are "off-line" functionally). An example of this state commonly occurs following cortical strokes in which the contralateral cerebellum is hypofunctional on PET or SPECT images even though it is structurally intact, a phenomenon referred to as cerebellar diaschisis (George et al. 1991).

SPECT involves the peripheral injection of a radiotracer into a vein, which then travels into the brain and is deposited into neurons and glia (George et al. 1991). The gamma rays (or photons) that these radiotracers emit are then detected by rotating cameras and reconstructed into a three-dimensional image. Various radiotracers bind to different structures and have different half-lives that determine when the image can be acquired. The most popular current tracer is 99Tcm-hexamethylpropylamine oxine (HMPAO), which distributes to the brain in a fashion roughly equivalent to blood flow (Devous et al. 1986; Ell et al. 1985). The tracer can be injected in the patient anywhere in the hospital; it "sets" within the active brain regions within 2–5 minutes. The patient can then be transported to the nuclear medicine suite for actual image acquisition. If necessary, tranquilizing medications (which do not affect the actual image because the HMPAO pattern has already been deposited) can be given to sedate the patient for scanning. The ability to inject while subjects are away from the nuclear medicine suite and outside of the camera makes SPECT imaging particularly useful for studying diseases such as epilepsy or mania. Those areas of the brain that are more active demand either more blood flow, the basis of HMPAO SPECT and oxygen (O^{15}) PET, or more glucose, the basis of glucose (fluorodeoxyglucose; FDG) PET (Sokoloff 1977, 1978). Functional images thus change as a result of alterations in brain activity due to differences in subjects' behavior during tracer uptake.

PET involves the peripheral injection of radiotracers that, as they degrade, emit positrons. These are highly unstable particles that travel a short distance and then collide with an electron (Itturalde 1990). This reaction releases two photons traveling in exactly the opposite direction (180 degrees apart). These photons are then detected by rotating cameras outside of the head and computer reconstructed. In PET, as opposed to SPECT, the cameras are instructed to include for final analysis only those particles that are recorded simultaneously in a detector and in its 180-degree counterpart, thus enabling a more precise reconstruction of exactly where the photon originated. In general, this gives PET a higher image resolution than SPECT.

The majority of PET imaging in mania has been done using glucose (FDG) or oxygen (O^{15}). They are necessarily produced in a cyclotron. O^{15} image acquisition takes approximately 1–5 minutes, whereas FDG requires on the order of one-half hour. Both PET and SPECT offer the possibility of imaging more selective pharmacological systems in the brain with selective radiotracers. Examples in SPECT include dopamine receptors with 123-iodobenzamide (IBZM), acetylcholine with 3-quinuclidnyl-4-[123] iodobenzilate (IQNB), and benzodiazepine receptors with flumazenil (George et al. 1991). To date, specific ligands with PET have imaged dopamine, opiates, and acetylcholine receptors. PET radiotracers have also been made by attaching a labeled carbon atom to various neuroactive compounds such as labeled deprenyl or fluoxetine.

The newest functional neuroimaging technology is functional MRI, or fMRI (M. S. Cohen and Bookheimer 1994; David et al. 1994; George et al. 1994a; Kwong et al. 1992; Rosen et al. 1994; Stehling et al. 1991; Turner et al. 1991). There are basically two techniques that use the imaging power of MRI systems to image functional brain changes rather than brain structure: injecting a bolus of a magnetic compound and watching its distribution through the brain over a short time, or taking very fast images (on the order of 1 image per second) to distinguish the differences between activity at rest and during a specific behavior. This latter technique capitalizes on the fact that oxyhemoglobin is nonmagnetic and deoxyhemoglobin is paramagnetic. Brain areas with high demand, therefore, will have a different ratio of oxyhemoglobin to deoxyhemoglobin and thus give off a different magnetic signal (a technique that is blood oxygenation level dependent [BOLD]).

For PET and SPECT, to assess whether there are differences in regional activity across tasks or between groups, various regions are typically sampled, and the results of mean activity are averaged and compared across tasks or groups. This is the region of interest analysis. The placement of regions can be guided by an atlas, performed semi-automatically, or the images coregistered with the patient's structural MRI. In an alternative method that has been developed, images are nonlinearly fitted into a standard atlas of the brain and then comparisons are done on a point-by-point (pixel-by-pixel) basis (Friston et al. 1989, 1991). With echoplanar BOLD functional MRI, the images are typically mapped onto the subject's structural MRI, and, for a given individual, the statistical significance of regions that change with different tasks can be determined (see Figure 11–1).

Within the short span of 25 years, therefore, we have progressed from having practically no useful methods of examining the brains of living manic patients to having two methods for looking at brain structure and at least three methods for examining brain function. These methods have essentially opened up windows into the brain, providing preliminary glimpses into the neuroanatomy of mania. Even though findings to date have not been definitive, important clues have been

Brain structure   Brain function

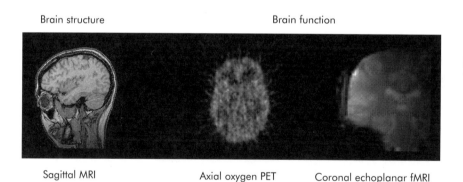

Sagittal MRI   Axial oxygen PET   Coronal echoplanar fMRI

Figure 11–1.   New imaging technologies. Diagram of the key differences between structural scanners (magnetic resonance imaging [MRI]) (left) and functional imaging scanners (positron-emission tomography [PET] and function MRI [fMRI]). Each of these methods has unique attributes as well as problems.

uncovered that promise to make the next 25 years much more enlightening and productive in understanding the neural substrates underlying mania.

▶ Problems Unique to Using Functional Imaging to Study Mania

There are problems inherent to studying mania with functional imaging techniques, depending on whether trait issues (i.e., bipolar disorder) or the actual state of mania is being addressed. One of the main problems in studying bipolar I disorder revolves around determining the correct diagnosis. First, some bipolar I disorder subjects, who are incorrectly classified initially as recurrent unipolar depression, later develop a manic episode. Thus, almost by definition, imaging bipolar I disorder subjects requires that they have already had a manic episode. This requirement also makes it difficult to factor out trait abnormalities that are independent of the experience of having lived through an episode of mania. There is always the possibility that some recurrent unipolar subjects will later become bipolar I disorder or bipolar II disorder, thereby minimizing between-group differences. To some extent, these problems in diagnosis can be avoided through fastidious life-charting of the course of illness (Post et al. 1988; Roy-Byrne et al. 1985; Squillace et al. 1984); also, a thorough family history looking for relatives with bipolar disorder is helpful. Additionally, problems arise when attempting to distinguish primary from secondary mania. A thorough history and physical screening, along with laboratory work, course of illness, and high resolution structural imaging can help avoid this pitfall.

Another diagnostic problem is that most imaging studies assume all bipolar I disorder patients are the same. However, it may be that the bipolar affective disorder (BPAD) diagnosis is heterogeneous. For example, some have argued that there may be a dysphoric subset of mania, distinct from the rest of bipolar disorder (Post et al. 1989). It is becoming more apparent that bipolar disorder rarely exists on its own. There are high rates of comorbidity with alcohol and substance abuse, as well as with a host of other psychiatric diagnoses. Thus, "pure" bipolar patients usually included in studies are actually a very small subset of the total group of bipolar patients. Studies employing "pure" bipolar patients, although methodologically more exact because there are fewer variables to control for, may actually misrepresent the bipolar patient population as a whole. Neurobiological and neuroimaging findings in this group may or may not be applicable to the entire group of bipolar patients. Finally, imaging studies involving first-break manic patients are likely to include a subset of subjects who later develop schizophrenia.

In addition to problems in determining the correct diagnosis, it is increasingly difficult to image subjects in a medication-free state. Several studies have convincingly demonstrated that bipolar I disorder is a lifetime disorder and that chronic treatment with mood stabilizers can decrease the likelihood of recurrences (Post et al. 1993). Thus, most bipolar I disorder subjects are taking mood-stabilizing medications, and it is difficult to image them when they are medication free. This issue is further complicated by reports of treatment refractoriness induced by lithium discontinuation (Post et al. 1992). These bipolar subjects were typically doing well, had their medication discontinued and then relapsed, and did not re-respond to the mood stabilizer. Cases like these raise ethical issues about discontinuing medication in a bipolar subject who is doing well, just to obtain a "clean" imaging study. However, studies of nonresponders and those who have become tolerant to medication should be less problematic.

Additional problems arise that are unique to imaging subjects when they are actively manic—the manic state as opposed to the trait of mania. The signal achieved in functional imaging studies depends largely on the mental and physical activity of the subject during the exact moments of tracer uptake into the brain (George et al. 1991; Haxby et al. 1991; Ring et al. 1991). Indeed, this is the very basis of activation studies in which serial scans are performed and the behavior across scans is modified slightly, thereby demonstrating the brain regions responsible for the behavior. It can be difficult to image actively manic subjects while they are not on medications. Further, it is almost impossible to control completely for their behavior. Actively manic subjects by definition have racing thoughts, hyperactivity, problems paying attention, and performance differences from other pathological groups as well as healthy control subjects. Additionally, manic patients may hyperventilate and thus have changes in global blood flow rates in addition to their regional differences.

It is important to keep these problems in mind as the published studies to date attempting to identify the brain regions important in mania are reviewed in the following sections.

▶ IMAGING STUDIES OF BIPOLAR DISORDER (TRAIT OF MANIA)

Structural Studies

Studies of brain structure in mood disorders with MRI and CT have been done on heterogeneous patient groups and have used widely divergent image acquisition parameters and scanners. To date, there has been no consistent methodology of scan acquisition or region measuring, making comparisons across studies extremely difficult. Thus, with the exception of increased third ventricle size in manic patients, only a few of the abnormal findings in structural studies in depression have been replicated, due in part to differences in methodology as well as patient populations (for a summary of studies, see Tables 11–1 and 11–2).

Regional volumetric analysis. In general, the original studies of the structural anatomy of patients with affective illness were largely unremarkable (Jeste et al. 1988; Nasrallah et al. 1989; Schlegel and Kretzschmar 1987a, 1987b; Schlegel et al. 1989). More recently, however, well-designed studies employing advanced imaging techniques have found volumetric differences involving the prefrontal and temporal lobes in BPAD subjects compared with control subjects. Several investigators have found an increase in ventricular size in patients with BPAD compared with control subjects (Altshuler et al. 1991; Andreasen et al. 1990; Kellner et al. 1986; Nasrallah et al. 1982; Pearlson et al. 1984; M. L. Scott et al. 1983; Shima et al. 1984; Strakowski et al. 1993b), although others have not (Schlegel and Kretzschmar 1987a). In some but not all studies (Andreasen et al. 1990), increased ventricular size has been found more convincingly in BPAD men, in patients with more frequent hospitalizations, in patients with more

Table 11–1. Representative brain structure magnetic resonance imaging (MRI) studies in primary bipolar disorder

Investigator	Subjects	Findings: volumetric measurements and other structural anomalies
Temporal lobe reduction		
Hauser et al. 1989	15 BPAD, 2 unipolar, 21 control subjects	Decreased bilateral temporal lobe/cerebrum ratio
Altshuler et al. 1991	10 (6 from above) BPAD, 10 control subjects	Decreased temporal lobe volume in BPAD
Rossi et al. 1991	16 BPAD, 10 schizophrenic	Schizophrenic patients have decreased left and right temporal lobe volume
Increased ventricular size (VBR)		
Strakowski et al. 1993b	17 BPAD (first episode), 16 control subjects	Increased third ventricle size; different gray/white matter distribution in BPAD
Swayze et al. 1992	48 BPAD, 54 schizophrenic, 47 control subjects	Decreased size of right hippocampus in BPAD versus control subjects; normal basal ganglia size
Schlegel and Kretzschmar 1987a, 1987b	60 mood disorders, 60 control subjects	No difference in VBR

Study	Subjects	Findings
Weinberger et al. 1982	23 mood disorders, 27 other illness, 17 control subjects, 35 first-episode schizophrenia, 17 chronic schizophrenia	Increased VBR in schizophrenia than in mood disorders or with control subjects
Shima et al. 1984	46 major depression, 11 control subjects, 35 patient control subjects	Increased VBR in mood subjects; correlation with poor outcome, age
Nasrallah et al. 1982	24 young manic males, 27 control subjects, 55 chronic schizophrenia	Increased VBR in both patient groups compared with control subjects; no differences between patient groups
Basal ganglia size		
Aylward et al. 1994	30 BPAD, 30 control subjects	Male bipolar subjects had larger caudate volumes than male control subjects
Krishnan et al. 1992	50 major depression, 50 control subjects	Depressed subjects had smaller caudate volume than control subjects
Husain et al. 1991	41 major depression, 44 control subjects	Depressed subjects had smaller putamen

(continued)

Table 11–1. Representative brain structure magnetic resonance imaging (MRI) studies in primary bipolar disorder (*continued*)

Investigator	Subjects	Findings: volumetric measurements and other structural anomalies
Dolan et al. 1990	14 BPAD, 10 unipolar, 10 control subjects	Increased frontal T1 signal; unipolar versus control subjects; BPAD normal
McDonald et al. 1991	12 BPAD, 12 age-matched control subjects	Increased subcortical hyperintensities in manic subjects with onset after > age 50
Jurjus et al. 1993	63 schizoaffective, 67 schizophrenia, 37 control subjects	No difference in major brain anomalies in either patient group from control subjects
Strakowski et al. 1993a	18 BPAD (first hospitalization), 15 control subjects	Twice as many subcortical white matter hyperintensities in BPAD; nonsignificant

Note.   BPAD = bipolar affective disorder. VBR = ventricle/brain ratio.

Table 11–2. Studies of brain structure in primary bipolar disorder

Investigator	Subjects	Findings: correlations between brain size and clinical parameters
Computed tomography		
Kellner et al. 1983	10 mixed	Increased ventricular ratio correlates with urinary free cortisol
Kellner et al. 1986	21 mixed	Increased ventricular size correlates with impaired cognition
Mukherjee et al. 1993	15 BPAD (manic)	Increased third ventricle size correlates with dexamethasone suppression test nonsuppression
Magnetic resonance imaging		
Coffman et al. 1990	30 BPAD, 52 control subjects	Decreased cognitive performance in BPAD; deficits correlate with decreased midsagittal area
Andreasen et al. 1990	24 BPAD, 27 unipolar, 108 schizophrenia, 75 control subjects	Increased ventricular size in male BPAD subjects; no relation to clinical correlates, treatment response, or cognitive impairment
Pearlson et al. 1984	27 BPAD, 27 control subjects	BPAD larger VBR than control subjects; increased VBR with more hospitalizations, persistent unemployment

Note. BPAD = bipolar affective disorder. VBR = ventricle/brain ratio.

frequent psychotic depressions, and in patients with persistent unemployment (Pearlson et al. 1984). The interpretation of these studies is unclear, however, because numerous pathophysiological processes may result in ventricular enlargement. However, atrophy of periventricular white matter regions, particularly the prefrontal and temporal lobes, is one possible mechanism. At least two studies have supported this notion that the ventricular enlargement is due to focal atrophy of surrounding tissue, particularly the temporal lobes. Hauser et al. (1989) reported bilateral decreased temporal lobe volume in 15 BPAD subjects, and Altshuler et al. (1991) found decreased temporal lobe volume in 10 BPAD subjects compared with control subjects. Small temporal lobes and increased ventricular size have also been found in numerous studies of schizophrenic subjects, raising the question of the uniqueness of this finding for BPAD. Some comparison studies have found differences in cerebral ventricular volume between BPAD subjects and those with schizophrenia (Weinberger et al. 1982), but others did not find this difference (Nasrallah et al. 1982; Reider et al. 1983; Rossi et al. 1991). Swayze et al. (1990) found enlarged ventricles in 54 schizophrenic subjects compared with 47 control sujbects. Interestingly, there was a trend for increased ventricular volume in 48 BPAD subjects compared with control subjects, particularly in men with BPAD. These studies imply that both BPAD subjects (especially BPAD men) and schizophrenic subjects have small temporal lobes compared with control subjects and that schizophrenic subjects may have even smaller temporal lobes (or greater atrophy) than BPAD subjects.

Finally, Swayze et al. (1992) found abnormally small right hippocampal volume in 48 BPAD subjects compared with 47 control subjects. Conflicting studies have found larger (Aylward et al. 1994), normal (Swayze et al. 1992), and smaller (Husain et al. 1991; Krishnan et al. 1992) basal ganglia volume in BPAD (Aylward et al. 1994) and mixed mood disorders (Krishnan et al. 1992; Swayze et al. 1992).

Structural anomalies. MRI has also been used to investigate whether the brains of BPAD subjects have increased rates of structural anomalies. Jurjus et al. (1993) examined MRI scans of 67 schizophrenic, 63 BPAD, and 37 healthy control subjects. They found no difference between the groups when examining for 23 developmental anomalies recognizable on MRI. However, their control group had a 23% rate of these anomalies, which is very high for the general population. This high rate in control subjects differs from other studies, which looked for and found high levels of midline MRI developmental anomalies in schizophrenia (George et al. 1989; T. F. Scott et al. 1993).

Two early studies have examined the T1 relaxation time in specific brain regions. Rangel-Guerra et al. (1983) found increased T1 values in frontal and temporal white matter, which normalized with lithium therapy. Dolan et al. (1990) used MRI to examine 14 medicated patients with BPAD, 10 medicated patients with unipolar depression, and 10 control subjects. Interestingly, they also found increases in T1 signal intensity in the frontal white matter; however, this was true only of unipolar depressed subjects compared with control subjects, and it was not seen in the BPAD subgroup. The significance of increased T1 values is unclear, but possibly reflects shifts in water distribution, which may in turn represent changes in metabolism. It is unclear whether these results represent a change in brain structure or function or both.

Several studies have examined the frequency of white matter lesions in patients with BPAD. These white matter lesions, formerly known as unidentified bright objects (UBOs), occur with increasing frequency as people age and occur with higher than expected frequency in certain populations (e.g., post-ischemia, multiple sclerosis, vascular disease). McDonald et al. (1991) noted increased subcortical UBOs in a special population of manic subjects who had onset of disease after age 50. Strakowski et al. (1993a) imaged 18 BPAD subjects at the time of their first hospitalization. BPAD subjects had twice as many subcortical UBOs as did control subjects, although this difference failed to reach statistical significance. Aylward et al. (1994) examined 30 BPAD subjects and 30 control subjects and found increased white matter hyperintensities in the BPAD group, especially in older subjects. The significance and the meaning of these increased rates of UBOs in BPAD subjects are unclear.

Correlations Between Brain Structure and Clinical Parameters

Numerous studies have sought to compare the degree of brain changes in BPAD subjects with clinical parameters. In one of the first studies of this type, Kellner et al. (1986) used CT scans in 21 mixed mood disorder subjects and found that the degree of ventricular enlargement correlated positively with cognitive impairment. In another study, Kellner et al. (1983) found that ventricular volume increased as urinary free cortisol levels rose. High levels of circulating corticosteroids are often found in depressed subjects, and exogenous steroid administration is used clinically to shrink brain tissue in edematous states such as with brain tumors or following a stroke. In a more recent study using MRI and BPAD subjects in the manic state, Mukherjee et al. (1993) reported that the size of the third ventricle was correlated with nonsuppression on the dexamethasone suppression test, a method of assessing corticosteroid tone. Finally, in a provocative study indirectly confirming the earlier Kellner et al. finding, Coffman et al. (1990) scanned 30 BPAD subjects and 52 control subjects. Within the BPAD group, the degree of cognitive deficits correlated with decreased size of midsagittal structures.

In summary, several studies have suggested that BPAD subjects have smaller temporal lobes as well as larger ventricles. Additionally, these abnormalities in volume may be indirectly affected by serum cortisol levels, which are known to be abnormal in BPAD, particularly during depressive and manic states. Furthermore, several studies have now revealed that BPAD subjects have increased rates of nonspecific subcortical white matter abnormalities (UBOs). This result and studies that have found increased cerebrospinal fluid (CSF) protein in BPAD males raise the interesting possibility that at least some forms of BPAD may be characterized by a subcortical disease process involving release of excess proteins and some other disease process including apoptosis or demyelination. It seems clear that further studies looking for volumetric as well as developmental abnormalities, and involving larger numbers of patients with well-documented life histories, would help settle many of these issues raised in the studies to date.

Brain Regions Involved in Secondary Mania

Mania can sometimes result from strokes, closed head injuries, or brain tumors (secondary mania). In general, secondary mania has been seen to occur significantly more in association with right than left hemisphere lesions (Robinson et al. 1988; Ross and Rush 1981; Ross et al. 1994; Starkstein et al. 1991). These lesions typically involve either the right basal frontal or right temporal cortex, the right head of the caudate, or the right thalamus (Starkstein et al. 1987, 1988, 1989, 1990, 1991). The involvement of the right hemisphere in mania is even more interesting in light of numerous studies that have documented that left hemisphere lesions, particularly in the prefrontal cortex, cause secondary depression (George et al. 1994d; Jorge et al. 1993; Robinson and Szetela 1981; Robinson et al. 1984; Stern and Bachman 1991). In one of the more enlightening studies of secondary mania, Starkstein et al. (1990) imaged three actively manic patients with PET FDG who developed mania after a stroke or trauma (secondary mania). All had metabolic deficits in the right basotemporal cortex (for a summary of studies, see Table 11–3).

Additional information about the neuroanatomical structures involved in mania comes from case reports of patients with focal epilepsy who develop manic symptoms in relation to their seizures. Numerous studies (Barczak et al. 1988; Drake 1988; Gillig et al. 1988) have found that secondary mania develops in patients with focal epilepsy

Table 11–3. Brain regions and diseases that produce secondary mania

Investigators	Clinical syndrome	Brain region
Strokes and brain trauma		
Jorge et al. 1993;		
Robinson and Szetela 1981;		
Robinson et al. 1984, 1988;		
Stern and Bachman 1991	Depression	Left frontal lobe
Starkstein et al. 1987, 1988,		
1989, 1990, 1991	Mania	Right hemisphere
Focal epilepsy		
Barczak et al. 1988;		
Drake 1988;		
Gillig et al. 1988;		
Pakalnis et al. 1987	Mania	Right temporal lobe
Arroyo et al. 1993	Laughter, mirth	Anterior cingulate
Bromfield et al. 1992;		
Robertson and Trimble 1983	Depression	Left hemisphere

originating from the right temporal lobe. Functional imaging with PET and SPECT has documented that in the minutes to hours following a focal epileptic discharge, the seizure site is hypometabolic and has decreased regional cerebral blood flow (Marks et al. 1992). The functions subsumed by that area of cortex are thus temporarily taken off-line. When this occurs in the motor strip, the temporary paralysis that follows is known as a "Todd's paralysis." It is unclear if the epileptic right temporal lobe discharge is temporarily taking off-line the regions in the right temporal lobe needed to prevent mania. This line of reasoning would account for both the lesion and epilepsy cases of secondary mania arising with right temporal lobe damage.

Thus, structural studies in mania to date uniformly implicate the temporal lobes and subcortical structures, particularly on the right, in the pathogenesis of manic states. This information has come from volumetric studies and studies examining anomalies in primary BPAD, as well as from imaging secondary manias induced by stroke and epilepsy. However, studies to date have provided only a mere sketch of the relevant neuroanatomy, and the evidence is not totally compelling. Further work with more refined diagnostic groups (both primary and secondary mania) and rigorous and reproducible image analysis programs are clearly warranted.

Overview of Functional Studies in Unipolar Depression

As discussed, even if brain structure is normal, there can be marked abnormalities in the function of that region and the behavior that it normally subserves. In general, more information about regional neuroanatomy has emerged from functional than structural studies in mood disorders. Numerous investigators using PET and SPECT have demonstrated that depressed patients have decreased metabolism or flow in the prefrontal lobes, particularly in the left anterolateral prefrontal cortex (ALPFC) (Austin et al. 1992; Baxter et al. 1985, 1989; Bench et al. 1992; Dolan et al. 1992; Drevets et al. 1992; Ketter et al. 1993c; Mayberg et al. 1991) (see Table 11–4). In one of the landmark articles in this area, Baxter et al. (1989) used FDG PET to study 10 patients with unipolar depression, 10 patients with bipolar depres-

Table 11–4. Functional imaging studies in primary depression

Investigators	Subjects	Findings
Single photon emission computed tomography		
Mayberg et al. 1991	7 unipolar, 10 control subjects	Decreased regional cerebral blood flow in frontal, temporal cingulate and left caudate
Austin et al. 1992	40 unipolar, 20 control subjects	1) Decreased frontal, anterior temporal, and right thalamus 2) Endogenous depression had increased anterior cingulate activity compared with nonendogenous
Positron-emission tomography		
Baxter et al. 1985	10 unipolar, 10 bipolar, 10 obsessive-compulsive disorder (depressed), 10 obsessive-compulsive disorder (euthymic), 10 control subjects	1) Decreased left dorsal ALPFC in all forms of depression, not in control subjects or subjects with pure obsessive-compulsive disorder 2) Correlation between depression severity and decreasing frontal metabolism 3) After treatment, 12 subjects had normalization of left ALPFC
Martinot et al. 1990	10 depressed, 10 control subjects	1) Decreased left/right prefrontal cortex during depression that normalized after treatment 2) Decreased left prefrontal cortex metabolism in depression that did not recover

(continued)

Table 11–4. Functional imaging studies in primary depression *(continued)*

Investigators	Subjects	Findings
Positron-emission tomography *(continued)*		
Bench et al. 1992	33 depressed, 23 control subjects	Decreased left anterior cingulate gyrus and left ALPFC in depression
Dolan et al. 1992	33 depressed, 10 cognitive impairment, 10 normal cognition	1) Decreased left anteromedial prefrontal cortex 2) Increased cerebellar vermis in cognitively impaired
Drevets et al. 1992	13 depressed, 33 control subjects	1) Frontal and prefrontal hypermetabolism 2) Correlation between worsening severity of depression and decreasing left prefrontal flow
Ketter et al. 1993b	9 mood disorder; 18 control subjects	Decreased left > right ALPFC, superior temporal, supra-marginal, right anterior cingulate in depression

Note. ALPFC = anterolateral prefrontal cortex.

sion, 10 patients with obsessive-compulsive disorder with secondary depression, and 12 control subjects. Glucose metabolism in the left ALPFC in all depressed subjects was significantly lower than in control subjects or nondepressed subjects with obsessive-compulsive disorder. The researchers also found a significant negative correlation between Hamilton Rating Scale for Depression (HRSD) (Hamilton 1960) scores and ALPFC metabolism. That is, the more severe the depression, the lower the left prefrontal cortex metabolism. Interestingly, in responders to drug therapy, left frontal hypometabolism normalized as patients improved (see Figure 11–2).

Bench et al. (1992) used oxygen-15 PET to study 33 patients with primary depression compared with 23 age-matched control subjects. The depressed group as a whole had reduced blood flow in the left anterior cingulate and the left ALPFC. In a subgroup analysis of this study, Dolan et al. (1992) discovered that depressed subjects with cognitive impairment had decreased activity in the left anteromedial frontal cortex and increased activity in the cerebellar vermis when compared with noncognitively impaired subjects. This finding implies that depressed subjects with cognitive impairment show deficits not only in the left ALPFC, but also in more medial areas of the frontal lobes. This same group has extended this work with 40 depressed subjects and found that the depression subtype of the individual (psychomotorically slow, anxious, or cognitively impaired) determines which brain regions are most highly affected (Bench et al. 1993). For example, psychomotor slowing is highly correlated with decreased flow in the left ALPFC. Cognitive impairment involves decreased activity in the left medial prefrontal region; prominent anxiety in depression is associated with increased activity in the right posterior cingulate and bilateral inferior parietal regions.

In our National Institute of Mental Health (NIMH) laboratory, O^{15}-water PET has been used to study nine medication-free inpatients with mood disorders (mostly bipolar II disorder) and 18 age- and sex-matched control subjects (Ketter et al. 1993c). Depressed subjects, compared with healthy control subjects, had significantly lower resting blood flow in the ALPFC (left more than right), left mesial temporal lobe, right anterior cingulate gyrus, and bilateral supramarginal gyrus.

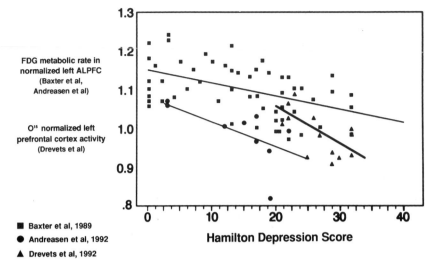

Figure 11–2. Summary graph compiling data from several different studies. The graph demonstrates the inverse relationship between prefrontal activity and Hamilton Rating Scale for Depression (HRSD) scores in numerous studies. In unipolar depression, a fairly consistent finding across studies in primary and secondary depression has been a relative decrease in mesial and lateral prefrontal activity as subjects were more depressed. Some have argued that this is a central aspect of understanding the pathophysiology and phenomenology of unipolar depression. Others have maintained that this decreased prefrontal activity is a mere correlation of the symptom of psychomotor slowing. This prefrontal hypoactivity has not been found as consistently in studies involving bipolar depressed subjects. FDG = fluorodeoxyglucose. ALPFC = anterolateral prefrontal cortex. *Squares* = Baxter et al. 1989; *circles* = Andreasen et al. 1992; *triangles* = Drevets et al. 1992. *Source.* Reprinted from George MS, Ketter TA, Post RM: "SPECT and PET Imaging in Mood Disorders." *Journal of Clinical Psychiatry* 54:6–13, 1993. Used with permission. Copyright 1993 Physicians Postgraduate Press, Inc.

Drevets et al. (1992) conducted one of the few studies in this field with discordant results, although they also found that the left ALPFC was abnormal. Using O^{15} PET to study 23 patients with familial pure depressive disorder compared with 33 control subjects, they found that the patients had absolute increases in blood flow in the left ALPFC, although they again found an inverse relationship between left prefrontal flow and severity of depression on the HRSD. The authors speculated that the increased left frontal activity in the depressed patients might have existed either because of the use of a particular subset of depressed patients (familial pure depressive disorder) or because the subjects were actively ruminating about sad thoughts during the scan. Studies in our NIMH laboratory (George et al. 1995) and elsewhere (Pardo et al. 1993) have confirmed this idea that thinking sad thoughts activates the left medial and orbital prefrontal regions. Thus ruminating about sadness during the scan, as well as differences in patient population, may account for the different findings in the Drevets et al. study. Interestingly, within the group of depressed subjects in the Drevets et al. study, worsening depression correlated with a drop in left prefrontal flow, similar to the other studies discussed.

To date, at least three published studies of primary depression have been carried out with SPECT (Austin et al. 1992; Mayberg et al. 1991, 1994). Mayberg et al. (1991) studied 7 medicated depressed subjects compared with 10 age-matched control subjects. Relative cerebral blood flow was decreased in the frontal, temporal, and cingulate regions in the depressed subjects. Austin et al. (1992) imaged 59 depressed subjects and 52 control subjects with HMPAO SPECT. They found a 3% reduction in left frontal metabolism in depressed subjects compared with control subjects. This difference was most pronounced in elderly depressed subjects. Interestingly, a subgroup of patients with endogenous depression had increased activity in the cingulate gyrus compared with other depressed patients. This study demonstrates the possibility of clinical heterogeneity within the mood disorders and argues for the strict need to subtype patients.

Blunted activation. It is possible to look beyond differences between depressed subjects and control subjects during passive mental tasks (resting). Neuropsychological and neuropharmacological activation tasks may be used in conjunction with imaging to explore whether certain regions differ in depression compared with control subjects in terms of their degree of activation during specific tasks (George et al. 1994d; Haxby et al. 1991; Ring et al. 1991). Cardiac stress tests are a common clinical example of this concept of stressing an organ and then being able to "see" the extent of pathology. A heart that appears normal at rest may be damaged or pathological when activated. Weinberger, Berman, and colleagues have pioneered the use of the Wisconsin Card Sorting Test to demonstrate that schizophrenic subjects fail to activate the left dorsolateral prefrontal cortex (DLPFC) in the same manner as control subjects during this task (Berman and Weinberger 1990; Berman et al. 1988; Weinberger et al. 1986, 1991). In a head-to-head study, mood disorder subjects, who are not known to have performance difficulties with this task, showed normal activation of the left ALPFC while performing the Wisconsin Carding Sort Test (Berman et al. 1993). In our NIMH laboratory, it has been shown that a group of mixed mood disorder subjects (unipolar, bipolar I disorder, bipolar II disorder) have blunted activation of the anterior limbic system (the amygdala and its afferents) when given a dose of intravenous procaine, despite having a similar experiential response to the drug (Ketter et al. 1993a). Similarly, mood disorder subjects failed to activate the right insula compared with control subjects while matching faces for their emotional content (George et al. 1993a). Mood disorder subjects had a selective performance deficit with this task (Gur et al. 1993; Rubinow and Post 1992). Further, mood disorder subjects compared with control subjects failed to activate the left midcingulate when selecting a response despite interference (the Stroop task) (George et al. 1993b, 1994c). Thus, three studies (two different neuropsychological tasks and one pharmacological probe) have demonstrated a lack of activation of limbic structures (amygdala, anterior cingulate, midcingulate, and insula) in a group of medication-free, diagnostically mixed mood disorder subjects who were largely depressed at the time of the scan. As a contradistinction, mood disorder subjects appear to have normal to above-normal regional activation in tasks involving mostly cortical activity, such as the Wisconsin Card Sorting Test (the left DLPFC) and a spatial matching task (parietal cortex) (George et al. 1994d).

These pilot activation studies have raised many interesting questions, and further work is clearly needed to assess whether these findings are true for other tasks, are restricted to one mood subgroup versus another, or are more state than trait dependent. However, in general, the bulk of studies to date have indicated that depressed mood disorder subjects at rest have decreased activity in the left prefrontal cortex (more medial than lateral) and fail to activate limbic and paralimbic regions during specific pharmacological and neuropsychological tasks.

Functional Studies in Bipolar Disorder at "Rest"

Studies involving pure bipolar subjects, or in which results for BPAD subjects were reported separately, are fewer in number and in general have different findings than the studies in predominantly unipolar patients. A fairly consistent finding of the depressed state within unipolar subjects has been that they have decreased left ALPFC activity at rest that worsens when the depression becomes more severe. The results from functional imaging studies in BPAD subjects are less clear and consistent.

Silfverskiöld and Risberg (1989) used xenon-133 SPECT to study 43 medication-free depressed subjects and 30 actively manic subjects who were on medication. There were no differences between the two groups; however, within the BPAD group, as neuroleptic dosage increased, global regional cerebral blood flow decreased. The BPAD subjects were rescanned when euthymic while taking medications, and no differences were found. However, this study is limited because the xenon method has a very low spatial resolution and is weighted toward cortical, as opposed to subcortical, activity.

At least three studies have used FDG PET to study bipolar disorder. Baxter et al. (1985) scanned 11 unipolar depressed and 13 BPAD subjects (5 depressed, 5 manic, 3 mixed) as well as 9 healthy control subjects. The BPAD depressed subjects had decreased whole brain metabolism compared with control subjects. The manic group had increased whole brain metabolism compared with control subjects, with the largest regional increases in the frontal and temporal cortex, thalamus, and anterior cingulate. In a later extension of this same study, Schwartz et al. (1987) reported on 12 unipolar depressed subjects and 9 BPAD subjects, all of whom were depressed at the time of the scan. The unipolar group had a decreased left caudate/hemisphere ratio compared with the BPAD group. This difference could have been accounted for by increased hemispheric activity or decreased left caudate activity in the unipolar group, or by increased left caudate activity in the BPAD group. This possibility is interesting in the light of work that has shown that as the personality trait of novelty-seeking increases, left caudate activity increases at rest in a series of healthy volunteers (George et al. 1994b).

Post et al. (1987) used 18-FDG to examine 13 affectively ill subjects (5 depressed, 6 euthymic, 2 manic), 18 control subjects, and 17 patients with schizophrenia. Scanning was done during somatosensory stimulation of the right forearm. The actively depressed subjects had decreased activity in the temporal lobes bilaterally. Finally, pilot data in our NIMH group hint that BPAD subjects, as compared with control subjects, may have increased activity at rest in the right temporal lobe (Ketter et al. 1994b). Additionally, tentative pilot findings hint that these right temporal hyperactive areas normalize after treatment with carbamazepine, in those patients who responded to treatment (Ketter et al. 1994a).

Migliorelli et al. (1993) used HMPAO SPECT to image five acutely manic patients (all women) compared with seven age-matched healthy control subjects. Using an region of interest method of analysis, they found that manic patients had significantly lower cerebral blood flow of the right basotemporal cortex than did control subjects. All subjects had a normal-screening CT scan. The task was to sit quietly in a dark room with eyes open and ears unplugged. Interestingly, the investigators noted a trend that higher mania rating scales were correlated with significantly lower basotemporal blood flow, although this trend was noted using only three subjects. Unfortunately, the authors did not scan these subjects again after treatment of the manic episode to determine whether the abnormality was state dependent.

Finally, several studies have used the new imaging technologies to look at pharmacological subsystems in mania. Suhara et al. (1992) used a dopamine (D1) ligand and PET to image 10 BPAD subjects (1 manic, 3 depressed, and 6 euthymic) and 21 healthy control subjects. They found decreased D1 binding in the BPAD group in a region encompassing the prefrontal cortex. Kato et al. (1993) used phosphorus magnetic resonance spectroscopy to image 17 BPAD subjects, while both manic and euthymic, and 17 control subjects. The BPAD manic subjects had an increase in the phosphomonoester peak in the frontal cortex and a decreased peak when euthymic, as compared with the control group. These novel specific neuropharmacologic images hold much promise for future investigation of BPAD brain abnormalities but are still in their infancy in terms of understanding all the factors (e.g., activity at time of the scan, diet, effect of medications) that may cause between-group or within-group differences over time. (For a summary of these studies, see Table 11–5.)

Recently our team at the Medical University of South Carolina (MUSC) has worked to develop a noninvasive MRI technique that images brain perfusion (Bohning et al. 1996, 1997). In this sequence, one magnetically tags or labels hydrogen atoms in the bloodstream in a given slice of brain and then images how many of these tagged atoms have flowed or perfused into another brain slice. This technique is called *spin-labeling and inversion recovery* and has the advantages of MRI spatial resolution on the order of 1–2 mm, provides absolute measurements of blood perfusion without using an arterial line as in PET, uses no radiation, and does not require an iv line or tracer injection.

In pilot work, our group at MUSC has begun to use this sequence to serially scan subjects with rapid-cycling BPAD. Paying close attention to repositioning of the brain, and trying to keep all other variables constant (time of day, medications, sleep), we have now begun applying this technique to understanding mania (Figure 11–3 *(a), (b),* and *(c)*.

In this patient, global flow increased during states of hypomania, but only if the mania was pure or euphoric (consistent with Baxter et al. 1985). When the subject was scanned during dysphoric manic episodes, global flow was reduced and resembled perfusion patterns seen in the depressed state. Examination of regional changes is under way. Analysis of the regional changes across various time points in this patient, as well as in others, will, it is hoped, allow further testing of many of the hypotheses generated in the literature review in this chapter.

This patient demonstrates the power of these new noninvasive MRI techniques to discern longitudinal changes in BPAD. For example, in 11–3 *(a)*, perfusion scans 5 and 8 were both taken during a mild depression. In conventional imaging, these scans would be treated the

Table 11–5. Functional imaging studies in bipolar disorder (state and trait)

Investigators	Type of study	Subjects	Findings
Silfverskiöld and Risberg 1989	Xenon 133	40 depressed (medication free), 30 manic (medicated)	BPAD: increasing neuroleptic dose associated with decreased regional cerebral blood flow; no change after treatment when euthymic
Baxter et al. 1985	FDG PET	11 unipolar depression; 5 BPAD, depressed; 5 BPAD, manic; 3 BPAD, mixed; 9 control subjects	Within the BPAD group, decreased whole brain metabolism; increased whole brain metabolism; largest increases in frontal, temporal thalamus, and anterior cingulate
Schwartz et al. 1987	FDG PET (extension of above)	12 unipolar depressed; 9 BPAD, depressed	Increased left caudate/hemisphere ratio in bipolar compared with unipolar
Post et al. 1987	FDG PET	13 mood disorder (5 depressed, 6 euthymic, 2 manic)	Decreased temporal lobe activity bilaterally
Migliorelli et al. 1993	HMPAO SPECT	5 BPAD (manic and medication-free), 7 control subjects	Decreased regional cerebral blood flow in right temporal lobe in manic versus control subjects
Suhara et al. 1992	Dopamine SPECT	21 control subjects, 10 BPAD (1 manic, 3 depressed, 6 euthymic)	Decreased frontal cortex dopamine binding in BPAD

| Kato et al. 1993 | Phosphorus magnetic resonance spectroscopy | 17 BPAD (manic and euthymic), 17 control subjects | Increased phosphomonoester peak in mania; decreased phosphomono-ester when euthymic |

Note. BPAD = bipolar affective disorder. FDG = fluorodeoxyglucose. PET = positron-emission tomography. HMPAO = hexamethylpropylamine oxine. SPECT = single photon emission computed tomography.

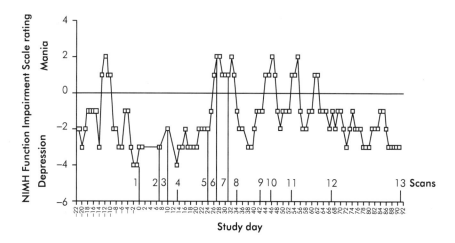

Figure 11-3 *(a)*. This graph depicts daily mood ratings over 4 months on the NIMH Functional Impairment Scale (Squillace et al. 1984) in a 30-year-old man with rapid-cycling bipolar disorder. Vertical numbered lines extending up from the *x* axis denote days on which he underwent a perfusion MRI scan.

same for data analysis. Serial imaging allows one to recognize and directly test for differences due to the clinical course, past, present, and future. For example, in scan 5, the patient is going from depression to mania, and in scan 8 the patient is going from mania to a depressed state. Serial imaging may allow examination of the dynamic nature of bipolar disorder.

In summary, the functional imaging studies to date have revealed that global metabolism may increase in mania. Within the global changes, there may be persistent hyperactivity in the right temporal lobe when euthymic, which becomes hypoactive during states of acute mania. Serial scanning of subjects as they cycle into and out of manic states, preferably while medication free, will definitely help expand on these interesting but speculative findings.

Imaging the Phenomenology of Mania

An alternative method of exploring the neural networks associated with mania is to produce manic-like symptoms in healthy control sub-

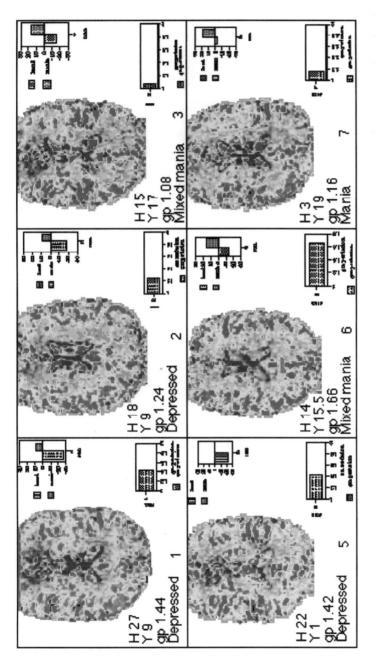

Figure 11–3 (*b*). Representative perfusion MRI scans in this individual on separate days. At the upper right of each scan is depicted mood on the day of the scan, measured by the Young Mania Scale (red) (Young et al. 1978) and the Hamilton Rating Scale for Depression (black, inverted) (Hamilton 1960). At the lower right of each scan is graphed global gray-matter perfusion.

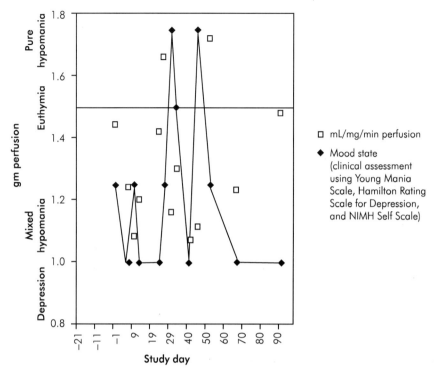

Figure 11–3 *(c)*.   Graph of global mood, on the *y* axis, from a combination of rating scales (Young Mania Scale [Young et al. 1978], Hamilton Rating Scale for Depression [Hamilton 1960], and NIMH Self-Rating Scale [Squillace et al. 1984]), condensed into pure hypomania, euthymia, or dysphoric or mixed hypomania. On the *x* axis are the days on which the patient underwent an MRI perfusion scan at the level of the anterior cingulate and medical prefrontal cortex (app. AC-PC line plus 14) (see Figure 11–3 *(b)*). This graph shows that global gray matter perfusion correlates with mood state so that during euphoric manic states, there is increased perfusion, and during dysphoric manic spells and depressed states, there is decreased global perfusion.
Note.   Dr. George acknowledges the help of Dr. Vidya Upadhyaya with this patient in particular and with the research project in general.

jects and image the resultant global and regional brain changes. To the extent that the symptoms produced are similar to the symptoms experienced in mania, the results can then be extrapolated back to understanding the functional neuroanatomy of mania. This approach of looking at regional brain changes on symptom- rather than disease-based grounds has also been applied to understanding the left DLPFC hypoactivity of depression. Dolan et al. (1993) imaged regional cerebral blood flow with PET in 40 depressed and 30 schizophrenic subjects, then examined which brain regions correlated with the symptom of psychomotor slowing, ignoring diagnosis. Interestingly, left DLPFC activity decreased with worse psychomotor slowing in both patient groups, regardless of diagnosis. The researchers argued that the functional image change in left DLPFC activity was due to the behavior (psychomotor slowing) and not necessarily the disease (schizophrenia or BPAD).

How can one begin to apply this behavioral or phenomenological approach to understanding mania? The symptom of euphoria is commonly, although not always, seen in mania. Euphoria, whether induced by morphine (S. R. Cohen et al. 1991; London et al. 1990b, 1991), cocaine (London et al. 1990a), or procaine (Ketter et al. 1993b, 1994c), appears to involve a relative deactivation of secondary association cortex. This finding is interesting in light of the cases discussed earlier of secondary mania resulting from ablative or destructive lesions of the right hemisphere, particularly the right anterio-mesial temporal cortex and the orbit-frontal lobe. These studies would predict that euphoric mania, compared with dysphoric mania or euthymia, is characterized by relatively decreased activity in secondary association cortex, in addition to other brain changes associated with mania (see Figure 11–4).

Similarly, some manic subjects experience dysphoric states or exhibit mixed states with both manic and depressive symptoms. At NIMH, we carried out a study using O^{15} PET to image the brain regions activated in healthy control subjects during a state of transient sadness (George et al. 1995). Compared with the neutral state, transient sadness activates the anterior temporal cortex, the anterior cingulate, and the left mesial prefrontal cortex. This pattern involves activation of the anterior limbic system, defined as the projections of the amygdala. The George et al. study and a study by Pardo et al. (1993) predict that patients with irritable or dysphoric mania would have relatively more activity in anterior cingulate, amygdala, and orbital and medial prefrontal cortex than would euphoric manic subjects or BPAD subjects in the euthymic or depressed states (see Figure 11–5).

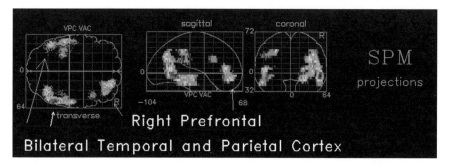

Figure 11–4. Decreased activity during transient happiness predominantly in the right hemisphere. A look-through (like a chest X ray) statistical parametric map (SPM) of the brain areas that are significantly decreased during transient self-induced happiness compared with a neutral emotion control task. Note that large areas of cortex, particularly on the right side, have decreased activity during happiness. In general, euphoric states induced by several different compounds have as a common feature this relative deactivation of secondary cortex, as compared with a neutral baseline. These studies predict that euphoric mania would have relatively decreased activity in these areas. These euphoria-induced positron-emission tomography (PET) studies are also interesting because ablative or destructive lesions of the right basal ganglia and temporal cortex sometimes produce secondary mania. Thus, destruction of function in these areas, either temporarily or on a more permanent basis, may dysregulate a system held in check by these cortical and subcortical regions. All points graphed are areas that significantly differ at $P < .01$ significance from the resting state. VPC = ventral posterior commissure. VAC = ventral anterior commissure.

Imaging the regional activation that occurs in conjunction with phenomenology, and then reasoning back to the brain regions involved in mania, is fraught with assumptions that may not hold. However, utilizing refined pharmacologic agents and neuropsychologic tasks in studies represents an interesting new way to begin to understand the brain in mania. These studies can serve as useful adjuncts to the more conventional studies of BPAD subjects in various stages of the illness—especially because they can control for one variable and often generate testable hypotheses about brain function in various stages of BPAD.

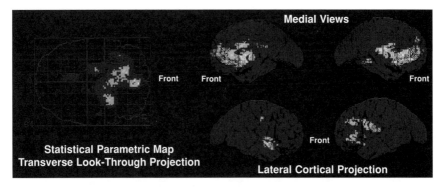

Figure 11–5. Regional brain activity during sadness (increased activity in anterior limbic structures). In contrast to the brain picture in euphoria, two studies have now demonstrated that self-induced dysphoria or sadness is associated with increased activity in the left medial and orbital prefrontal cortex, as well as the anterior limbic loop. Thus dysphoric mania may be associated with increased activity in these areas. The increased activity in these regions may provide an explanation of why states of depression or mania sometimes occur after states of prolonged grief or sadness, when these regions are highly activated.

▶ REGIONAL BRAIN CHANGES THAT OCCUR IN RESPONSE TO TREATMENT

One final method of examining the brain regions associated with BPAD involves imaging BPAD subjects before and after various treatments. To date, this imaging has been done in only a handful of pure BPAD groups. Nevertheless, it is worthwhile to review the treatment effect studies in mixed mood disorder groups. Three studies have now determined that a subset of mood disorder patients who will respond to sleep deprivation exhibit hyperactivity in the cingulate gyrus. Furthermore, this cingulate hyperactivity resolves after effective sleep deprivation. Wu et al. (1992) originally reported that hyperactivity in the cingulate cortex predicts which clinically depressed subjects will get a mood lift from a night of sleep deprivation. FDG PET scans taken before and after a night of total sleep deprivation in actively depressed subjects and healthy control subjects revealed that only the subgroup of depressed patients who had cingulate hyperactivity prior to sleep deprivation responded with a mood lift after sleep deprivation. Further, staying awake all night reduced the cingulate hyperactivity in this sub-group; the other depressed subjects and healthy control subjects showed virtually no changes. Ebert et al. (1991, 1994) in Germany used HMPAO SPECT and found results from an initial and follow-up study to be virtually identical to the Wu et al. study. Preliminary work using FDG PET in our NIMH laboratory is also consistent with this finding. Thus, in three separate studies by two groups, cingulate hy-peractivity in the pre-sleep deprivation scan predicted whether a de-pressed subject would improve after sleep deprivation. In susceptible individuals, sleep deprivation can trigger episodes of hypomania or mania. It would be interesting to examine the functional brain changes associated with sleep deprivation in nondepressed BPAD subjects who progress into hypomania or mania.

Similarly, the mechanism or mechanisms of action of electroconvul-sive therapy (ECT) are not known. However, Sackeim et al. (1992) used xenon SPECT to demonstrate that in some patients, transient changes in frontal lobe function following ECT may be crucial to eventual antidepressant treatment response. They performed SPECT scans prior to, and within an hour after, ECT in a group of depressed subjects and then followed their clinical response. In virtually all sub-jects, ECT resulted in decreased brain activity in many regions. Inter-estingly, depressed subjects with the best clinical response to ECT also had the largest decrease in frontal lobe activity immediately following ECT. Put another way, a large transient decrease in frontal lobe activity immediately after ECT was positively correlated with a good clinical response to ECT. A similar study in BPAD subjects undergoing ECT would be most revealing.

Finally, in the area of treatment response, preliminary work in the our NIMH laboratory has shown that BPAD subjects who respond to treatment with carbamazepine have increased activity in their right temporal lobes while they are medication free. Following treatment with carbamazepine, this right temporal lobe activity was reported to normalize (Ketter et al. 1994a).

In summary, numerous functional neuroimaging studies have dem-onstrated both resting abnormalities and deficient activation of the limbic, temporal, and prefrontal lobes in mood disorder subjects as compared with control subjects. Further, four imaging studies have

shown that abrupt changes in prefrontal or cingulate activity is associated with response to either ECT or sleep deprivation. These studies
implicate the prefrontal region as abnormal and important in the
pathophysiology of unipolar depression. In bipolar depression, in contrast, structural and functional studies have repeatedly implicated the
temporal lobes as pathological, particularly on the right.

More studies specifically addressing brain changes in BPAD as a
function of treatment must be carried out. The hypothesis generated
from the resting studies in BPAD would be that hypoactive regions in
the right temporal cortex during a manic state normalize or even become hyperactive during euthymia. The Post studies and Migliorelli
studies have supported this notion.

▶ SUMMARY, CONCLUSIONS, AND FUTURE CLINICAL DIRECTIONS

This review of structural and functional imaging studies in BPAD has
highlighted the lack of large, well-controlled imaging studies in mania. Despite the problems inherent in imaging manic subjects, these
studies have demonstrated that it is possible to conduct meaningful
studies at certain centers using the appropriate modalities.

Additionally, specific brain regions have repeatedly been implicated
in these studies (see Table 11–6). The temporal cortex has been found
to have small volume (two studies), to be hyperactive when euthymic
(one study), to be hypoactive during acute mania (two studies), and
possibly to predict response to carbamazepine treatment (one pilot
study). Imaging studies of secondary mania have hinted that subcortical structures, particularly on the right, are also involved in mania.
However, it is unlikely that any one region (e.g., the right temporal
lobe) is the only site of pathology in mania. Some diseases, such as
Parkinson's disease and the basal ganglia do involve relatively discrete regions of the brain. However, BPAD—specifically the state of
mania—likely involves distributed neural networks that involve both
cortical and subcortical structures in both hemispheres, with an emphasis on the right (see Figure 11–6). Thus, although the studies in
mania are too early to define a true neuroanatomy of mania, they are
beginning to implicate the brain regions that are either primarily or

Table 11–6. Summary of brain regions implicated in mania and depression

Brain region	Action	Result
Temporal lobe		
Right	Stimulate	Increased FDG PET activity during depression in BPAD subjects compared with control subjects. In responders, carbamazepine cools off this abnormality
	Ablate	Strokes, lesions cause secondary mania; decreased activity during acute mania in HMPAO SPECT
Prefrontal		
Left	Ablate	Strokes cause secondary depression; decreased activity seen in numerous studies of depression with functional neuroimaging
Right	Ablate	Strokes cause secondary mania

FDG = fluorodeoxyglucose. PET = positron-emission tomography. BPAD = bipolar affective disorder. HMPAO = hexamethylpropylamine oxine. SPECT = single photon emission computed tomography.

secondarily involved in mania pathogenesis.

This review should highlight the need for a structural brain scan (either CT or MRI) in patients with new-onset mania or psychosis to exclude other treatable brain diseases. Although research studies using functional imaging (PET, SPECT, fMRI) have begun to note differences in depression subtypes from healthy control subjects and from each other, both at rest and during activation, the field awaits large-scale studies examining their use in clinical settings to make diagnoses or predict treatment response. Functional MRI scanning, with its exquisite temporal and spatial resolution and lack of radiation exposure, holds great promise in this area. Perhaps, in the not too distant future, we may be able to use functional neuroimages either at rest or activated, both to diagnose and help treat mania and depression. Imaging studies, either ongoing or in the planning stages, will undoubtedly shed more light on the emerging neuroanatomy of mania.

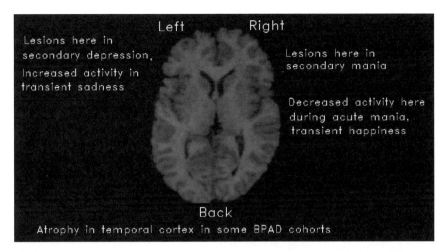

Figure 11–6.   Summarized neuroanatomy of mania. The field is still too immature to enable an entire neuroanatomy of mania to be painted. However, several key structures have been repeatedly implicated by both structural and functional scans in both primary and secondary mania, as illustrated on this axial magnetic resonance imaging (MRI) scan. These structures include the mesial temporal lobe and other subcortical structures on the right. Hypoactivity in these areas during a manic episode has been found in functional studies of primary and secondary mania. Some studies have found increased activity in these same regions during depression in bipolar affective disorder (BPAD) subjects.

▶ REFERENCES

Altshuler LL, Conrad A, Hauser P: Reduction of temporal lobe volume in bipolar disorder: a preliminary report of magnetic resonance imaging (letter). Arch Gen Psychiatry 48:482–483, 1991

Andreasen NC, Swayze V, Flaum M, et al: Ventricular abnormalities in affective disorder: clinical and demographic correlates. Am J Psychiatry 147:893–900, 1990

Arroyo S, Lesser RP, Gordon B, et al: Mirth, laughter and gelastic seizures. Brain 116:757–780, 1993

Austin MP, Dougall N, Ross M, et al: Single photon emission tomography with 99mTc-exametazime in major depression and the pattern of brain activity underlying the psychotic/neurotic continuum. J Affect Disord 26:31–43, 1992

Aylward EH, Roberts-Twillie JV, Barta PE, et al: Basal ganglia volumes and white matter hyperintensities in patients with bipolar disorder. Am J Psychiatry 151:687–693, 1994

Barczak P, Edmunds E, Betts T: Hypomania following complex partial seizures: a report of three cases. Br J Psychiatry 152:137–139, 1988

Baxter LR Jr, Phelps ME, Mazziotta JC, et al: Cerebral metabolic rates for
glucose in mood disorders: studies with positron emission tomography
and fluorodeoxyglucose F18. Arch Gen Psychiatry 42:441–447, 1985

Baxter LR Jr, Schwartz JM, Phelps ME, et al: Reduction of prefrontal cortex
glucose metabolism common to three types of depression. Arch Gen
Psychiatry 46:243–250, 1989

Bench CJ, Friston KJ, Brown RG: The anatomy of melancholia: focal abnormalities of cerebral blood flow in major depression. Psychol Med
22:607–615, 1992

Bench CJ, Friston KJ, Brown RG, et al: Regional cerebral blood flow in
depression measured by positron emission tomography: the relationship
with clinical dimensions. Psychol Med 23:579–590, 1993

Berman KF, Weinberger DR: The prefrontal cortex in schizophrenia and
other neuropsychiatric diseases: in vivo physiological correlates and
other cognitive deficits, in Progress in Brain Research, Vol 85. Edited by
Uylings HBM, Van Eden CG, De Bruin JPC, et al. Amsterdam, Netherlands, Elsevier Science Publishers, 1990, pp 521–537

Berman KF, Illowsky BP, Weinberger DR: Physiological dysfunction of dorsolateral prefrontal cortex in schizophrenia, IV: further evidence for regional and behavioral specificity. Arch Gen Psychiatry 45:616–622,
1988

Berman KF, Doran AR, Pickar D, et al: Is the mechanism of prefrontal hy-
pofunction in depression the same as in schizophrenia? regional cerebral
blood flow during cognitive activation. Br J Psychiatry 162:183–192,
1993

Bohning DE, Wright AC, Pecheny AP, et al: Repeatability of spin-labeled in
vivo perfusion maps. Paper presented at the 2nd International Conference on Functional Mapping of the Human Brain, Boston, MA, June
17–21, 1996

Bohning DE, Speer AM, Pecheny AP, et al: Acetazolamide-induced perfusion changes measured with MR spin-labeling. Paper presented at 5th
Scientific Meeting of the International Society for Magnetic Resonance
in Medicine, Vancouver, BC, Canada, April 1997

Bromfield EB, Altshuler L, Leiderman DB, et al: Cerebral metabolism and
depression in patients with complex partial seizures. Arch Neurol
49:617–623, 1992

Coffman JA, Bornstein RA, Olson SC, et al: Cognitive impairment and cerebral structure by MRI in bipolar disorder. Biol Psychiatry 27:1188–
1196, 1990

Cohen MS, Bookheimer SY: Localization of brain function using magnetic
resonance imaging. Trends Neurosci 17:268–277, 1994

Cohen SR, Kimes AS, London ED: Morphine decreases cerebral glucose utilization in limbic and forebrain regions while pain has no effect. Neuropharmacology 30:125–134, 1991

David A, Blamire A, Breiter H: Functional magnetic resonance imaging: a new technique with implications for psychology and psychiatry. Br J Psychiatry 164:2–7, 1994

Devous MD, Stokely EM, Chehabi HH, et al: Normal distribution of regional cerebral blood flow measured by dynamic single-photon emission tomography. J Cereb Blood Flow Metab 6:95–104, 1986

Dolan RJ, Poynton AM, Bridges PK, et al: Altered magnetic resonance white-matter T1 values in patients with affective disorder. Br J Psychiatry 157:107–110, 1990

Dolan RJ, Bench CJ, Brown RG, et al: Regional cerebral blood flow abnormalities in depressed patients with cognitive impairment. J Neurol Neurosurg Psychiatry 55:768–773, 1992

Dolan RJ, Bench CJ, Liddle PF, et al: Dorsolateral prefrontal cortex dysfunction in the major psychoses: symptom or disease specificity? J Neurol Neurosurg Psychiatry 56:1290–1294, 1993

Drake ME: Episodic depression and hypomania with temporal EEG paroxysms. Psychosomatics 29:354–357, 1988

Drevets WC, Videen TO, Preskorn SH, et al: A functional anatomical study of unipolar depression. J Neurosci 12:3628–3641, 1992

Ebert D, Feistel H, Barocka A: Effects of sleep deprivation on the limbic system and the frontal lobes in affective disorders: a study with Tc-99m-HMPAO SPECT. Psychiatry Res 40:247–251, 1991

Ebert D, Feistel H, Barocka A, et al: Increased limbic flow and total sleep deprivation in major depression with melancholia. Psychiatry Res 55:101–109, 1994

Ell PJ, Cullum I, Costa DC: Regional cerebral blood flow mapping with a new Tc-99m-labelled compound. Lancet 1:50–51, 1985

Engel J: Seizures and Epilepsy. Philadelphia, PA, FA Davis, 1989

Friston KJ, Passingham RE, Nutt JG, et al: Localisation in PET images: direct fitting of the intercommissural (AC-PC) line. J Cereb Blood Flow Metab 9:690–695, 1989

Friston KJ, Frith CD, Liddle PF, et al: Comparing functional (PET) images: the assessment of significant change. J Cereb Blood Flow Metab 11:690–699, 1991

George MS, Scott T, Kellner CH, et al: Abnormalities of the septum pellucidum in schizophrenia: two case reports and a discussion. J Neuropsychiatry Clin Neurosci 1:385–390, 1989

George MS, Ring HA, Costa DC, et al: Neuroactivation and Neuroimaging With SPECT. London, England, Springer-Verlag, 1991

George MS, Ketter TA, Gill DS, et al: Blunted CBF with emotion recognition in depression (abstract). American Psychiatric Association 1993 Annual Meeting New Research Program and Abstracts (NR 114). Washington, DC, American Psychiatric Association, 1993a, p 88

George MS, Ketter TA, Parekh PI, et al: Differences in performance and regional brain activation in controls and mood-disordered subjects while performing a classic and emotional Stroop (abstract). American College of Neuropsychopharmacology (ACNP) Abstracts of Panels and Posters, 1993b

George MS, Ketter TA, Post RM: SPECT and PET imaging in mood disorders. J Clin Psychiatry 54:6–13, 1993c

George MS, Kellner CH, Bernstein H, et al: An MRI investigation into mood disorders in multiple sclerosis: a pilot study. J Nerv Ment Dis 180:410–412, 1994a

George MS, Ketter TA, Parekh PI, et al: Personality traits correlate with resting rCBF (abstract). American Psychiatric Association 1994 Annual Meeting New Research Program and Abstracts (NR450). Washington, DC, American Psychiatric Association, 1994b, p 173

George MS, Ketter TA, Parekh PI, et al: Regional brain activity when selecting a response despite interference: an H215O PET study of the Stroop and an emotional Stroop. Human Brain Mapping 1:194–208, 1994c

George MS, Ketter TA, Parekh PI, et al: Spatial ability in affective illness: differences in regional brain activation during a spatial matching task (H215O PET). Neuropsychiatry, Neuropsychology, and Behavioral Neurology 7:142–153, 1994d

George MS, Ketter TA, Parekh PI, et al: Brain activity during transient sadness and happiness in healthy women. Am J Psychiatry 152:341–351, 1995

Gillig P, Sackellares JC, Greenberg HS: Right hemisphere partial complex seizures: mania, hallucinations and speech disturbances during ictal events. Epilepsia 29:26–29, 1988

Gur RC, Erwin RJ, Gur RE, et al: Facial emotion discrimination, II: behavioral findings in depression. Psychiatry Res 42:241–251, 1993

Hamilton M: A rating scale for depression. J Neurol Neurosurg Psychiatry 23:56–62, 1960

Hauser P, Altshuler L, Berrettini W: Temporal lobe measurement in primary affective disorder by magnetic resonance imaging. Journal of Neuropsychiatry 1:128–134, 1989

Haxby JV, Grady CL, Ungerleider LG, et al: Mapping the functional neuroanatomy of the intact human brain with brain work imaging. Neuropsychologia 29:539–555, 1991

Husain MM, Mcdonald WM, Doraiswamy PM, et al: A magnetic resonance imaging study of putamen nuclei in major depression. Psychiatry Res 40:95–99, 1991

Itturalde MP: Dictionary and Handbook of Nuclear Medicine and Clinical Imaging. Boston, MA, CRC Press, 1990

Jackson JH: Observations on the localisation of movements in the cerebral hemispheres. West Riding Lunatic Asylum Medical Reports 3:175–190, 1873

Jackson JH: On temporary mental disorders after epileptic paroxysms. West Riding Lunatic Asylum Medical Reports 5:103–129, 1874

Jeste DV, Lohr JB, Goodwin FK: Neuroanatomical studies of major affective disorders: a review and suggestions for further research. Br J Psychiatry 153:444–459, 1988

Jorge RE, Robinson RG, Starkstein SE, et al: Depression and anxiety following traumatic brain injury. J Neuropsychiatry Clin Neurosci 5:369–374, 1993

Jurjus GJ, Nasrallah HA, Brogan M, et al: Developmental brain anomalies in schizophrenia and bipolar disorder: a controlled MRI Study. J Neuropsychiatry Clin Neurosci 5:375–378, 1993

Kato T, Takahashi S, Shioiri T, et al: Alterations in brain phosphorous metabolism in bipolar disorder detected by in vivo 31P and 7Li magnetic resonance spectroscopy. J Affect Disord 27:53–60, 1993

Kellner CH, Rubinow DR, Gold PW, et al: Relationship of cortisol hypersecretion to brain CT scan alterations in depressed patients. Psychiatry Res 8:191–197, 1983

Kellner CH, Rubinow DR, Post RM: Cerebral ventricular size and cognitive impairment in depression. J Affect Disord 10:215–219, 1986

Ketter TA, Andreason PJ, George MS, et al: Blunted CBF response to procaine in mood disorders (abstract). American Psychiatric Association 1993 Annual Meeting New Research Program and Abstracts (NR297). Washington, DC, American Psychiatric Association, 1993a, p 134

Ketter TA, Andreason PJ, George MS, et al: Paralimbic rCBF increases during procaine-induced psychosensory and emotional experiences (abstract). Biol Psychiatry 33:66A, 1993b

Ketter TA, Andreason PJ, George MS, et al: Reduced resting frontal lobe CBF in mood disorders (abstract). Paper presented at the 146th annual meeting of the American Psychiatric Association, San Francisco, CA, May 22–27, 1993c

Ketter TA, George MS, Andreason PJ, et al: Carbamazepine decreases regional cerebral glucose metabolism in affective disorders and has complex relationships with mood state (abstract). CINP [Collegium Internationale Neuro-Psychopharmacologicum] Abstracts, 1994a

Ketter TA, George MS, Andreason PJ, et al: CMRglu in unipolar versus bipolar depression (abstract). Paper presented at the 147th annual meeting of the American Psychiatric Association, Philadelphia, PA, May 21–26, 1994b

Ketter TA, George MS, Andreason PJ, et al: Positive correlations between procaine-induced paralimbic rCBF increases and psychosensory and emotional experiences (abstract). CINP Abstracts, 1994c

Krishnan KRR, McDonald WM, Escalona PR, et al: Magnetic resonance imaging of the caudate nuclei in depression. Arch Gen Psychiatry 49:553–557, 1992

Kwong KK, Belliveau JW, Chesler DA, et al: Dynamic magnetic resonance imaging of human brain activity during primary sensory stimulation. Proc Natl Acad Sci U S A 89:5675–5679, 1992

London ED, Cascella NG, Wong DF, et al: Cocaine-induced reduction of glucose utilization in human brain. Arch Gen Psychiatry 47:567–574, 1990a

London ED, Broussolle EPM, Links JM, et al: Morphine-induced metabolic changes in human brain: studies with positron emission tomography and [fluorine-18]fluorodeoxyglucose. Arch Gen Psychiatry 47:73–81, 1990b

London ED, Morgan MJ, Phillips RL, et al: Mapping the metabolic correlates of drug-induced euphoria. NIDA Res Monogr 105:54–60, 1991

Marks DA, Katz A, Hoffer P, et al: Localization of extratemporal epileptic foci during ictal single photon emission computed tomography. Ann Neurol 31:250–255, 1992

Martinot JL, Harley P, Fulcic A, et al: Left prefrontal glucose hypometabolism in the depressed state: a confirmation. Am J Psychiatry 147:1313–1317, 1990

Mayberg HS, Jeffery PJ, Wagner HN, et al: Regional cerebral blood flow in patients with refractory unipolar depression measured with TC-99m HMPAO SPECT (abstract). J Nucl Med 32:951, 1991

Mayberg HS, Lewis PJ, Regenold W, et al: Paralimbic hypoperfusion in unipolar depression. J Nucl Med 35:929–934, 1994

McDonald WM, Krishnan KRR, Doraiswamy PM, et al: Occurrence of subcortical hyperintensities in elderly subjects with mania. Psychiatry Res 40:211–220, 1991

McHenry LC: Garrison's History of Neurology. Springfield, IL, Charles C Thomas, 1969

Migliorelli R, Starkstein SE, Teson A, et al: SPECT findings in patients with primary mania. J Neuropsychiatry Clin Neurosci 5:379–383, 1993

Mukherjee S, Schnur DB, Lo ES, et al: Post-dexamethasone cortisol levels and computerized tomographic findings in manic patients. Acta Psychiatr Scand 88:145–148, 1993

Nasrallah HA, McCalley-Winters M, Jacoby CG: Cerebral ventricular enlargement in young manic males: a controlled CT study. J Affect Disord
4:15–19, 1982

Nasrallah HA, Coffman JA, Olson SC: Strucutral brain-imaging findings in
affective disorders: an overview. J Neuropsychiatry Clin Neurosci 1:21–
26, 1989

Pakalnis A, Drake ME, Kuruvilla J, et al: Forced normalization: acute psychosis after seizure control in seven patients. Arch Neurol 44:289–292,
1987

Pardo JV, Pardo PJ, Raichle ME: Neural correlates of self-induced dysphoria.
Am J Psychiatry 150:713–719, 1993

Pearlson GD, Garbacz DJ, Tompkins RH, et al: Clinical correlates of lateral
ventricular enlargement in bipolar affective disorder. Am J Psychiatry
141:253–256, 1984

Penfield W, Jasper H: Epilepsy and the Functional Anatomy of the Human
Brain. Boston, MA, Little, Brown, 1954

Post RM, Delisi LE, Holcomb HH, et al: Glucose utilization in the temporal
cortex of affectively ill patients: positron emission tomography. Biol Psychiatry 22:46–54, 1987

Post RM, Roy-Byrne PP, Uhde TW: Graphic representation of the life course
of illness in patients with affective disorder. Am J Psychiatry 145:844–
848, 1988

Post RM, Rubinow DR, Uhde TW: Dysphoric mania: clinical and biological
correlates. Arch Gen Psychiatry 46:353–358, 1989

Post RM, Leverich GS, Altshuler L, et al: Lithium discontinuation-induced
refractoriness: preliminary observations. Am J Psychiatry 149:1727–
1729, 1992

Post RM, Ketter TA, Pazzaglia PJ, et al: New developments in the use of
anticonvulsants as mood stabilizers. Neuropsychobiology 27:132–137,
1993

Rangel-Guerra RA, Perez-Payan H, Minkoff L, et al: Nuclear magnetic resonance in bipolar affective disorders. American Journal of Neuroradiol-
ogy 4:229–231, 1983

Reider RO, Mann LS, Weinberger DR, et al: Computed tomographic scans
in patients with schizophrenia, schizoaffective, and bipolar affective disorder. Arch Gen Psychiatry 40:735–739, 1983

Ring HA, George M, Costa DC, et al: The use of cerebral activation procedures with single photon emission tomography. Eur J Nucl Med
18:133–141, 1991

Robertson MM, Trimble MR: Depressive illness in patients with epilepsy: a
review. Epilepsia 24:S109–S116, 1983

Robinson RG, Szetela B: Mood change following left hemisphere brain injury. Ann Neurol 9:447–453, 1981

Robinson RG, Kubos KL, Starr LB, et al: Mood disorders in stroke patients: importance of location of lesion. Brain 107:81–93, 1984

Robinson RG, Boston JD, Starkstein SE, et al: Comparison of mania and depression after brain injury: causal factors. Am J Psychiatry 145:172–178, 1988

Rosen BR, Belliveau JW, Aronen HJ, et al: Functional neuroimaging, in Magnetic Resonance Neuroimaging. Edited by Kucharczyk J, Moseley M, Barkovich AJ. Boca Raton, FL, CRC Press, 1994

Ross ED, Rush AJ: Diagnosis and neuroanatomical correlates of depression in brain-damaged patients. Arch Gen Psychiatry 38:1344–1354, 1981

Ross ED, Homan RW, Buck R: Differential hemispheric lateralization of primary and social emotions: implications for developing a comprehensive neurology for emotions, repression and the subconscious. Neuropsychiatry, Neuropsychology, and Behavioral Neurology 7:1–19, 1994

Rossi A, Stratta P, Di Michele V, et al: Temporal lobe structure by magnetic resonance in bipolar affective disorders and schizophrenia. J Affect Disord 21:19–22, 1991

Roy-Byrne PP, Post RM, Uhde TW, et al: The longitudinal course of recurrent affective illness: life chart data from research patients at NIMH. Acta Psychiatr Scand (suppl) 71:5–34, 1985

Rubinow DR, Post RM: Impaired recognition of affect in facial expression in depressed patients. Biol Psychiatry 31:947–953, 1992

Sackeim HA, Devanand DP, Prudic J: Medication resistance as a predictor of ECT outcome and relapse (abstract). American College of Neuropsychopharmacology (ACNP) Abstracts of Panels and Posters 51, 1992

Schlegel S, Kretzschmar K: Computed tomography in affective disorders, part I: ventricular and sulcal measurements. Biol Psychiatry 22:4–14, 1987a

Schlegel S, Kretzschmar K: Computed tomography in affective disorders, part II: brain density. Biol Psychiatry 22:15–23, 1987b

Schlegel S, Frommberger U, Buller R: Computerized tomography (CT) in affective disorders: relationship with psychopathology. Psychiatry Res 29:271–272, 1989

Schwartz JM, Baxter LR, Mazziotta JC, et al: The differential diagnosis of depression: relevance of positron emission tomography studies of cerebral glucose metabolism to the bipolar-unipolar dichotomy. JAMA 258:1368–1374, 1987

Scott ML, Golden CJ, Ruedrich SL, et al: Ventricular enlargement in major depression. Psychiatry Res 8:91–93, 1983

Scott TF, Price TRP, George MS, et al: Midline cerebral malformations and schizophrenia. J Neuropsychiatry Clin Neurosci 5:287–293, 1993

Shima S, Shikano T, Kitamura T, et al: Depression and ventricular enlargement. Acta Psychiatr Scand 70:275–277, 1984

Silfverskiöld P, Risberg J: Regional cerebral blood flow in depression and mania. Arch Gen Psychiatry 46:253–259, 1989

Sokoloff L: Relation between physiological function and energy metabolism in the central nervous system. J Neurochem 29:13–26, 1977

Sokoloff L: Local energy metabolism: its relationship to local functional activity and blood flow, in Cerebral Vascular Smooth Muscle and Its Control. Edited by Purves MJ, Elliott L. Amsterdam, Netherlands, Elsevier, 1978, pp 171–197

Squillace K, Post RM, Savard R, et al: Life directing of the longitudinal course of recurrent affective illness, in Neurobiology of Mood Disorders. Edited by Post RM, Ballenger JC. Baltimore, MD, Williams & Wilkins, 1984, pp 38–59

Starkstein SE, Pearlson GD, Boston J, et al: Mania after brain injury: a controlled study of causative factors. Arch Neurol 44:1069–1073, 1987

Starkstein SE, Boston JD, Robinson RG: Mechanisms of mania after brain injury: 12 case reports and review of the literature. J Nerv Ment Dis 176:87–100, 1988

Starkstein SE, Robinson RG, Honig MA, et al: Mood changes after right-hemisphere lesions. Br J Psychiatry 155:79–85, 1989

Starkstein SE, Mayberg HS, Berthier ML, et al: Mania after brain injury: neuroradiological and metabolic findings. Ann Neurol 27:652–659, 1990

Starkstein SE, Fedoroff P, Berthier ML, et al: Manic-depressive and pure manic states after brain lesions. Biol Psychiatry 29:149–158, 1991

Stehling MK, Turner R, Mansfield P: Echo-planar imaging: magnetic resonance imaging in a fraction of a second. Science 254:43–50, 1991

Stern RA, Bachman DL: Depressive symptoms following stroke. Am J Psychiatry 148:351–356, 1991

Strakowski SM, Woods BT, Tohen M, et al: MRI subcortical signal hyperintensities in mania at first hospitalization. Biol Psychiatry 33:204–206, 1993a

Strakowski SM, Wilson DR, Tohen M, et al: Structural brain abnormalities in first-episode mania. Biol Psychiatry 33:602–609, 1993b

Suhara T, Nakayama K, Inoue O, et al: D1 dopamine receptor binding in mood disorders measured by positron emission tomography. Psychopharmacology (Berlin) 106:14–18, 1992

Swayze VW, Andreasen NC, Alliger RJ, et al: Structural brain abnormalities in bipolar affective disorder. Arch Gen Psychiatry 47:1054–1058, 1990

Swayze VW, Andreasen NC, Alliger RJ, et al: Subcortical and temporal structures in affective disorder and schizophrenia: a magnetic resonance imaging study. Biol Psychiatry 31:221–240, 1992

Taylor J: Selected Writings of John Hughlings Jackson. New York, Basic Books, 1958

Temkin O: The Falling Sickness: A History of Epilepsy From the Greeks to the Beginnings of Modern Neurology. Baltimore, MD, Johns Hopkins University Press, 1945

Turner R, Le Bihan D, Moonen CT, et al: Echo-planar time course MRI of cat brain oxygenation changes. Magn Reson Med 22:159–166, 1991

Weinberger DR, Delisi LE, Perman GP, et al: Computed tomography in schizophreniform disorder and other acute psychiatric disorders. Arch Gen Psychiatry 39:778–783, 1982

Weinberger DR, Berman KF, Zec RF: Physiologic dysfunction of dorsolateral prefrontal cortex in schizophrenia, I: regional cerebral blood flow evidence. Arch Gen Psychiatry 43:114–124, 1986

Weinberger DR, Berman KF, Daniel DG: Prefrontal cortex dysfunction in schizophrenia, in Frontal Lobe Function and Dysfunction. Edited by Levin HS, Eisenberg HM, Benton AL. New York, Oxford University Press, 1991, pp 275–287

Wu JC, Gillin JC, Buchsbaum MS, et al: Effect of sleep deprivation on brain metabolism of depressed patients. Am J Psychiatry 149:538–543, 1992

Young RC, Biggs JT, Ziegler VE, et al: A rating scale for mania: reliability, validity and sensitivity. Br J Psychiatry 133:428–435, 1978

SECTION

3

Treatment

CHAPTER 12

LITHIUM

Raymond L. Ownby, M.D., Ph.D., and
Paul J. Goodnick, M.D.

I n this chapter, we provide a general review of recent research on
the use of lithium in the treatment of mania. This research
ranges across a wide variety of topics, which are organized in
this chapter under the general rubrics of clinical use and basic pharmacologic mechanisms.

The topic of clinical use includes studies that have reviewed the use
of lithium in pregnancy and have concluded that lithium may not be
as hazardous as previously thought. Other investigators have studied
the effects of various dosing and discontinuation schedules on relapse.
Several studies have focused on predictors of response to lithium; others have reviewed the effects of lithium on granulopoiesis and the
clinical uses of this effect. Still other studies have investigated other
secondary effects of lithium. A few studies have investigated the phenomenological presentation of patients in manic states, potentially
relevant in determining which patients may respond to lithium.

One study focused on exactly how lithium works in a naturalistic
setting (such as a clinic) and found that relapse rates may be considerably higher than in more controlled settings. Other researchers criticized this study, however, on its methodological grounds. The final
topic on clinical use deals with the increased interest in geriatric psychiatry and consequently the incidence of geriatric mania and the use
of lithium for its treatment.

In the second portion of this chapter, we focus on the basic pharmacology of lithium. There has been a great deal of research in this area during the last few years, with exciting results. Researchers have investigated possible molecular mechanisms of lithium action, and several avenues of investigation seem promising. Perhaps the most promising of these is the focus on the role of G protein-mediated intracellular signaling. Lithium has been shown to affect this process at several sites, perhaps in close relation to the effects of calcium in this same signaling process. Other research has focused on the effects of lithium on the cell membrane, including its downstream effect on beta-adrenoreceptors and the activity of several enzymes. Several studies have focused on lithium's effects on choline and inositol metabolism, which may have relevance for lithium's effects on mood via second-messenger as well as cholinergic systems. A particularly interesting recent finding is that lithium may stabilize intracellular actin filaments, affecting second-messenger systems by stabilizing the intracellular skeleton of filaments. A number of others studies have examined lithium's effects on other biological parameters as well.

▶ CLINICAL STUDIES

Lithium and Pregnancy

Lithium has traditionally been considered a potent teratogen, especially being implicated in cardiac defects such as Ebstein's anomaly. Reports made during the 1970s, based on admittedly biased reporting of abnormalities (e.g., Nora et al. 1974), suggested that lithium might be associated with an unusually high incidence of birth defects. During the last several years, however, several reviews have once again pointed out the biased nature of these early reports and have challenged the prevailing viewpoint.

Ananth (1993b) reviewed the use of lithium during pregnancy and lactation. Review of the evidence concerning the teratogenicity of lithium suggests that the use of lithium may be related to an increased incidence of birth defects. Originally, Ananth reviewed the report of September 1980, in which the lithium registry indicated 25 malformed of 225 cases, with 6 cases of Ebstein's anomaly. A later study (Linden and Rich 1983) indicated cardiac defects in 7% (3/41) of children according to another registry. However, a more recent prospective study (Jacobson et al. 1992) recruited 148 women using lithium during the first trimester of pregnancy. This study showed a total malformation rate not significantly different from control subjects. Despite earlier data indicating an overall rate of 8% of cardiac malformations in patients taking lithium in pregnancy, with a particular focus on the increased rate of Epstein's malformation (an overall rate of 1 in 20,000 births, but perhaps 1 in 60 births when on lithium), these data may be overstated. Some series of studies have specifically looked at Epstein's anomaly but have not detected any lithium use. In utero exposure to lithium was reviewed; several cases were presented that indicate the neonate developed complications despite a normal or therapeutic level in the mother. The physical symptoms in the neonate include cyanosis, lethargy, shallow respirations, and poor sucking. These symptoms can be due to a lithium level in the infant that is two or three times higher than the mother's "normal" level—for example, the newborn becomes lithium toxic with a level of 2.2–2.4 mEq/L. In terms of lactation, care must also be considered. Although the concentration of lithium in the breast milk is generally only 30%–50% of that in maternal plasma, the effect of this amount of lithium is unknown. Furthermore, even a level of only 0.6 mmol/L in the baby may produce cyanosis, floppy muscles, and electrocardiographic changes. Furthermore, the onset of a cold in the baby can lead to a sudden rise in lithium from a level half that of that of the mother (approximately 0.3 mEq/L) to one that is twice that of the mother (1.4 mmol/L), leading to lithium intoxication.

Cohen et al. (1994) reviewed studies on the use of lithium during pregnancy, reporting on two cohort and six case-control studies. They found that in contrast to earlier studies that may have overestimated the incidence of congenital heart defects due to the way data were collected, later more systematic studies showed no large increase in the incidence of such congenital defects, including Epstein's anomaly. In reviewing the two most recent cohort studies on lithium teratogenicity, Cohen et al. reported a rate of all congenital anomalies for lithium versus control subjects of either 7/59 (12%) versus 9/228 (4%) with a risk ratio of 3.0 or 4/106 (4%) versus 3/123 (2%) with a risk ratio of 2.0. Similar results for cardiac malformations (lithium versus control subjects) were either 4/59 (6.8%) versus 2/228 (0.9%) with a risk ratio of 7.7 or 1/106 (0.9%) versus 1/123 (0.8%) with a risk ratio of 1.2. Also, in reviewing four case control studies for Epstein's anomaly, no cases were seen to be associated with lithium intake.

Cohen et al. (1994) also briefly reported on animal studies on the teratogenicity of lithium and noted that increased incidence of birth defects had been seen only with toxic levels of lithium and at concentrations at which many substances are teratogenic. Especially important is the finding in animal studies that even at toxic levels, no increased incidence of cardiac defects was found with lithium.

These authors went on to argue that although there was relatively little evidence to suggest that pregnancy helps stabilize bipolar disorder patients' moods, "far more compelling is the evidence suggesting significant morbidity associated with untreated bipolar disorder" (Cohen et al. 1994, p. 148). Therapeutic guidelines for bipolar patients who become pregnant were then offered, emphasizing the importance of preconception counseling and brief discontinuation of lithium for patients at risk of relapse. They suggested that it may be worth the risk to maintain high-risk patients on lithium throughout the pregnancy, although no specific guidelines to determine which patients are high, medium, or low risk are provided.

Birch et al. (1993; see additional discussion later) came to a similar conclusion, noting "recent evidence suggests that the incidence of fetal abnormality during lithium treated pregnancy is no higher than normal" (p. 228). They suggested that risks and benefits should be discussed with patients and noted "there may be extremely powerful psychiatric arguments for the continuation of lithium, particularly where there is a high risk of severe mood disturbance or suicide attempts" (p. 228).

Dosing, Relapse, and Discontinuation

A number of studies have investigated the effectiveness of various dosing regimens and methods of lithium discontinuation. These studies provide at least some empirical support for attempts to simplify dosing regimens and to standardize practice for long-term lithium maintenance and its discontinuation. For example, Abraham et al.

(1992) studied the effects of once- versus twice-daily lithium dosing for patients with mood disorders. This study was considered particularly important in light of studies that have shown that once-daily dosing may reduce long-term effects on the kidney. Twenty patients were studied in a nonblind crossover design in which each patient was maintained on each dosing schedule for at least 1 month, but no difference in clinical efficacy was found. Patients with once-daily dosing had higher white cell counts, increased serum ionized calcium, and increased serum phosphate, but were otherwise not different from the twice-daily dosing group.

Birch et al. (1993) reported results of a consensus committee on the use of lithium for the prophylaxis of recurrent mood disorders. They discussed practical issues such as patient selection, medical workup prior to beginning therapy, and initiation and adjustment of lithium therapy. They also discussed monitoring of laboratory values during therapy as well as possible signs and symptoms of lithium intoxication. In one section of the article, Birch et al. discussed the use of lithium with other medications, including other psychotropics and several nonpsychotropic medications (diuretics, nonsteroidal anti-inflammatory medications, and angiotensin-converting enzyme [ACE] inhibitors). The need for long-term lithium therapy for prophylaxis and strategies for discontinuation were also discussed.

Faedda et al. (1993) reported a comparison of several strategies for discontinuation of lithium. In this study, there were 64 patients with DSM-III-R (American Psychiatric Association 1987) diagnoses of bipolar disorder who had been controlled on lithium alone for periods ranging from 1 ½ to 5 years. Rapid discontinuation was defined as occurring over a period of less than 2 weeks; gradual discontinuation occurred over a period of 2–4 weeks. Faedda et al. found that within 5 years, 75% of the patients had a recurrence of their disorder; bipolar I patients were somewhat more likely to have a recurrence than bipolar II patients. Risk of new manic or depressive episodes was significantly greater after a rapid rather than a gradual discontinuation. The rate of recurrence was more elevated within the first year after rapid discontinuation (Larck ratio of 5.4), after which relapse rates became nearly equal.

Klein et al. (1992) followed 10 patients with bipolar disorder in remission as their lithium treatment was discontinued under placebo-controlled conditions. They observed that changes in sleep pattern and levels of motor activity often presaged a manic or depressive episode and suggested that study of physical activity levels might be an index of such changes. Patients wore actigraphs on their wrists, devices designed to measure their physical activity levels. Of the 10, 7 relapsed into mania or hypomania during the first 3 months after discontinuation. Those patients who relapsed were found to have had higher levels of physical activity than those who did not relapse, even when both groups were euthymic and maintained on lithium treatment; this difference increased in magnitude as the relapsing patients became symptomatic.

Kukopulos et al. (1992) reported on the relationship of changes in lithium levels and observed mood. Serum lithium levels of 29 inpatients and outpatients were obtained in two different mood states, and patients' moods were blindly rated by psychiatrists on a six-point scale. Statistical analysis showed that patients' depressed moods were associated with levels somewhat higher than those obtained when patients were euthymic, whereas hypomania and mania were associated with lower levels. The investigators concurrently collected data on lithium clearance to assess whether increased diuresis could account for the observed fluctuations in the patients' lithium levels, but there was no evidence of any change in lithium diuresis during the observed fluctuations in their moods. The investigators concluded that lithium must have shifted to another unknown body compartment and suggested that, in light of the association of mood state fluctuations with level fluctuations, it may be of considerable clinical importance.

Suppes et al. (1991) reviewed studies on results of lithium discontinuation in bipolar I disorder and were able to locate 14 studies that met their criteria. With data on 257 patients, this study found that greater than 50% of new episodes of either mania or depression occurred within 10 weeks of lithium discontinuation. Data were available for 124 cases, which allowed calculation of survival analysis statistics. For these cases, the time to 50% chance of relapse was 5 months. There were significant differences between time to recurrence of depression and time to recurrence of mania: time to a 25% chance of recurrence of mania was 2.7 months, and time to a 25% chance of recurrence of depression was 14 months. These authors concluded that the discontinuation of lithium treatment carries a substantial risk of recurrence of mood symptoms and suggested that this risk may be greater than that seen in the natural course of the illness, arguing for caution in the discontinuation of previously successful lithium treatment.

Goodwin (1994) briefly reviewed the results of studies on relapse after lithium discontinuation and argued that available data suggest it may be counterproductive to maintain patients on lithium for less than 2 years. Given a 50% risk of relapse within 3 months after discontinuation of lithium treatment and a 50% probability of relapse after 2 years without lithium maintenance, discontinuation of lithium treatment may actually increase the likelihood of a manic episode if done before 2 full years on lithium. It should be noted that Goodwin's conclusions are based on limited data, but they should provoke closer scrutiny of the use of lithium and perhaps better patient education about the need for long-term lithium compliance to obtain better outcomes.

Terao (1993) reported on the use of a patient self-administration technique in recurrent, possibly bipolar, depression; in two cases, patients had lithium available for self-administration at the first signs of a recurrence of depression (in both cases, a "leaden" feeling in their legs). In both of these cases, early self-administration of lithium by these older patients (a 67-year-old and a 56-year-old) appeared effective in aborting the full recurrence of their depressions.

Terao et al. (1994) discussed the use of lithium level to dose ratio as a means of determining patient compliance. Using this measure, Terao et al. were able to identify patient compliance both while patients were in inpatient units and when they returned from home passes. The criterion suggested for maintaining good compliance after discharge was a lithium level to dose ratio expressed as a percentage of mean basal lithium level to dose ratio between 75% and 125%. With this criterion, the investigators were able to judge that 20/45 patients (44%) were in poor compliance either on the ward or on leave. They argued for the use of this measure in assessing patient compliance in the future.

Thau et al. (1993) reviewed studies on the use of high doses of lithium in the acute treatment of mania. They noted that some evidence exists to suggest that an alternative to the use of combination lithium and neuroleptics, anticonvulsants, or electroconvulsive therapy (ECT) in acute mania is to use increasing levels of lithium. This study reported four uncontrolled trials and case reports of high-dose lithium. The majority of these patients (22/27, 81%) improved on high-dose lithium, often after minimal response was observed at lower levels. Eighteen controlled studies have investigated the use of lithium in acute mania, with the great majority of patients finding it effective. Many of these studies used doses resulting in serum levels as high as 2.0 mmol/L. Thau et al. concluded that the use of high-dose lithium therapy should be considered when the patients display violence or poor impulse control, hyperactivity even when treated with adequate doses of neuroleptics, and other conditions suggesting treatment resistance to more conventional approaches.

Perhaps the most controversial of recent publications is that which has been interpreted as showing the deleterious effect of discontinuation without evident need (e.g., toxicity or severe renal effects). Post et al. (1993) showed that such withdrawal can lead to future refractoriness to lithium therapy. In one case, a 43-year-old woman who stopped lithium because she had been doing well for 7 years developed continual cycling of severe depression to hypomania 1 year later; this time she did not respond to reinstitution of lithium. The National Institute of Mental Health case series shows that 13.6% of lithium-refractory patients acquired this phenomenon after a period of lithium discontinuation. Another problem reported is that of lithium tolerance—that is, that 25 of 49 patients chosen specifically to be followed because of "excellent initial responses to lithium" later showed new episodes in the follow-up period of prophylaxis. Thus, lithium should be discontinued only with great caution and patient consent; even in this situation, the patient may lose benefit over long-term follow-up, requiring other treatments. The importance and effectiveness of long-term lithium maintenance is echoed by Schou (1997).

Prediction of Response

Dilsaver et al. (1993) reviewed studies that have investigated factors that may predict patients' response to lithium versus the anticonvulsants carbamazepine and valproate. They noted that these studies have shown that 80%–90% of all patients with classic manic symptomatology may respond to lithium, but fewer than 40% of rapid-cycling or dysphoric manic patients may respond to lithium. These patients, in contrast, may have a better response to anticonvulsants. The authors suggested that prospective studies might further clarify these issues as well as the relative effectiveness of these agents in prophylaxis of manic recurrences. A later review by Calabrese et al. (1996) supports these conclusions.

Miller et al. (1991) reviewed records of 53 manic patients and hypothesized that behavioral variables such as elation, grandiosity, paranoia, irritability, delusions, and hallucinations would predict response to lithium treatment. Of the 53 patients, 40 (75%) were described as responders to lithium as evidenced by global assessment of functioning scores over 60 with at least a 20-point increase during hospitalization. None of the clinical variables predicted response, although it is unclear from the report in the article precisely how ability to predict was assessed statistically.

Barton et al. (1993) studied the effect of lithium on the moods of persons without psychiatric disorders. Thirty volunteers were randomly assigned to 5 weeks of either placebo or lithium treatment with a midstudy crossover. Lithium levels were maintained at a mean serum level of 0.54 mEq/L, and mood was assessed with visual analogue scales and the Profile of Mood States. None of the measures showed a mood-improving or mood-stabilizing effect in these nonpsychiatric volunteers.

Granulopoiesis

Ananth and Johnson (1993) reported on the "practical applications" of lithium. Beginning with the well-known effect of lithium increasing numbers of granulocytes, they noted that this effect results through multiple mechanisms, including humoral effects on colony-stimulating activity, stimulation of the pluripotent stem cell, and stimulation of granulocyte colonies in the marrow. They also reviewed evidence that shows that this effect is not limited to granulocytopoiesis; there are also an increased number of progenitor cells for both megakaryocytes and erythrocytes. Eosinophilia and thrombocytosis may thus be observed among patients on lithium. The effect of lithium on granulocytes has been used in various leukopenic conditions, including plastic anemia, Fealty's syndrome, various forms of leukemia, and drug-induced leukopenic disorders.

Gallicchio and Hughes (1992) reported on the mechanism of lithium action in and effect of lithium administration on central and peripheral areas of bone marrow. After lithium treatment, both areas showed an increased number of pluripotential stem cells. They noted that the number of erythrocyte precursors was reduced from marginal areas after lithium administration, whereas other types of immature cells showed no spatial distribution differences.

Rybakowski et al. (1993) compared various measures of hematologic functioning during an episode of depression among three groups of patients: one group of euthymic mood disorder patients was receiving lithium, a second group was receiving fluoxetine, and a third group was medication free. There were no differences in erythrocyte measures between the groups, but patients on lithium had increased number of total leukocytes and neutrophils. Patients on lithium also had higher numbers of T_4 and B lymphocytes than patients on fluoxetine. The authors interpreted these results in the context of data that have suggested that lithium may have an immunomodulatory effect in some patients.

Side Effects

Aberg-Wistedt et al. (1993) monitored electrolyte and hormone measures during lithium prophylaxis as a means of investigating lithium's effects on water metabolism and kidney function. Their results suggest that patients' initial weight gain during the first 6 months of treatment may be related to changes in water and electrolyte homeostasis. Patients' blood pressures and pulse rates were lowered, a finding that the authors suggested may be related to decreased metabolic rate and thus also to weight gain. Serum creatinine was increased over time, consistent with the possible onset of decreases in kidney function. Blood pressure and other changes were reversed over a 1-year use of lithium, a finding the authors interpreted as reflecting different mechanisms of lithium action early and late in lithium use.

Ananth (1993a) provided a detailed review of the effects of lithium on memory. He reported that patients often complained of memory loss when on lithium and that this effect was also seen in control subjects who were given therapeutic doses of lithium. Ananth also reported several possible reasons for lithium's effects on memory—it is a potent inhibitor of acetylcholine release and has effects on the thyroid and vasopressin functions, which may be related to memory dysfunction. Despite these reasons for concern, however, studies of the effects of lithium on memory function are mixed. Lithium is often associated with the subjective sensation of memory loss and of psychomotor slowing, but objective memory deficits are not always demonstrated. Ananth concluded that much of the variability in study results was due to differences in populations studied and how they were studied. Thus, there is little evidence that lithium causes memory disorders, and, although it is quite possible that some patients develop memory dysfunction on lithium, there is little evidence to suggest that it is clinically significant or progressive.

In an apparent retrospective study without random assignment of patients to study groups, Axelsson and Lagerkvist-Briggs (1993) investigated a variety of differences between patients with acute mania treated with neuroleptics alone or with a combination of lithium and neuroleptics. Fifteen patients received neuroleptics only, and 19 received the combination. These authors noted some clinical differences between the groups. Those who received combination treatments had an earlier onset of illness, longer duration of illness, more aggressiveness, more paranoid ideation, and more frequent episodes of mood disturbances. They concluded that there is no objective evidence in favor of a combination of treatments for acute mania over neuroleptic monotherapy. This study, however, suffers from nonrandom assignment of patients to treatment groups and the presence of relevant differences between the groups. These differences appear particularly relevant in that they suggest the patient group that received combination therapy may have had more severe illnesses, thus masking any differences in efficacy between treatments.

Kingsbury and Salzman (1993) provided a concise review of lithium's effects on the parathyroid gland and its role in causing hypercalcemia. They reported that lithium has four effects related to the parathyroid and hypercalcemia: 1) lithium alters the set point of the parathyroid gland, necessitating higher calcium levels to decrease hormone production; 2) it directly stimulates parathyroid tissue to produce parathyroid hormone; 3) it interferes with renal cyclic adenosine monophosphate (cAMP), which is regulated by the parathyroid; and 4) elevated levels of magnesium have been observed in lithium-treated patients with hyperparathyroidism. Kingsbury and Salzman stated that minor elevations of calcium, magnesium, or parathyroid hormone levels that do not cause symptoms should not be a cause of abandonment of lithium treatment. If high calcium levels do not return to baseline 1 month after discontinuation of lithium, however, medical or surgical consultation should be obtained. The authors also noted that hypertension or depression that develops after the institution of lithium treatment should cause concern about kidney or parathyroid function changes and should be investigated.

In patients with long-term lithium treatment, Linder et al. (1993) studied calcium and magnesium levels in serum and in erythrocytes. They found that long-term lithium treatment was associated with increased extra- and intracellular magnesium levels. Patients' plasma calciums were increased, with levels greater than 2.6 mmol/L in almost 21% of the patients and greater than 2.8 mmol/L in 4.6% of the patients. These results have implications for the mechanism of lithium action (see the section on pharmacology later in this chapter), but it is worth noting that patients may present with elevated calcium levels (for the clinical significance of these elevations, see Kingsbury and Salzman 1993).

McHenry and Racke (1993) also reviewed the effects of lithium on parathyroid function. They noted that lithium-related hyperparathyroidism was first reported in 1973 and found reports of 42 other cases of hyperparathyroidism since then. They noted that lithium induces increases in parathyroid hormone in vivo in humans as well as in vitro with both human and animal cells. It also affects intracellular calcium-related signaling, but the exact site of lithium action is unknown.

Musa and Tripuraneni (1993) reported on the use of potassium supplements as a treatment for lithium-induced polyuria. They gave results from a pilot study in which four patients with lithium-induced polyuria were treated with oral potassium supplementation of 20 mmol/day. The patients' 24-hour urine volumes decreased significantly over pretreatment values, whereas their urine osmolalities showed a significant increase. They suggested that potassium supplementation may be a safer and cheaper alternative to treatment with antihypertensives.

Sperling et al. (1993) reviewed reports of lithium-related cardiac dysrhythmias. They noted that there have been multiple studies of lithium-associated adverse cardiac effects and reported that most of these studies occurred in the context of high or toxic lithium levels or when lithium was combined with other psychotropics, especially tricyclics. They found that cardiac disturbances associated with lithium included atrioventricular (AV) block, T-wave changes, and tachycardias. They also found, however, that in some cases these adverse effects were not associated with toxic lithium levels, suggesting that there may be important interindividual variations in their susceptibility to these effects.

Naturalistic Study and Comment

Harrow et al. (1990) reported a naturalistic follow-up study of manic patients treated with lithium. They argued that the usual well-controlled drug study may not have accurately reflected the typical result of the use of a drug in the real world and that "the best way to study manic outcome in typical clinical practice is to follow up a large random sample of manic patients from several different settings, in typical treatment with a variety of clinicians" (Harrow et al. 1990, p. 665). They followed 73 manic and 66 unipolar depressed patients for a mean of 1.7 years after hospitalization and found that 1) manic patients had difficulty in posthospital functioning, and 2) manic patients on lithium did not show a better outcome overall than those not on lithium. Harrow et al. argued that manic patients may have a more severe and recurrent illness than previously appreciated and that further study of other treatments for mania, such as the anticonvulsant carbamazepine, may be warranted.

On the other hand, Schou (1993) took issue with this type of study, arguing that it did not really address issues of the efficacy of lithium treatment but of those factors that may influence its success in actual clinical practice. Schou suggested that "the studies provide some, but limited, evidence of lowered efficacy of lithium treatment, probably caused by failing compliance, possibly also by selection of patients on too loose diagnostic criteria" (p. 79). He also argued, after reviewing a number of such studies, that "the main reason for the patients' poor fate was that so many of them discontinued the treatment, usually against medical advice" (p. 79). He emphasized the importance of better patient education, increased levels of social and psychological support, and closer supervision of patients on lithium.

Geriatric Mania

Consistent with increasing interest in issues in geriatric psychiatry, several discussions on the use of lithium in geriatric mania have appeared. Charron et al. (1991) noted that mania is often believed to be rare among the elderly, but reported on six cases they had contact with over 2 years. In these cases, no obvious etiological factor could be identified, and their clinical presentations were similar to those of younger patients with mania. Several of the patients had strong family histories of mood disorder (e.g., alcoholism, depression, suicide), and in one case the patient's sister had presented with late-onset mania at age 66 years. Charron et al. treated five of these six cases with lithium and reported good response in these cases; follow-up for as long as 2.5 years has not shown the appearance of dementia or other organic etiology.

In Young (1992) and Young and Klerman (1992), studies related to geriatric mania are reviewed. These reports noted the importance of determining whether organic factors are related to late-onset mania, especially medical disorders and drugs. They also reported that the phenomenology of late-onset mania is similar to that of earlier-onset mania and that it responds similarly well to lithium.

▶ PHARMACOLOGY

In the last several years, there have been a number of advances in understanding the mechanism of lithium action. These advances are important not only to the understanding of the basic mechanism but also to the possible development of other medications with similar mechanisms. Most of these advances have focused on the understanding of lithium's effects at the level of cell and molecular biology. Lithium has been shown to have effects on cell membranes; the internal structure of the cell; and, most importantly, the operations of several components of the system that translates the external effects of neurotransmission into changes in the cell itself. These second-messenger systems operate to process the signal initiated by the receipt of a neurotransmitter at the cell membrane into changes in cell physiology.

Overview

Advances in understanding lithium's effects focus on two components of the second-messenger systems. Although difficult to review briefly all these systems here (for more complete reviews, see Birnbaumer 1990; Dubovsky et al. 1992; Johnson et al. 1993; Lenox and Watson 1994), it is important to note that the second-messenger system of the cell depends on several different forms of signaling; the most clinically relevant to lithium depends on G protein signaling and phosphoinositol-diphosphate cycling in the signaling system. G proteins are located in or near the cell membrane (see Figure 12–1); when the neuroreceptor is activated by a transmitter, the protein's configuration changes so that its subunits dissociate. There is substantial evidence that these G proteins may be abnormally active in patients with bipolar disorder and that lithium may act to normalize their level of activity.

The dissociated subunit of the G protein in turn initiates a cascade of further reactions, one of which is dependent on the presence of inositol as a substrate. Because inositol poorly penetrates the blood-brain barrier, the neuron is dependent on recycled inositol for continued activity of this signaling system. Lithium has been shown to inhibit the activity of one key enzyme in this cycle, causing a depletion of free inositol and a decrease in signaling activity. In addition to these two central effects, lithium has also been shown to act on the cytoskeleton of the cell and may act directly on the cell membrane as well.

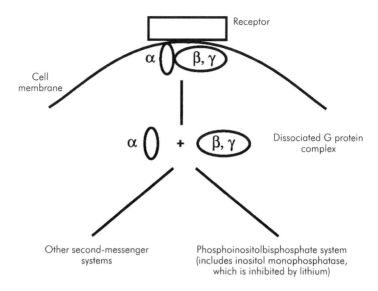

Figure 12–1.   G protein–mediated second-messenger systems.

G Proteins and Related Topics

Avissar and Schreiber (1992) presented a lengthy review of their work on the role of G proteins in mood disorders. They observed that the proteins have a central role in intracellular signaling. They found that lithium treatment inhibited G protein coupling to muscarinic cholinergic and beta-adrenergic receptors. Mean levels for percentage increase in the binding capacity of ^{3}H-Gpp(NH)p (a GTP analog) after carbamylcholine and isoproterenol, respectively, were 60% and 63% for untreated manic patients, 18% and 25% for lithium-treated bipolar patients, and 28% and 23% for control subjects. These findings were interpreted to suggest that lithium's effects on G proteins may be the mechanism of both its antidepressant and antimanic effects.

Avissar and Schreiber (1992) went on to compare the effects of other antibipolar therapies (lithium, anticonvulsants, and ECT) with effects of antidepressants on G protein function. Antibipolar therapies inhibited stimulatory and other G proteins, whereas antidepressants altered only stimulatory G protein function. Hyperactive G proteins were found in untreated manic patients, whereas the G proteins of lithium-treated euthymic patients were normally active. Avissar and Schreiber developed a mathematical model that accounts for unstable oscillations in intracellular signaling due to altered G protein functioning. They related this model to clinically observed manic and depressive symptomatology as well as to the phenomena of manic switching and rapid cycling.

In a study discussed in Avissar and Schreiber's (1992) review, Schreiber et al. (1991) reported finding hyperfunctional G proteins in untreated bipolar patients. They also noted that lithium-treated bipolar patients showed G protein response to agonist stimulation that was similar to that observed in control subjects.

Friedman et al. (1993) noted that protein kinase C activity stimulated by serotonin was twice as high in 12 untreated bipolar patients than in groups of schizophrenic patients and control subjects. This increased platelet protein kinase C activity was reduced by approximately 50% over 2 weeks after treatment with lithium. The time course of the change, according to this study, paralleled that observed with lithium's clinical effects on acute mania.

Li et al. (1993) investigated possible effects of lithium and carbamazepine on G proteins by assaying messenger ribonucleic acid (RNA) levels for G protein subunits in rat cortex. Chronic lithium treatment decreased the levels of messenger RNA for several G protein subunits; carbamazepine did not show this effect. Li et al. suggested that lithium may modify G protein function by acting on the processes that regulate gene expression. Despite these lithium effects to reduce G proteins, levels found in lithium-treated bipolar euthymic patients remain higher than those found in control subjects (Mitchell et al. 1997).

cAMP and Membrane Effects

Mork et al. (1993) studied the effects of lithium and rubidium on cAMP function in human T lymphocyte culture. Rubidium had been previously shown to lengthen and increase the severity of episodes of mania: "the administration of rubidium has generally been found to induce emotional and behavioral effects that are in the opposite direction to those observed after administration of lithium" (Mork et al.

1993, p. 109). In T cell culture, isoprenaline stimulated cAMP production, and incubation of cells with lithium inhibited by 25% isoprenaline's stimulation of cAMP production, whereas rubidium augmented it by 50%. Rubidium therapy for 14 days also decreased by 25% the beta-adrenergic–stimulated cAMP production in rat cortex. This study made an analogy between this effect and the downregulation of beta-adrenergic receptor function by antidepressants and suggested that this cAMP effect might be a mechanism of rubidium's reported antidepressant effects. They concluded that T cell culture may be a useful medium by which to model lithium-induced changes in intracellular second-messenger systems.

Kofman and Belmaker (1993) extensively reviewed the significance of inositol in lithium's clinical effects on mood disorders. They commented on the well-known finding that lithium inhibits inositol monophosphate, thereby depleting brain inositol level. They reviewed animal data that showed that the intrathecal administration of inositol may abolish some behavioral effects of lithium, suggesting that depletion of brain inositol is, in fact, closely related to lithium's observed clinical effects. Agam et al. (1993) reported that, in contrast to the finding that lithium reduces inositol levels in rat brain, no decrease in cerebrospinal fluid inositol levels was detected in 9 schizophrenic patients treated with 1,200 mg of lithium for 3–7 days.

Wilson et al. (1993) noted that lithium has been reported to affect immune function of patients treated with it and that it also been shown to affect B and T lymphocyte function in tissue culture. They further observed that lithium has been reported to attenuate the cAMP increase typically induced by stimulation of lymphocytes with pokeweed mitogen and speculated that this effect might be closely related to lithium's effects on immune functioning. Wilson et al. (1993) found that lithium decreased cAMP production by lymphocytes in culture to stimulation by pokeweed mitogen. Inositol phosphate and inositol lipid production were increased after 3–4 days. Because previous work had shown that the lithium-induced proliferation of lymphocytes occurred in this time range (also 3–4 days), Wilson et al. speculated that the inositol changes may be related to lithium's effects on immune system function.

Finally, two articles dealt with lithium's effect on the actin filaments, which are important constituents of the cytoskeleton. DalleDonne et al. (1993) observed that actin filament bundling was enhanced in the presence of lithium. Colombo et al. (1993) called the effects of lithium on actin an "intriguing interaction" and suggested that lithium's effects on clinical symptoms in mood disorders as well as its teratogenic effects may be related to its effects on actin. Increased bundling, for example, might affect intracellular transport processes in patients and might affect cell migration during embryogenesis. It should be noted, however, that these data are preliminary and that there is little evidence for a specific association of lithium's effects on actin and its clinical use in mood disorders.

▶ Conclusion

In this chapter, we focused on both clinical and biological issues. Some of the most important new findings in recent years, in terms of treatment issues, have been that 1) lithium may not be teratogenic as previously believed, but may be more a threat to the newborn through lactation; 2) if a patient is to be discontinued from treatment, it should be done over a course of weeks; 3) a patient's lithium level while at a constant dose may be influenced by mood state—increasing in depression and decreasing in mania; and 4) lithium may have significant influence on the parathyroid gland to affect blood and bone calcium concentrations. Our knowledge concerning lithium's mechanism of action has gone beyond its effects on neurochemicals to the effects it has on subcellular units, including G proteins and second-messenger cAMP. It is hoped that the continued explosion of information on the biological basis and clinical use of lithium will lead both to a further understanding of the basis of bipolar disorder and improved basic treatment for its treatment and prevention.

▶ References

Aberg-Wistedt A, Eneroth P, Malmgren R, et al: Studies on some hormone and electrolyte changes during one year of lithium therapy in depression. Lithium 4:261–266, 1993

Abraham G, Delva N, Waldron J, et al: Lithium treatment: a comparison of once- and twice-daily dosing. Acta Psychiatr Scand 85:65–69, 1992

Agam G, Shapiro J, Levine J, et al: Short-term lithium treatment does not reduce human CSF inositol levels. Lithium 4:267–269, 1993

American Psychiatric Association: Diagnostic and Statistical Manual of Mental Disorders, 3rd Edition, Revised. Washington, DC, American Psychiatric Association, 1987

Ananth J: Does lithium affect memory? Lithium 4:167–179, 1993a

Ananth J: Lithium during pregnancy and lactation. Lithium 4:231–237, 1993b

Ananth J, Johnson KM: Lithium and granulopoiesis: practical applications. Lithium 4:13–23, 1993

Avissar S, Schreiber G: The involvement of guanine nucleotide binding proteins in the pathogenesis and treatment of affective disorders. Biol Psychiatry 31:435–459, 1992

Axelsson R, Lagerkvist-Briggs M: Clinical and neurobiological findings during treatment with neuroleptics alone and combined with lithium: a comparative study of patients with bipolar disorder in acute manic phase. Lithium 4:45–52, 1993

Barton CD, Dufer D, Monderer R, et al: Mood variability in normal subjects on lithium. Biol Psychiatry 34:878–884, 1993

Birch NJ, Groft P, Hullin RP, et al: Lithium prophylaxis: proposed guidelines for good clinical practice. Lithium 4:225–230, 1993

Birnbaumer L: G proteins in signal transduction. Annu Rev Pharmacol Toxicol 30:675–705, 1990

Calabrese JR, Fatemi H, Kujawa M, et al: Predictors of response to mood stabilizers. J Clin Psychopharmacol 16:245–325, 1996

Charron M, Fortin L, Opaquette I: De novo mania among elderly people. Acta Psychiatr Scand 84:503–507, 1991

Cohen LS, Friedman JM, Jefferson JW, et al: A reevaluation of risk of in utero exposure to lithium. JAMA 271:146–150, 1994

Colombo R, DalleDonne I, Milzani A: Lithium and actin: an intriguing interaction. Lithium 4:1–11, 1993

DalleDonne I, Milzani A, Colombo R: Lithium supports actin bundle formation. Lithium 4:285–291, 1993

Dilsaver SC, Swann AC, Shoaib AM, et al: The manic syndrome: factors which may predict a patient's response of lithium, carbamazepine and valproate. J Psychiatry Neurosci 18:61–66, 1993

Dubovsky SL, Murphy J, Christiano J, et al: The calcium second messenger system in bipolar disorders: data supporting new research directions. Journal of Neuropsychiatry and Clinical Neurosciences 4:3–14, 1992

Faedda GL, Tondo L, Baldessarini RJ, et al: Outcome after rapid vs gradual discontinuation of lithium treatment in bipolar disorder. Arch Gen Psychiatry 50:448–455, 1993

Friedman E, Wang HY, Levinson D, et al: Altered platelet protein kinase C activity in bipolar affective disorder, manic episode. Biol Psychiatry 33:520–525, 1993

Gallicchio VS, Hughes NK: Lithium stimulation of hematopoiesis: demonstration that lithium influences the spatial distribution of hematopoietic progenitor cells with endosteal bone marrow. Lithium 3:117–124, 1992

Goodwin GM: Recurrence of mania after lithium withdrawal. Br J Psychiatry 164:149–152, 1994

Harrow M, Goldberg JF, Grossman LS, et al: Outcome in manic disorders. Arch Gen Psychiatry 47:665–671, 1990

Jacobson SJ, Jones K, Johnson X, et al: Prospective multicenter study of pregnancy outcome after lithium exposure during the first trimester. Lancet 339:530–533, 1992

Johnson FN, Birch NJ, Carstens M, et al: Mechanisms of lithium action. Rev Contemp Pharmacother 4:287–318, 1993

Kingsbury SJ, Salzman C: Lithium's role in hyperparathyroidism and hypercalcemia. Hosp Community Psychiatry 44:1047–1048, 1993

Klein E, Lavie P, Meiraz R, et al: Increased motor activity and recurrent manic episodes: predictors of rapid relapse in remitted bipolar disorder patients after lithium discontinuation. Biol Psychiatry 31:279–284, 1992

Kofman O, Belmaker RH: Biochemical, behavioral, and clinical studies of the role of inositol in lithium treatment and depression. Biol Psychiatry 34:839–852, 1993

Kukopulos A, Reginaldi D, Johnson FN: Fluctuations in serum lithium levels as a function of mood state. Lithium 3:195–201, 1992

Lenox RH, Watson DG: Lithium and the brain: a psychopharmacological strategy to a molecular basis for manic depressive illness. Clin Chem 40:309–314, 1994

Li PP, Young LT, Tam YK, et al: Effects of chronic lithium and carbamazepine treatment on G-protein subunit expression in rat cerebral cortex. Biol Psychiatry 34:162–170, 1993

Linden S, Rich CC: The use of lithium during pregnancy and lactation. J Clin Psychiatry 44:358–360, 1983

Linder J, Levin K, Saaf J, et al: Influence of lithium treatment on calcium and magnesium in plasma and erythrocytes. Lithium 4:115–123, 1993

McHenry CR, Racke FK: Lithium effects on parathyroid function. Lithium 4:87–94, 1993

Miller F, Tanenbaum JH, Griffin A, et al: Prediction of treatment response in bipolar, manic disorder. J Affect Disord 21:75–77, 1991

Mitchell PB, Manji HK, Chen G, et al: High level of Gsα in platelets of euthymic patients with bipolar affective disorder. Am J Psychiatry 154:218–223, 1997

Mork A, Hansen ER, Geisler A, et al: Effects of rubidium and lithium on isoprenaline-induced cyclic AMP formation in human T lymphocyte cultures and rat brain. Lithium 4:109–113, 1993

Musa M, Tripuraneni BR: Lithium-induced polyuria ameliorated by potassium supplementation. Lithium 4:199–203, 1993

Nora JJ, Nora AH, Toews WH: Lithium, Epstein's anomaly and other congenital defects. Lancet 2:594–595, 1974

Post RM, Leverich GS, Pazzaglia PJ, et al: Lithium tolerance and discontinuation as pathways to refractoriness, in Lithium in Medicine and Biology. Edited by Birch NJ, Padgham C, Hughes MS. Carnforth, UK, Marius Press, 1993, pp 71–84

Rybakowski JK, Amsterdam JD, Prystowsky MB: Blood cell indices in affective patients during lithium prophylaxis. Lithium 4:205–209, 1993

Schou M: Lithium prophylaxis: about "naturalistic" or "clinical practice" studies. Lithium 4:77–81, 1993

Schou M: Forty years of lithium treatment. Arch Gen Psychiatry 54:9–13, 1997

Schreiber G, Avissar S, Danon A, et al: Hyperfunctional G proteins in mononuclear leukocytes of patients with mania. Biol Psychiatry 29:273–280, 1991

Sperling W, Wiesmann M, Boning J: Cardiac dysrhythmias under lithium therapy. Lithium 4:161–165, 1993

Suppes T, Baldessarini RJ, Faedda GL, et al: Risk of recurrence following discontinuation of lithium treatment in bipolar disorder. Arch Gen Psychiatry 48:1082–1088, 1991

Terao T: Prodromal symptoms of depression and self-administration of lithium. Biol Psychiatry 34:198–199, 1993

Terao M, Terao T, Kumashiro M, et al: Lithium compliance study of inpatients using serum level-to-dose ratio. Lithium 4:181–188, 1994

Thau K, Meszaros K, Simhandl C: The use of high dosage lithium carbonate in the treatment of acute mania: a review. Lithium 4:149–159, 1993

Wilson R, Fraser WD, Wakeham M, et al: The effect of lithium on the intracellular mediators cAMP, inositol phosphate and inositol lipid. Lithium 4:135–138, 1993

Young RC: Geriatric mania. Clin Geriatr Med 8:387–399, 1992

Young RC, Klerman GL: Mania in late life: focus on age of onset. Am J Psychiatry 149:867–876, 1992

CHAPTER 13

CARBAMAZEPINE

Terence A. Ketter, M.D., F.R.C.P.C., Robert M. Post, M.D.,
Kirk Denicoff, M.D., Peggy J. Pazzaglia, M.D.,
Lauren B. Marangell, M.D., Mark S. George, M.D., and
Ann M. Callahan, M.D.

C arbamazepine (CBZ) is a unique tricyclic compound used in the treatment of seizure disorders, pain syndromes, and mood disorders (Post 1988). The multiple actions of CBZ and its putative mechanisms have been reviewed elsewhere (Post 1988; Post et al. 1994). In this chapter, we review the use of CBZ in the acute treatment and prophylaxis of mania, with a special emphasis on its pharmacology and pharmacokinetics, to provide clinicians with background information needed to use this medication effectively.

▶ UTILITY OF CBZ IN ACUTE MANIA

Nineteen controlled studies indicate the acute antimanic efficacy of CBZ or its keto-cogener oxcarbazepine by various methodologies (Table 13–1) (Ballenger and Post 1978; D. Brown et al. 1989; Desai et al. 1987; Emrich 1990; Emrich et al. 1985; Goncalves and Stoll 1985; Grossi et al. 1984; Klein et al. 1984; Lenzi et al. 1986; Lerer et al. 1987; Lusznat et al. 1988; Möller et al. 1989; Müller and Stoll 1984; Okuma et al. 1979, 1988, 1990; Post et al. 1987; Small et al. 1991; Stoll et al. 1986). Several trials involved placebo-controlled B-A-B-A designs, some used parallel designs in comparison with neuroleptics, and others were augmentation studies. Although some individual stud-

Table 13–1. Controlled studies of carbamazepine (CBZ) and oxcarbazepine (OXCBZ) in acute mania

Investigators	N	Diagnosis	Design	Doses (mg/day) [blood level]	Other drugs	Duration	Results
Ballenger and Post 1978; Post et al. 1987	19 CBZ, 19 placebo	Manic-depressive	Double-blind (B-A-B-A)	600–2,000 CPZ [7–15.5 µg/mL]	None	11–56 days	12/19 improved—time course similar to neuroleptics; frequent relapses on placebo substitution
Okuma et al. 1979	32 CBZ, 28 CPZ	Manic-depressive psychosis	Blind versus CPZ	300–900 CBZ [2.7–11.7 µg/mL; mean, 7.2 ± 3.4]; 150–450 CPZ	Bedtime hypnotics	3–5 weeks	21/23 improved on CBZ (marked to moderate); 15/28 improved on CPZ
Grossi et al. 1984	18 CBZ, 19 CPZ	Manic-depressive	Blind versus CPZ randomized	200–1,200 CBZ; 200–500 CPZ	?	3 weeks	10/15 improved on CBZ; 13/17 improved on CPZ; CBZ fewer side effects than CPZ
Klein et al. 1984	14 CBZ, 13 placebo	Manic/excited schizoaffective	Randomized blind versus placebo addition to haloperidol	600–1600 CBZ [6–18 µg/mL]	Haloperidol, 14–45 mg all patients	5 weeks	10/14 improved on CBZ plus haloperidol; 7/13 improved on placebo plus haloperidol
Müller and Stoll 1984; Goncalves and Stoll 1985	6 CBZ, 6 placebo	Manic, schizoaffective	Blind versus placebo	600–1,200 CBZ	Haloperidol and hypnotics	3 weeks	6/6 CBZ better than placebo ($P < .01$)
Müller and Stoll 1984	10 OXCBZ, 10 haloperidol	Manic-depressive	Randomized blind versus haloperidol	900–1,200 OXCBZ; 15–20 haloperidol	Haloperidol and hypnotics	2 weeks	No significant difference

Study	Sample	Diagnosis	Design	Dose	Concomitant	Duration	Results
Emrich et al. 1985	7 OXCBZ, 7 placebo	Manic psychosis	Double-blind (B-A-B)	1,800–2,100 OXCBZ	None	Variable	6/7 (> 25% improvement on Inpatient Multi-dimension Rating Scale)
Lenzi et al. 1986	11 CBZ, 11 lithium	Manic-depressive and schizo-affective	Blind versus lithium	400–1,600 CBZ [7–12 µg/mL]; 900 lithium [0.6–1.2 mEq/L]	CPZ all patients	19 days	CBZ = lithium efficacy; CBZ group required less CPZ; CBZ less paranoia and extrapyramidal side effects
Stoll et al. 1986	14 CBZ, 18 haloperidol	Manic	Randomized versus halo-peridol	600–1,200 CBZ; 5–30 haloperidol	CPZ	3 weeks	12/14 improved on CBZ; 12/18 improved on haloperidol
Desai et al. 1987	5 CBZ, 5 placebo	Manic	Blind versus placebo addi-tion to lithium	400 fixed-dose CBZ	Lithium all patients	4 weeks	CBZ plus lithium better on Bech-Raefelson Mania Scale than lithium (P < .05)
Lerer et al. 1987	14 CBZ, 14 lithium	Manic	Blind versus lithium random-ized	1,400–2,600 CBZ [4.7–14 µg/mL]; 900–3,900 lithium [0.54–1.7 mEq/L]	Chloral hydrate, barbiturates hs	4 weeks	4/14 improved on CBZ; 11/14 im-proved on lithium; lithium Clinical Global Impression better (P < .05); no significant differ-ence on Brief Psych-iatric Rating Scale

(continued)

Table 13–1. Controlled studies of carbamazepine (CBZ) and oxcarbazepine (OXCBZ) in acute mania (*continued*)

Investigators	N	Diagnosis	Design	Doses (mg/day) [blood level]	Other drugs	Duration	Results
Lusznat et al. 1988	22 CBZ, 22 lithium	Manic	Blind versus lithium randomized	CBZ dose not stated [6–12 µg/mL]; lithium dose not stated [0.6–1.4 mmol/L]	CPZ, haloperidol, remazepam	6 weeks	No significant difference
Okuma et al. 1988	103 CBZ, 98 placebo	Schizoaffective, schizophrenic, atypical psychosis	Blind versus placebo	400–1,200 CBZ	Neuroleptics		50% improved on CBZ
Brown et al. 1989	8 CBZ, 9 haloperidol	Manic	Blind versus haloperidol	400–1,600 CBZ; 20–80 haloperidol	CPZ, in 3 patients on CBZ and in 7 patients on haloperidol	4 weeks	6/8 marked improvement on CBZ; 3/9 marked improvement on haloperidol; CBZ slower onset, higher completion rate (75% versus 22%), fewer extrapyramidal side effects, less procyclidine required
Möller et al. 1989	11 CBZ, 9 placebo	Manic or schizoaffective	Blind versus placebo	600 CBZ	Haloperidol 24 mg all patients, levomepromazine	3 weeks	No significant difference; CBZ needed less levomepromazine
Emrich 1990	17 OXCBZ, 20 haloperidol	Manic	Blind versus haloperidol	2,400 OXCBZ; mean haloperidol, 42	?	15 days	16/17 improved on OXCBZ (excellent or good); 15/20 improved on haloperidol (excellent or good)

Study	Subjects	Type	Design	Dose	Comparator	Duration	Results
Emrich 1990	29 OXCBZ, 24 lithium	Manic	Blind versus lithium	1,400 OXCBZ		15 days	27/29 improved on OXCBZ (excellent or good); 22/24 improved on lithium (excellent or good)
Okuma et al. 1990	50 CBZ, 51 lithium	Manic	Blind versus lithium	400–1,200 CBZ [CBZ mean, 7.3 µg/mL]; 400–1,200 lithium [lithium mean, 0.46 mEq/L]	Neuroleptics	4 weeks	31/50 improved on CBZ; 30/51 improved on lithium; no significant difference; CBZ onset earlier
Small et al. 1991	24 CBZ, 24 lithium	Manic	Blind versus lithium	700–1,036 CBZ [30–37 µmol/L]; 1,035–1,275 lithium [0.6–0.9 mmol/L]	Hypnotics	6–8 weeks	8/24 improved on CBZ; 8/24 improved on lithium; CBZ better than lithium in weeks 2 and 3; no significant difference after 8 weeks
Total of all 19 studies	351 CBZ, 63 OXCBZ, 146 lithium, 104 neuroleptics, 157 placebo						171/290 (59.0%) improved on CBZ; 49/53 (92.45%) improved on OXCBZ[a]; 71/113 (62.83%) improved on lithium; 58/92 (63.04%) improved on neuroleptics

Note. CPZ = chlorpromazine; Li = lithium; OXCBZ = oxcarbazepine.
[a]All from Emrich 1990 and Emrich et al. 1985.

ies may be criticized for methodological shortcomings, taken together this group of clinical trials provides substantial evidence of the acute antimanic efficacy of CBZ. Indeed, this body of data is greater than that initially utilized by the U.S. Food and Drug Administration to approve lithium for the treatment of acute mania.

Overall antimanic response rates are comparable with those seen with lithium or valproate (about two-thirds of patients). Although CBZ has weaker antidepressant than antimanic properties, some evidence suggests that it may provide antidepressant benefit in about one-third of refractory patients (Post et al. 1986). CBZ has a rapid onset of antimanic efficacy, similar to that of neuroleptics (Figures 13–1 and 13–2). Thus, lack of clinical improvement after 7–10 days may be an indication to consider augmentation or alternative strategies. In the few studies that have examined the relationships between blood CBZ levels and acute antimanic or antidepressant responses, these relationships have been weak and resemble the nonlinear relationship between blood CBZ levels and anticonvulsant responses. However, specific studies to determine a therapeutic window in the treatment of mania have not been conducted. Thus, titrating CBZ dose to clinical efficacy in the absence of side effects, or to a side-effect threshold, may be more useful than adhering to fixed dosage or blood level ranges.

The efficacy of CBZ in acute mania is also supported by a substantial open treatment literature. It has been suggested that patients with severe, psychotic, or dysphoric mania; rapid cycling; inadequate response to lithium; and no family history of bipolar disorder may respond better to CBZ than to lithium (Post et al. 1987). However, those with a history of psychosensory symptoms (which have been hypothesized to be due to limbic dysfunction) do not appear to be preferentially responsive to CBZ compared with patients without such symptoms. CBZ is frequently used in combination with other medications in the acute treatment of mania, as described later.

▶ Utility of CBZ in Mania Prophylaxis

As summarized in Table 13–2, a series of doubled-blind, randomized, open-randomized, or otherwise partially controlled studies (Ballenger

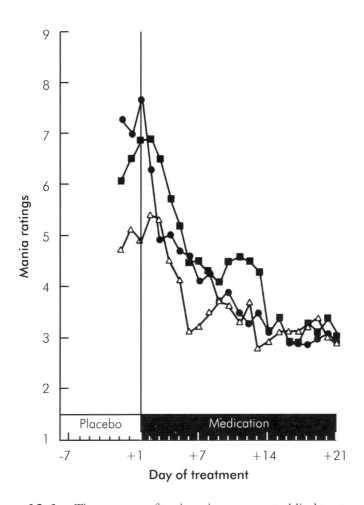

Figure 13–1. Time course of antimanic response to blind treatment with carbamazepine (squares, (N = 19) compared with neuroleptics (*circles*, N = 17) and lithium (*triangles*, N = 19).
Source. Reprinted from Post RM, Ballenger JC, Uhde TW, et al: "Efficacy of Carbamazepine in Manic-Depressive Illness: Implications for Underlying Mechanisms," in *Neurobiology of Mood Disorders.* Edited by Post RM, Ballenger J. Baltimore, MD, Williams & Wilkins, 1984a, pp 777–816. Used with permission.

and Post 1978; Bellaire et al. 1988; Cabrera et al. 1986; Coxhead et al. 1992; Di Costanzo and Schifano 1991; Elphick et al. 1988; Kishimoto and Okuma 1985; Lusznat et al. 1988; Mosolov 1991; Okuma

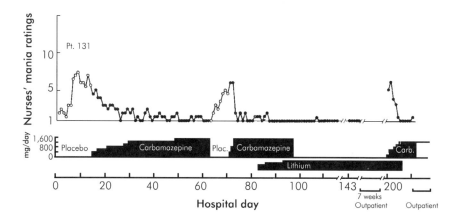

Figure 13-2. Repeated acute antimanic responses to carbamazepine in an individual patient. This female bipolar patient had broken through lithium prophylaxis with manic episodes on numerous occasions before hospitalization at the National Institute of Mental Health and did not require rehospitalization during more than 2 years of subsequent carbamazepine prophylaxis.
Source. Reprinted from Post RM, Ballenger JC, Uhde TW, et al: "Efficacy of Carbamazepine in Manic-Depressive Illness: Implications for Underlying Mechanisms," in *Neurobiology of Mood Disorders.* Edited by Post RM, Ballenger J. Baltimore, MD, Williams & Wilkins, 1984a, pp 777–816. Used with permission.

et al. 1981; Placidi et al. 1986; Post et al. 1983b; Watkins et al. 1987) are consistent with a very substantial open literature suggesting that CBZ may be effective in preventing episodes of both mania and depression when administered during long-term prophylaxis, either alone or in combination with lithium in previous lithium nonresponders. Although some of these trials may have methodological shortcomings, the B-A-B-A design studies and trials of CBZ in rapid cycling and lithium-refractory patients constitute compelling evidence of the efficacy of CBZ (Prien and Gelenberg 1989). The double-blind, randomized trials are at least supportive of the clinical efficacy of CBZ, usually to a degree similar to that of lithium. The open studies suggesting efficacy of CBZ, if anything, report lower response rates than the controlled studies, further supporting the efficacy of CBZ in patients with lithium-refractory illness. CBZ may be effective in some

Table 13-2. Controlled and quasi-controlled studies of carbamazepine (CBZ) and oxcarbazepine prophylaxis in manic-depressive illness

Investigators	Design	Placebo	CBZ responders	D/C	Response (%)	Lithium responders	D/C	Response (%)
Ballenger and Post 1978; Post et al. 1983b	B, M		6/7		86	—		—
Okuma et al. 1981	B, R	2/9	6/10		60	—		—
Kishimoto and Okuma 1985	C		?/18		decreased number hospitalized versus lithium	—		—
Cabrera et al. 1986[a]	R		—		50	3/6		50
Placidi et al. 1986	B, R		21/29	12	72	20/27	13	74
Watkins et al. 1987	B, R		16/19		84	15/18		83
Bellaire et al. 1988	R		?/50		CBZ not significantly greater than lithium	—		—
Elphick et al. 1988	B, C		3/8		38	8/11		73

(continued)

Table 13–2. Controlled and quasi-controlled studies of carbamazepine (CBZ) and oxcarbazepine prophylaxis in manic-depressive illness (continued)

Investigators	Design	Placebo	CBZ responders	D/C	Response (%)	Lithium responders	D/C	Response (%)
Di Costanzo and Schifano 1991	R[b]		?/16		—	?/16	?/16	—
Lusznat et al. 1988	B, R		9/16	11	56	5/17	10	29
Mosolov 1991	R?		22/30		73	21/30		70
Coxhead et al. 1992	B, R		7/13		54	7/15		47
All controlled studies			90/132		68	79/124		64
All open studies			390/629[c]		62			

Note.   B = blind. M = mirror image. — = not stated. R = randomized. C = crossed-over. D/C = discontinued.
[a] Oxcarbazepine only.
[b] Pseudo-randomized to lithium versus CBZ plus lithium; CBZ plus lithium greater antimanic and antidepressant efficacy in first year versus lithium alone.
[c] Includes CBZ combination therapies.

Source.   Adapted from Post RM: "Anticonvulsants and Novel Drugs," in *Handbook of Affective Disorders*, 2nd Edition. Edited by Paykel ES. London, Churchill Livingstone, 1992, p. 396. Used with permission.

individuals with valproate-refractory illness (Post et al. 1984c), and the CBZ-plus-valproate combination may be effective in patients with little or no response to either agent alone (Keck et al. 1992; Ketter et al. 1995b).

Clinical predictors of CBZ response have not been adequately elucidated. Although the initial studies of Okuma and colleagues (Okuma 1983; Okuma et al. 1981, 1988) indicated that some rapid cycling patients were highly if not preferentially responsive to CBZ, their later work reported lower response rates (similar to lithium) in rapid cycling compared with nonrapid cycling illness (Okuma 1993). However, even these rapid cycling patients had a CBZ response rate (40%) that was higher than rates reported with other agents in other studies. Himmelhoch (1987) suggested that patients with comorbid neurological or substance abuse problems and inadequate lithium responses may respond to CBZ or valproate. Although several investigators have suggested that psychosensory symptoms may indicate preferential response to CBZ and other anticonvulsants, such a trend has not been observed in acute therapy, and the relationship to prophylactic response remains to be delineated. Several studies have indicated that patients with a history of affective illness in first-degree relatives may have preferential responses to lithium, whereas the converse may be the case for CBZ (Ballenger and Post 1978; Post et al. 1987).

CBZ appears to have equal prophylactic antimanic and antidepressant efficacy, in contrast to its more potent acute antimanic compared with antidepressant effects. Loss of CBZ prophylactic efficacy over time has been observed (Figure 13–3), and Post et al. (1990) suggested that this may be due to a pharmacodynamic loss of efficacy related to a unique form of contingent tolerance. In these instances, the optimal algorithm for recapturing CBZ response has not been determined. However, switching to another treatment regimen with a different mechanism of action or returning later to CBZ (after a period off CBZ) are worth considering, based on case reports and anecdotal observations. Systematic clinical trials are required to better determine the efficacy of this and other approaches to recapturing CBZ response.

In view of the limited literature regarding response predictors for CBZ versus other mood stabilizers, the varying side-effect profiles of these agents are often used to help determine the optimal agent(s) for

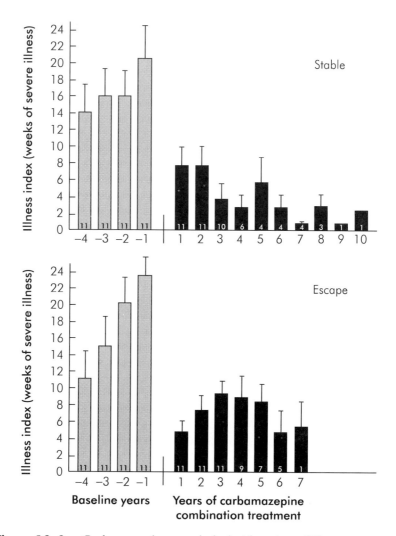

Figure 13–3. Carbamazepine prophylaxis (duration of illness × severity). Half of the patients showed persistent long-term prophylactic response to carbamazepine (top, stable, black bars), whereas the other half began to lose response in the second, third, and fourth years of treatment (bottom, escape, black bars). A more rapidly escalating course of illness before carbamazepine treatment (bottom, escape, gray bars) was related to the tolerance pattern.
Source. Reprinted from Post RM, Leverich GS, Rosoff AS, et al: "Carbamazepine Prophylaxis in Refractory Affective Disorders: A Focus on Long-Term Follow-Up." *Journal of Clinical Psychopharmacology.* 10:318–327, 1990. Used with permission.

individual patients. Lithium and valproate share tremor, gastrointestinal disturbance, weight gain, and alopecia as side effects; CBZ is more likely to be associated with rashes, drug interactions, and hematological problems. Finally, patients may have preferences based on their prior subjective experiences of receiving each of the mood stabilizers; any preferences should be integrated into the long-term treatment plan to help enhance compliance.

▌ CLINICAL PHARMACOLOGY OF CBZ

CBZ has a tricyclic structure similar to that of imipramine. It is approved in the United States for the treatment of trigeminal neuralgia and temporal lobe epilepsy. Although CBZ is approved in Canada for the treatment of bipolar disorder, the manufacturer has not submitted for such approval in the United States. CBZ is available in the United States as a proprietary product, Tegretol, in 200 mg tablets, 100 mg chewable tablets, and 100 mg/5 mL suspension (Mehta 1994). A slow-release formulation has recently become available in the United States. CBZ is also available in a generic formulation. The absorption of CBZ is slow and somewhat erratic, and differences have been observed in the bioavailability of the proprietary and generic formulations (Meyer et al. 1992). CBZ should not be exposed to humidity, because this can decrease its bioavailability (Nightingale 1990). CBZ plasma half-lives vary widely, with the average half-life of a single dose of CBZ being about 24 hours; because of autoinduction of metabolism, however, the average half-life falls to about 12 hours with chronic administration.

In the treatment of acute mania there are two divergent clinical needs that influence the rate of dosage titration. First, there is a pressing need for rapid control of the manic syndrome, which suggests that faster titration to higher doses could provide more rapid attainment of therapeutic levels, potentially yielding quicker onset of not only nonspecific sedation but also of specific antimanic effects. On the other hand, there is a need not to burden patients excessively with the increased side effects associated with overly rapid escalation of CBZ dosage. Such side effects include neurotoxicity (sedation, diplopia, and ataxia) and gastrointestinal disturbances that can not only complicate acute management, but may also result in patients developing negative perceptions of the adverse effects of CBZ that later interfere with compliance in prophylactic therapy. Thus, although a loading dose strategy may be effective in the treatment of mania with valproate (Keck et al. 1993), neurotoxic side effects may preclude such an approach with CBZ.

Doses of CBZ not well tolerated due to side effects during the first 2 weeks of therapy may be readily used after a month of therapy once patients have developed tolerance to most side effects and autoinduction of CBZ metabolism has decreased blood levels (Cereghino 1975).

As dosage and blood and cerebrospinal fluid levels of CBZ fail to correlate with psychotropic efficacy (Post 1989; Post et al. 1983a, 1984a) (Figure 13–4), it is common practice to increase the dosage

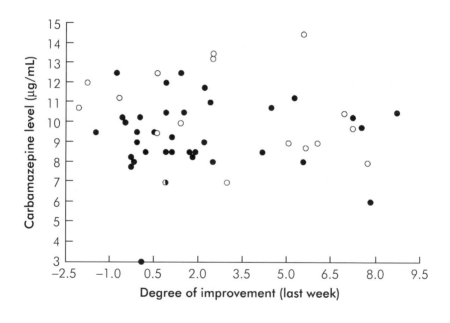

Figure 13–4. Lack of relationship between blood levels of carbamazepine and degree of clinical response in mood disorders. Closed circles indicate depressed patients, and open circles indicate manic patients. *Source.* Reprinted from Post RM: "Carbamazepine Treatment of Bipolar Affective Disorder." *Directions in Psychiatry* 9, lesson 19, 1989. Used with permission. Copyright 1989, Hatherleigh Company.

gradually as tolerated, monitoring both side effects and clinical efficacy until therapeutic efficacy is adequate, side effects supervene, or blood levels exceed 12 µg/mL. In contrast to the parent compound, cerebrospinal fluid levels of the active 10,11-epoxide metabolite (CBZ-E) may correlate with degree of clinical improvement in patients with mood disorders (Post et al. 1983a, 1984a, 1984b) (Figure 13–5). Analysis of an expanded sample on our clinical research unit indicated that although clinical improvement in depressed patients failed to correlate with blood CBZ levels, there was a trend toward a positive correlation with blood CBZ-E ratios, and a significant positive correlation with blood CBZ-E/CBZ ratios, suggesting a possible relationship between clinical response and the degree of enzyme induction (T. A. Ketter and R. M. Post, unpublished observations, August 1994).

In responders, a dose-response relationship may be evident (Figure 13–6), so that slowly increasing CBZ doses to maximize response in the absence of significant side effects is a clinically useful strategy, whereas increasing CBZ to high doses and side effects in the absence of any hint of therapeutic response is unlikely to be beneficial. CBZ is generally given in divided doses to minimize peak levels and side effects (Figures 13–7 and 13–8), although in some patients with insomnia or prominent daytime sedation the dosage can be weighted toward bedtime or given exclusively at bedtime to minimize side effects. Dizziness, ataxia, or diplopia emerging 1–2 hours after an individual dose is often a sign that the side effects threshold has been exceeded and that dose redistribution (spreading out the dose or giving more of the dose at bedtime) or dose reduction may be required.

Patients often develop benign alterations in serum chemistries, such as mild leukopenia and elevations of liver function tests that do not exceed three times the upper limit of normal. Obtaining baseline studies and careful clinical and laboratory monitoring is sufficient in these circumstances. However, rare but serious decreases in blood counts can occur, including aplastic anemia, with the risk estimated to be six per million (Mehta 1994). For this reason, it is important to alert patients to seek immediate medical evaluation and treatment if they develop signs and symptoms of possible hematological reactions, such as fever, sore throat, oral ulcers, and easy bruising or bleeding. In

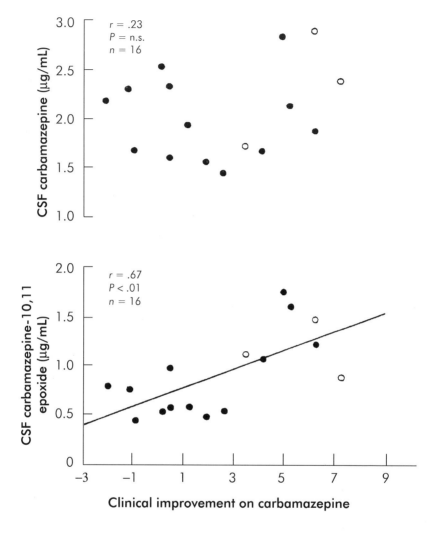

Figure 13–5.   Degree of clinical improvement in mood disorders is correlated with cerebrospinal fluid (CSF) levels of carbamazepine-10-11-epoxide, but not with CSF levels of carbamazepine itself. Closed circles indicate depressed patients, and open circles indicate manic patients. n.s. = not significant.

Source.   Reprinted from Post RM, Uhde TW, Ballenger JC, et al: "Carbamazepine and Its -10-11-Epoxide Metabolite in Plasma and CSF: Relationship to Antidepressant Response. *Archives of General Psychiatry* 40:673–676, 1983a.

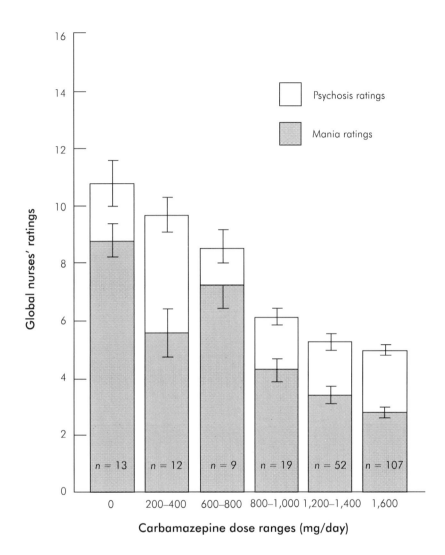

Figure 13–6. Dose-dependent antimanic and antipsychotic effects of carbamazepine in an individual patient during a prolonged manic episode. Numbers at bottoms of columns indicate numbers of days in various dosage ranges.

Source. Reprinted from Post RM, Ballenger JC, Uhde TW, et al: "Efficacy of Carbamazepine in Manic-Depressive Illness: Implications for Underlying Mechanisms," in *Neurobiology of Mood Disorders.* Edited by Post RM, Ballenger J. Baltimore, MD, Williams & Wilkins, 1984a, pp 777–816. Used with permission.

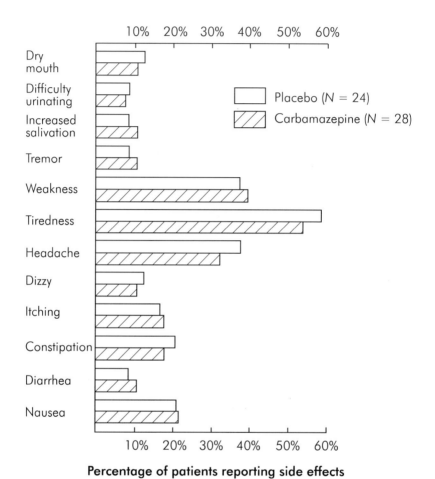

Figure 13-7. Side effects during carbamazepine treatment versus placebo in depressed patients.
Source. Reprinted from Ketter TA, Post RM: "Clinical Pharmacology and Pharmacokinetics of Carbamazepine," in *Anticonvulsants in Psychiatry.* Edited by Joffe RT, Calabrese JR. New York, Marcel Dekker, 1994, pp 147–187. By courtesy of Marcel Dekker, Inc. Used with permission.

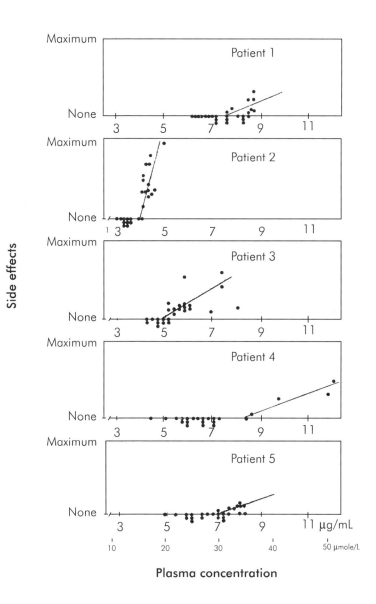

Figure 13–8.   Comparison of side-effects thresholds and slopes as a function of plasma drug concentration in individual patients. *Source.*   Adapted with permission from Tomson T: "Interdosage Fluctuations in Plasma Carbamazepine Concentration Determine Intermittent Side Effects." *Archives of Neurology* 41:830–834, 1984. Used with permission. Copyright 1984, American Medical Association.

general, CBZ should be discontinued if the white blood count falls below $2,000–3,000/mm^3$ or the absolute neutrophil count falls below $1,000/mm^3$. In the instance of benign leukopenia, the addition of lithium will increase the neutrophil count back toward normal (Kramlinger and Post 1990), but this strategy is not likely to be helpful for suppression of the red blood cell count, which is likely to be indicative of a more problematic process.

Similarly, because hepatitis can occur, patients should be advised to seek medical evaluation immediately if they develop malaise, abdominal pain, or other gastrointestinal symptoms. In general, CBZ is discontinued if liver function tests exceed three times the upper limit of the normal range.

Hypersensitivity reactions such as rashes are not uncommon (occurring in 10%–15% of patients), and patients should be instructed to seek a medical evaluation if they develop a rash. CBZ is generally discontinued if a rash occurs, because it can progress from a benign process to a more severe one that can include exfoliative dermatitis or Stevens-Johnson syndrome, which is potentially life threatening. However, in some patients with mood disorders refractory to all medications except CBZ, a repeat trial of CBZ with a course of prednisone in an effort to provide desensitization can be considered (Murphy et al. 1991; Vick 1983). If there is evidence of systemic allergy, fever, or malaise, prednisone cotreatment is less likely to be helpful. A substantial number of patients with CBZ-induced rashes may not have a rash on reexposure (even without prednisone coverage), but should a rash again develop, it usually appears more rapidly than the first occurrence. In view of these problems, CBZ is generally contraindicated in patients with histories of marrow suppression of hypersensitivity to CBZ or tricyclic antidepressants.

CBZ is teratogenic and is associated with low birth weight, craniofacial deformities, and spina bifida (Jones et al. 1989; Rosa 1991). Because it is present in breast milk, its use is generally avoided in pregnant women or breast-feeding mothers. In rare patients with severe mood disorders, clinicians may determine in consultation with a gynecologist that the benefits of treating with CBZ outweigh the risks as compared with other treatment options (Sitland-Marken et al. 1989).

▶ CBZ Pharmacokinetics and Drug Interactions

Patients with mood disorders often require treatment with more than one medication. The pharmacokinetic properties of CBZ are atypical among medications prescribed by psychiatrists and necessitate special care when treating patients concurrently with other medications (Ketter et al. 1991a, 1991b). In the past, mechanistic models were lacking to explain the diverse categories of drugs noted clinically to have interactions with CBZ.

Recent advances in molecular pharmacology characterizing the specific cytochrome P450 isoforms responsible for metabolism of CBZ and various other medications may allow the development of such mechanistic models (von Moltke et al. 1994).

Cytochrome P450 isoforms are specified in the format $CYPnXm$, where CYP denotes cytochrome P450, n the gene family number, X the gene subfamily letter, and m the gene number. In general, cytochromes within families have greater than 40% homology and within subfamilies have greater than 55% homology. Genes within subfamilies are clustered together on chromosomes. In humans, the majority of medications are metabolized by two isoforms, CYP2D6 and CYP3A4. Much attention has been focused on CYP2D6 because of to its role in the 2-hydroxylation of tricyclic antidepressants and increased tricyclic levels observed because of CYP2D6 inhibition by selective serotonin reuptake inhibitors (SSRIs) (Brosen and Kragh-Sorensen 1993). However, the CYP3A subfamily appears to be much more abundant in the human liver, representing more than 50% of total CYP in some samples (Gonzalez 1993). The isoform CYP3A4 appears particularly important as it mediates metabolism of a wide variety of medications, steroids, and carcinogens (Brian et al. 1990; Renaud et al. 1990). Thus, depending on their individual affinities and susceptibilities to induction or inhibition effects, substrates of CYP3A4 are at risk for kinetic interactions with a wide variety of drugs and steroids. Evidence suggests that the main metabolic pathway of CBZ (to its 10,11-epoxide) is mediated primarily by CYP3A4, with a minor contribution by CYP2C8 (Kerr et al. 1994).

These new molecular biochemical findings can be integrated with older clinical observations to begin to derive a mechanistic understanding of CBZ drug interactions. Three major principles (*A*, *B*, and *C*) make the effects of CBZ on the plasma levels of other drugs and the effects of other drugs on CBZ plasma levels more easily comprehensible.

A.   CBZ is a potent inducer of catabolic enzymes (including CYP3A4) and decreases the plasma levels of many medications, including CBZ itself (Rapeport et al. 1983).   Concurrent treatment with certain enzyme inducers can yield decreases in plasma CBZ levels and results in loss of CBZ efficacy (Figure 13–9, top left; Table 13–3, middle right). As mentioned, doses of CBZ not initially tolerated because of side effects will often be accepted after several weeks when induction of CBZ metabolism becomes prominent (Cereghino 1975).

B.   CBZ metabolism (which is primarily by CYP3A4) can be inhibited by certain enzyme inhibitors, yielding increases in plasma CBZ levels and CBZ intoxication (Figure 13–9, bottom left; Table 13–3, top right). If a patient is just below his or her side-effect threshold, the addition of drugs that inhibit CBZ metabolism (such as erythromycin, verapamil, or fluoxetine) may induce toxicity.

C.   CBZ has an active epoxide (CBZ-E) metabolite.   Because the active metabolite CBZ-E can yield therapeutic and adverse effects similar to those of CBZ (Pisani et al. 1987) and is not detected in conventional CBZ assays, the unwary clinician may misinterpret the significance of therapeutic or adverse effects associated with low or moderate plasma CBZ levels. With enzyme induction and certain drug interactions, the CBZ/CBZ-E plasma ratio decreases, and the potential for confounding effects of the "occult" CBZ-E increases.

In addition, CBZ and CBZ-E are bound to albumin, but not extensively, so that drug interactions due to binding are rare (Fleitman et al. 1980; Hooper et al. 1975; Lunde et al. 1970), with the important exception that valproic acid displaces CBZ from plasma proteins (Macphee et al. 1988; Moreland et al. 1984). This displacement results in an increase in free CBZ, which in combination with valproate-induced increases in CBZ-E can yield toxicity when utilizing CBZ-plus-valproate combination therapy.

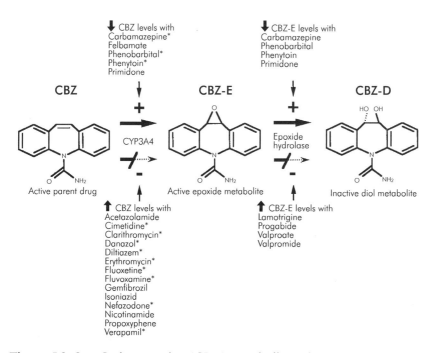

Figure 13–9. Carbamazepine (CBZ) metabolism. CBE-E = carbamazepine-10-11-epoxide. CBZ-D = carbamazepine-10,11-dihydro-dihydroxide. CYP3A4 = cytochrome P450 3A4 isoform. Asterisk indicates that molecular biochemical evidence supports CYP3A4. *Source.* Adapted from Ketter TA, Post RM, Worthington K: "Principles of Clinically Important Drug Interactions With Carbamazepine: Part I." *Journal of Clinical Psychopharmacology* 11:198–203, 1991a. Used with permission.

▶ CBZ INTERACTIONS WITH PSYCHOTROPIC DRUGS

CBZ has clinically significant drug interactions with various psychotropic drugs. (A more detailed review can be found in Ketter et al. 1991a, 1991b.)

Antidepressants

Care must be taken in the use of antidepressants in bipolar patients, because these agents have the potential to induce mania and rapid

Table 13–3. Carbamazepine (CBZ) drug interactions

CBZ → ↓ drug	Drug → ↑ CBZ
Alprazolam (?) 3A4ind(?)	**Acetazolamide**
Amitriptyline 3A4ind(?)	Baclofen (?)
Bupropion	Cimetidine 3A4inh
Clobazam 3A4ind(?)	**Clarithromycin** 3A4inh
Clomipramine (?)	**Danazol** 3A4inh(?)
Clonazepam 3A4ind	**Dextropropoxyphene**
Clozapine[a]	**Diltiazem** 3A4inh
Cyclosporine (?) 3A4ind	**Erythromycin** 3A4inh
Desipramine (?)	**Fluoxetine**
Dexamethasone (false-positive	Flurithromycin 3A4inh
dexamethasone suppression test)	**Fluvoxamine**
3A4ind	Gemfibrozil
Dicumarol (?)	**Isoniazid**
Doxacurium	Josamycin 3A4inh
Doxepin 3A4ind(?)	Lamotrigine (↑ CBZ-E[?])
Doxycycline	EHinh(?)
Ethosuximide 3A4ind	**Nefazodone** 3A4inh
Felbamate	Nicotinamide
Felodipine 3A4ind	Ponsinomycin 3A4inh
Fentanyl	**Propoxyphene**
Fluphenazine (?)	Terfenadine (↑ free CBZ[?])
Haloperidol	3A4inh
Hormonal contraceptives 3A4ind	**Triacetyloleandomycin** 3A4inh
Imidazole antifungals (?) 3A4ind	**Valproate** (↑ CBZ-E, ↑ free CBZ,
Imipramine 3A4ind	↑/↓/= CBZ) EHinh
Lamotrigine	**Verapamil** 3A4inh
Methadone	**Viloxazine**
Methylprednisolone 3A4ind	
Mianserin	Drug → ↓ CBZ
Nimodipine (?) 3A4ind	Adriamycin and cisplatin (?)
Nortriptyline (?)	**CBZ (autoinduction)** 3A4ind
Olanzapine	**Felbamate**
Oxiracetam (?)	Isoretinoin (?)
Pancuronium	**Phenobarbital** 3A4ind
Phenytoin (↓/↑/=)	**Phenytoin** 3A4ind
Prednisolone 3A4ind	**Primidone**
Praziquantel	Valproate (↑/↓/= CBZ)
Primidone	
Theophylline	CBZ → ↑ drug
Thiothixene (?)	False-negative pregnancy test
Valproate	Phenytoin (→/↑/=)
Vecuronium	
Warfarin 3A4ind	*(continued)*

Table 13–3.   Carbamazepine (CBZ) drug interactions *(continued)*

Note.   **Bold type** indicates risk of important drug inefficacy or CBZ intoxication. 3A4ind = CYP3A4 induction. 3A4inh = CYP3A4 inhibition. EHinh = epoxide hydrolase inhibition. ↑ = increased. ↓ = decreased. Equal sign = unchanged. (?) = slight or contradictory evidence.
[a]Combination with CBZ not advised due to risk of agranulocytosis.
Source.   Adapted from Ketter TA, Post RM, Worthington K: "Principles of Clinically Important Drug Interactions With Carbamazepine: Part 1." *Journal of Clinical Psychopharmacology* 11:198–203, 1991a. Used with permission.

cycling (Wehr et al. 1988). In general, antidepressants should be added to mood stabilizers and not used in monotherapy in bipolar patients, and antidepressant treatment-emergent mania or rapid cycling is an indication for discontinuation of the implicated agent. CBZ appears to induce the metabolism of tricyclic antidepressants, including amitriptyline (Leinonen et al. 1991), desipramine (Baldessarini et al. 1988), doxepin (Leinonen et al. 1991), and clomipramine (De la Fuente and Mendlewicz 1992); therefore, if patients fail to respond to standard doses of tricyclic antidepressants, tricyclic antidepressant and metabolite levels should be checked.

Case reports (Joffe et al. 1985; Yatham et al. 1990) and a series of 10 patients on our clinical research unit suggest that the addition of phenelzine or tranylcypromine to CBZ may be well tolerated, does not affect CBZ pharmacokinetics, and may provide relief of refractory depressive symptoms in some patients (Ketter et al. 1995a).

Patients receiving CBZ and bupropion have extremely low plasma bupropion levels and high hydroxybupropion (metabolite) levels (Ketter et al. 1992). The clinical impact of this dramatic decrease in the bupropion/hydroxybupropion ratio remains to be explored, but we have observed successful combination of CBZ and bupropion in many individuals, suggesting that it is not necessarily problematic.

Fluoxetine, fluvoxamine, and nefazodone (but not sertraline or paroxetine) may increase CBZ levels and cause clinical toxicity, possibly by inhibition of CYP3A4, rather than by inhibition of CYP2D6 or CYP1A2.

Antipsychotics

CBZ can be used effectively in combination with antipsychotics, although clinicians should be aware of potential drug interactions. CBZ increases haloperidol metabolism (Ereshefsky et al. 1986; Jann et al. 1989; Kahn et al. 1990), dramatically lowering its levels in the blood. There is weaker evidence that CBZ may increase the metabolism of other antipsychotic agents, including fluphenazine (Ereshefsky et al. 1986; Jann et al. 1989) and thiothixene (Ereshefsky et al. 1986), and that loxapine, chlorpromazine, and amoxapine may increase CBZ-E levels (Pitterle and Collins 1988). Also, animal studies suggest that promazine, chlorpromazine, perazine, chlorprothixene, and flupentixol may increase CBZ levels (Daniel et al. 1992). In view of these interactions, plasma antipsychotic medication levels should be checked if patients fail to respond to standard doses of antipsychotic agents during combined therapy with CBZ. As described in Chapter 15 of this volume, clozapine may be effective in the treatment of bipolar disorder. Combination of clozapine with CBZ is not recommended in view of the possibility of synergistic bone marrow suppression (Mehta 1997). However, these drugs have been used in combination in some European centers, one of which reported that CBZ decreases clozapine (a CYP1A2 and CYP2D6 substrate [Fischer et al. 1992]) levels (Raitasuo et al. 1993). Thus, clinicians wishing to combine a psychotropic anticonvulsant with clozapine should consider valproic acid rather than CBZ, except under unusual circumstances.

Benzodiazepines

High-potency anticonvulsant benzodiazepines, such as clonazepam or lorazepam, should be used in preference to others, because limited evidence implicates alprazolam and possibly even clorazepate in the induction of mania (Cole and Kando 1993). Although in general CBZ can be used effectively with these medications, CBZ may decrease plasma levels of clonazepam (Lai et al. 1978), alprazolam (Arana et al. 1988), and the anticonvulsant clobazam (Levy et al. 1983). CBZ-induced decreases in some benzodiazepine levels could be mediated by induction of CYP3A4.

Calcium-Channel Blockers

Clinicians should be aware of drug interactions between CBZ and these agents (especially with the nondihydropyridines) to provide optimal combination therapy. Enzyme-inducing anticonvulsants like CBZ appear to decrease nimodipine (Tartara et al. 1991) and felodipine (Capewell et al. 1988; Zaccara et al. 1993) levels, presumably by induction of CYP3A4, because this isoform mediates metabolism of nimodipine, felodipine, nifedipine, and nicardipine, as well as a variety of other dihydropyridines (Guengerich et al. 1991).

In addition, verapamil appears to be metabolized by CYP3A4 (Kroemer et al. 1993), and diltiazem metabolism also appears to occur within the CYP3A family (Pichard et al. 1990). Of clear clinical importance, elevated plasma CBZ levels and neurotoxicity have been reported during concurrent treatment with the nondihydropyridines verapamil and diltiazem, but not the dihydropyridine nifedipine (Brodie and Macphee 1986; Price and DiMarzio 1988).

Lithium

Lithium is a classic and traditional therapy of mania, and its use is described in Chapter 12 of this volume. However, lithium monotherapy can often result in inadequate efficacy. Thus, the combination of CBZ plus lithium is frequently used in bipolar disorder and may provide additive or synergistic antimanic (Kramlinger and Post 1989a) and antidepressant (Kramlinger and Post 1989b) effects. The combination is generally well tolerated, with merely additive neurotoxicity (McGinness et al. 1990), which can be minimized by gradual dose escalation. Pharmacokinetic interactions between these drugs do not occur, because lithium is excreted by the kidney with no hepatic metabolism. Also, CBZ will not reverse lithium-induced diabetes insipidus, but lithium may attenuate CBZ-induced hyponatremia (Klein 1987; Vieweg et al. 1987).

Thyroid Hormones

The thyroid-stimulating hormone response to thyrotropin-releasing hormone is blunted (Joffe et al. 1986) or unaltered (Connell et al.

1984) with CBZ therapy. However, clinical hypothyroidism during treatment with CBZ has been reported in only two patients (Aanderud and Strandjord 1980), despite use of CBZ in several hundred thousand neurological and psychiatric patients.

Valproate

As described in Chapter 14 of this volume, valproic acid appears effective in the treatment of mood disorders (McElroy et al. 1989). Several reports suggest that, in psychiatric patients, the combination of CBZ and valproic acid is not only tolerated but may show psychotropic synergy (Keck et al. 1992; Ketter et al. 1995b; Tohen et al. 1994). However, the effective use of these two medications together requires a thorough knowledge of their drug interactions.

As a general rule, clinicians should carefully monitor patients taking the combination of CBZ and valproic acid for side effects and consider decreasing the CBZ dose in advance (because of the expected displacement of CBZ from plasma proteins and increase in CBZ-E) and ultimately increasing the valproic acid dose (because of expected CBZ-induced decrements in valproic acid).

▌ CBZ INTERACTIONS WITH OTHER DRUGS

Drug interactions between CBZ and other (nonpsychotropic) drugs are also of substantial clinical importance. Many patients require long-term prophylactic CBZ treatment, during which emergent medical problems can result in the addition of other medications that may have drug interactions with CBZ. An overview of these interactions by drug category is included Table 13–3. For a review of these interactions, see Ketter et al. (1991a, 1991b).

▌ CONCLUSION

Lithium, CBZ, and valproic acid are the primary mood stabilizers used to treat bipolar disorder. Multiple factors, including phenomenology, family history, concurrent medications, medical status, and past history of therapeutic and adverse effects of psychotropics, influence the

Table 13-4. Suggestions for carbamazepine (CBZ) therapy

Getting started

Advise patient of signs and symptoms of common dose-related adverse effects and drug interactions.

Advise patient of signs and symptoms of hematological, hepatic, and allergic reactions.

Obtain baseline complete blood count, differential, liver function tests (± electrocardiogram if indicated).

Monitor toxicity clinically (± laboratories as indicated).

Discontinue if: rash, white blood cells < 2,000–3,000, neutrophils < 1,000, or liver function tests > 3 × upper limit of normal.

Dosage titration

In acute mania, start with 400–800 mg/day and ↑ by 200 mg/day q 2–4 days.

In less acute situations, start with 200–400 mg/day and ↑ by 200 mg/day q 4–7 days.

↑ dose clinically until therapeutic effect or supervening adverse effects.

↓ dose, spread out dose, or ↑ dose more gradually if adverse effects arise.

In first month, ↑ doses need to compensate for autoinduction.

Ultimate doses 600–2,000 mg/day in divided doses, with blood levels 4–12 µg/mL.

Combination therapy in general

May need to titrate doses of CBZ and other drugs more gradually to avoid adverse effects.

May need to lower peak doses of CBZ and concurrent drugs to avoid adverse effects.

Be alert for drugs that ↑ CBZ levels and yield toxicity (e.g., erythromycin, verapamil).

Check levels of CBZ (± CBZ-E, ± free CBZ), and concurrent drugs if toxicity occurs.

Be alert for CBZ ↓ ing levels of drugs and yielding inefficacy (e.g., contraceptives, warfarin).

Check levels of concurrent drugs if inefficacy occurs.

Combined with antidepressants

Tricyclics: Expect ↓ tricyclic levels, ↑ tricyclic metabolite levels.

Phenelzine, tranylcypromine: No pharmacokinetic interactions, combination tolerated (preliminary).

Bupropion: Expect ↓ bupropion levels, ↑ bupropion metabolite levels.

Fluoxetine, fluvoxamine, nefazodone: Expect ↑ CBZ levels.

(continued)

Table 13–4. Suggestions for carbamazepine (CBZ) therapy *(continued)*

Combined with antipsychotics
Haloperidol: Expect ↓ haloperidol levels. Therapeutic synergy?
Fluphenazine, thiothixine, and others: Expect ↓ antipsychotic levels?
Clozapine: **Not recommended due to agranulocytosis risk.**
 Expect ↓ clozapine levels.
Olanzapine: Expect ↓ olanzapine levels.

Combined with anxiolytics
Alprazolam, clonazepam: Expect ↓ anxiolytic levels.

Combined with calcium-channel blockers
Diltiazem, verapamil: Expect ↑↑ CBZ levels.
Nifedipine, nimodipine: No effect on CBZ levels. Expect ↓ nimodipine levels.

Combined with lithium
No pharmacokinetic interactions. Additive therapeutic effects.
Additive adverse effects (neurotoxicity, gastrointestinal, teratogenicity, antithyroid).
Opposing adverse effects (white blood cells, renal).

Combined with valproic acid
↓ CBZ dose (expect ↑ free CBZ and CBZ-E levels). ↑ valproate dose (expect ↓ valproate levels).
Additive adverse effects (neurotoxicity, hepatotoxicity, gastrointestinal, teratogenicity)?
Additive therapeutic effects?

Note. ↑ = increase, increased; ↓ = decrease, decreased. VPA = valproic acid.
Source. Adapted from Ketter TA, Post RM: "Clinical Pharmacology and Pharmacokinetics of Carbamazepine," in *Anticonvulsants in Psychiatry.* Edited by Joffe RT, Calabrese JR. New York, Marcel Dekker, 1994, pp. 147–187. By courtesy of Marcel Dekker, Inc. Used with permission.

choice of medication in individual patients. As CBZ is increasingly used in bipolar disorder and various other psychiatric disorders, as well as seizure and paroxysmal pain disorders, it is important for clinicians to be aware of its pharmacology and potential interactions with other drugs.

CBZ's complex pharmacology is more comprehensible in the context of the principles outlined in this chapter. Common problems with combination therapy include CBZ induction of metabolism of some drugs (such as hormonal contraceptives), undermining their efficacy; and other drugs (such as erythromycin or verapamil) inhibiting CBZ metabolism, causing CBZ toxicity. Knowledge of CBZ metabolism, as summarized in Figure 13–9, will aid in understanding the nature of interactions that involve its induction or inhibition. Important interactions discussed in this chapter and presented in bold type in Table 13–3 provide an outline to guide successful therapeutics. Instructing patients to alert their other caregivers that they are receiving CBZ may help avoid drug interactions. Informing patients of several of the common interactions can further assist in the warning process; other practitioners may inadvertently introduce commonly used drugs, such as erythromycin and nondihydropyridine calcium-channel blockers, with their attendant risks of toxicity.

Adjusting CBZ doses in anticipation of drug interactions or according to side effects will often alleviate problems and help to decrease the need for monitoring blood CBZ levels. Adjustments of doses of other agents such as birth control pills may also be necessary. Table 13–4 provides a summary of suggestions for CBZ therapy. Knowledge of CBZ pharmacology, pharmacokinetics, and drug interactions as described in this chapter is helpful for the safe and effective use of CBZ in bipolar disorder.

▶ REFERENCES

Aanderud S, Strandjord RE: Hypothyroidism induced by anti-epileptic therapy. Acta Neurol Scand 61:330–332, 1980

Arana GW, Epstein S, Molloy M, et al: Carbamazepine-induced reduction of plasma alprazolam concentrations: a clinical case report. J Clin Psychiatry 49:448–449, 1988

Baldessarini RJ, Teicher MH, Cassidy JW, et al: Anticonvulsant cotreatment may increase toxic metabolites of antidepressants and other psychotropic drugs (letter). J Clin Psychopharmacol 8:381–382, 1988

Ballenger JC, Post RM: Therapeutic effects of carbamazepine in affective illness: a preliminary report. Communications in Psychopharmacology 2:159–175, 1978

Bellaire W, Demish K, SToll KD: Carbamazepine versus lithium in prophylaxis of recurrent affective disorder (abstract). Psychopharmacology (Berlin) 96:287, 1988

Brian WR, Sari MA, Iwasaki M, et al: Catalytic activities of human liver cytochrome P-450 IIIA4 expressed in Saccharomyces cerevisiae. Biochemistry 29:1280–1292, 1990

Brodie MJ, Macphee GJ: Carbamazepine neurotoxicity precipitated by diltiazem. BMJ 292:1170–1171, 1986

Brosen K, Kragh-Sorensen P: Concomitant intake of nortriptyline and carbamazepine. Ther Drug Monit 15:258–260, 1993

Brown D, Silverstone T, Cookson J: Carbamazepine compared to haloperidol in acute mania. Int Clin Psychopharmacol 4:229–238, 1989

Cabrera JF, Muhlbauer HD, Schley J, et al: Long-term randomized clinical trial of oxcarbazepine vs lithium in bipolar and schizoaffective disorders: preliminary results. Pharmacopsychiatry 19:282–283, 1986

Capewell S, Freestone S, Critchley JA, et al: Reduced felodipine bioavailability in patients taking anticonvulsants. Lancet 2:480–482, 1988

Cereghino JJ: Serum carbamazepine concentration and clinical control, in Advances in Neurology. Edited by Penry JK, Daly DD. New York, Raven, 1975, pp 309–330

Cole JO, Kando JC: Adverse behavioral events reported in patients taking alprazolam and other benzodiazepines. J Clin Psychiatry 54:49–61, 1993

Connell JM, Rapeport WG, Gordon S, et al: Changes in circulating thyroid hormones during short-term hepatic enzyme induction with carbamazepine. Eur J Clin Pharmacol 26:453–456, 1984

Coxhead N, Silverstone T, Cookson J: Carbamazepine versus lithium in the prophylaxis of bipolar affective disorder. Acta Psychiatr Scand 85:114–118, 1992

Daniel W, Janczar L, Danek L, et al: Pharmacokinetic interaction between carbamazepine and neuroleptics after combined prolonged treatment in rats. Naunyn Schmiedebergs Arch Pharmacol 345:598–605, 1992

de la Fuente JM, Mendlewicz J: Carbamazepine addition in tricyclic antidepressant-resistant unipolar depression. Biol Psychiatry 32:369–374, 1992

Desai NG, Gangadhas BN, Channabasavanna SM, et al: Carbamazepine hastens therapeutic action on lithium in mania (abstract). Proceedings of the International Conference on New Directions in Affective Disorders, 1987, p 97

Di Costanzo E, Schifano F: Lithium alone or in combination with carbamazepine for the treatment of rapid-cycling bipolar affective disorder. Acta Psychiatr Scand 83:456–459, 1991

Elphick M, Lyons F, Cowen PJ: Low tolerability of carbamazepine in psychiatric patients may restrict its clinical usefulness. J Psychopharmacol 2:1–4, 1988

Emrich HM: Studies with (Trileptal) oxcarbazepine in acute mania. Int Clin Psychopharmacol 5:83–88, 1990

Emrich HM, Dose M, von Zerssen D: The use of sodium valproate, carbamazepine, and oxcarbazepine in patients with affective disorders. J Affect Disord 8:243–250, 1985

Ereshefsky L, Jann MW, Saklad SR, et al: Bioavailability of psychotropic drugs: historical perspective and pharmacokinetic overview. J Clin Psychiatry 47:6–15, 1986

Fischer V, Vogels B, Maurer G, et al: The antipsychotic clozapine is metabolized by the polymorphic human microsomal and recombinant cytochrome P450 2D6. J Pharmacol Exp Ther 260:1355–1360, 1992

Fleitman JS, Bruni J, Perrin JH, et al: Albumin-binding interactions of sodium valproate. J Clin Pharmacol 20:514–517, 1980

Goncalves N, Stoll KD: Carbamazepine in manic syndromes: a controlled double-blind study. Nervenarzt 56:43–47, 1985

Gonzalez FJ: Cytochrome P450 in humans, in Cytochrome P450, Vol 105. Edited by Schenkman JB, Greim H. Berlin, Springer-Verlag, 1993, pp 239–257

Grossi E, Sacchetti E, Vita A, et al: Carbamazepine versus chlorpromazine in mania: a double-blind trial, in Anticonvulsants in Affective Disorders. Edited by Emrich HM, Okuma T, Müller AA. Amsterdam, Netherlands, Excerpta Medica, 1984, pp 77–187

Guengerich FP, Brian WR, Iwasaki M, et al: Oxidation of dihydropyridine calcium channel blockers and analogues by human liver cytochrome P-450 111A4. J Med Chem 34:1838–1844, 1991

Himmelhoch JM: Cerebral dysrhythmia, substance abuse, and the nature of secondary affective illness. Psychiatric Annals 17:710–727, 1987

Hooper WD, Dubetz DK, Bochner F, et al: Plasma protein binding of carbamazepine. Clin Pharmacol Ther 17:433–440, 1975

Jann MW, Fidone GS, Hernandez JM, et al: Clinical implications of increased antipsychotic plasma condentrations upon anticonvulsant cessation. Psychiatry Res 28:153–159, 1989

Joffe RT, Post RM, Uhde TW: Lack of pharmacokinetic interaction of carbamazepine with tranylcypromine (letter). Arch Gen Psychiatry 42:738, 1985

Joffe RT, Post RM, Ballenger JC, et al: Neuroendocrine effects of carbamazepine in patients with affective illness. Epilepsia 27:156–160, 1986

Jones KL, Lacro RV, Johnson KA, et al: Pattern of malformations in the children of women treated with carbamazepine during pregnancy. N Engl J Med 320:1661–1666, 1989

Kahn EM, Schulz SC, Perel JM, et al: Change in haloperidol level due to carbamazepine: a complicating factor in combined medication for schizophrenia. J Clin Psychopharmacol 10:54–57, 1990

Keck PE Jr, McElroy SL, Vuckovic A, et al: Combined valproate and carbamazepine treatment of bipolar disorder. J Neuropsychiatry Clin Neurosci 4:319–322, 1992
Keck PE Jr, McElroy SL, Tugrul KC, et al: Valproate oral loading in the
treatment of acute mania. J Clin Psychiatry 54:305–308, 1993
Kerr BM, Thummel KE, Wurden CJ, et al: Human liver carbamazepine metabolism: role of CYP3A4 and CYP2C8 in 10,11-epoxide formation.
Biochem Pharmacol 47:1969–1979, 1994
Ketter TA, Post RM: Clinical pharmacology and pharmacokinetics of carbamazepine, in Anticonvulsants in Psychiatry. Edited by Joffe RT,
Calabrese JR. New York, Marcel Dekker, 1994, pp 147–187
Ketter TA, Post RM, Worthington K: Principles of clinically important drug
interactions with carbamazepine, part 1. J Clin Psychopharmacol
11:198–203, 1991a
Ketter TA, Post RM, Worthington K: Principles of clinically important drug
interactions with carbamazepine, part II. J Clin Psychopharmacol
11:306–313, 1991b
Ketter TA, Barnett J, Schroeder DH, et al: Carbamazepine induces bupropion metabolism (abstract NR 563). 145th Annual Meeting of the
American Psychiatric Association, Washington, DC, May 2–7, 1992
Ketter TA, Post RM, Parekh PI, et al: Addition of monoamine oxidase inhibitors to carbamazepine: preliminary evidence of safety and antidepressant efficacy in treatment-resistant deprssion. J Clin Psychiatry
56:471–475, 1995a
Ketter TA, Jenkins JB, Schroeder DH, et al: Carbamazepine but not valproate induces bupropion metabolism. J Clin Psychopharmacol 15:327–
333, 1995b
Kishimoto A, Okuma T: Antimanic and prophylactic effects of carbamazepine in affective disorders (abstract 506.4). 4th World Congress of Biological Psychiatry, September 8–13, 1985, p 363
Klein EM: Lithium and carbamazepine therapy in a patient with manic depressive illness: clinical effects, interactions and side effects. Isr J Psychiatry Relat Sci 24:295–298, 1987
Klein E, Bental E, Lerer B, et al: Carbamazepine and haloperidol v placebo
and haloperidol in excited psychoses: a controlled study. Arch Gen Psychiatry 41:165–170, 1984
Kramlinger KG, Post RM: Adding lithium carbonate to carbamazepine: antimanic efficacy in treatment-resistant mania. Acta Psychiatr Scand
79:378–385, 1989a
Kramlinger KG, Post RM: The addition of lithium to carbamazepine. antidepressant efficacy in treatment-resistant depression. Arch Gen Psychiatry 46:794–800, 1989b

Kramlinger KG, Post RM: Addition of lithium carbonate to carbamazepine: hematological and thyroid effects. Am J Psychiatry 147:615–620, 1990

Kroemer HK, Gautier JC, Beaune P, et al: Identification of P450 enzymes involved in metabolism of verapamil in humans. Naunyn Schmiedebergs Arch Pharmacol 348:332–337, 1993

Lai AA, Levy RH, Cutler RE: Time-course of interaction between carbamazepine and clonazepam in normal man. Clin Pharmacol Ther 24:316–323, 1978

Leinonen E, Lillsunde P, Laukkanen V, et al: Effects of carbamazepine on serum antidepressant concentrations in psychiatric patients. J Clin Psychopharmacol 11:313–318, 1991

Lenzi A, Lazzerini F, Grossi E, et al: Use of carbamazepine in acute psychosis: a controlled study. J Int Med Res 14:78–84, 1986

Lerer B, Moore N, Meyendorff E, et al: Carbamazepine versus lithium in mania: a double-blind study. J Clin Psychiatry 48:89–93, 1987

Levy RH, Lane EA, Guyot M, et al: Analysis of parent drug-metabolite relationship in the presence of an inducer: application to the carbamazepine-clobazam interaction in normal man. Drug Metab Dispos 11:286–292, 1983

Lunde PK, Rane A, Yaffe SJ, et al: Plasma protein binding of diphenylhydantoin in man. Interaction with other drugs and the effect of temperature and plasma dilution. Clin Pharmacol Ther 11:846–855, 1970

Lusznat RM, Murphy DP, Nunn CM: Carbamazepine vs lithium in the treatment and prophylaxis of mania. Br J Psychiatry 153:198–204, 1988

Macphee GJ, Mitchell JR, Wiseman L, et al: Effect of sodium valproate on carbamazepine disposition and psychomotor profile in man. Br J Clin Pharmacol 25:59–66, 1988b

McElroy SL, Keck PE Jr, Pope HG Jr, et al: Valproate in psychiatric disorders: literature review and clinical guidelines. J Clin Psychiatry 50:23–29, 1989

McGinness J, Kishimoto A, Hollister LE: Avoiding neurotoxicity with lithium-carbamazepine combinations. Psychopharmacol Bull 26:181–184, 1990

Mehta M: Physicians Desk Reference, 51st Edition. Montvale, NJ, Medical Economics, 1997

Meyer MC, Straughn AB, Jarvi EJ, et al: The bioinequivalence of carbamazepine tablets with a history of clinical failures. Pharm Res 9:1612–1616, 1992

Möller HJ, Kissling W, Riehl T, et al: Doubleblind evaluation of the antimanic properties of carbamazepine as a comedication to haloperidol. Prog Neuropsychopharmacol Biol Psychiatry 13:127–136, 1989

Moreland TA, Chang SL, Levy RH: Mechanisms of interaction between sodium valproate and carbamazepine in the rhesus monkey and in the isolated perfused rat liver, in Metabolism of Antiepileptic Drugs. Edited by Levy RH et al. New York, Raven, 1984, pp 53–60

Mosolov SN: Comparative effectiveness of preventive use of lithium carbonate, carbamazepine and sodium valproate in affective and schizoaffective psychoses. Zh Nevropatol Psikhiatr 91:78–83, 1991

Müller AA, Stoll KD: Carbamazepine and oxcarbazepine in the treatment of manic syndromes: studies in Germany, in Anticonvulsants in Affective Disorders. Edited by Emrich HM, Okuma T, Müller AA. Amsterdam, Netherlands, Excerpta Medica, 1984, pp 139–147

Murphy JM, Mashman J, Miller JD, et al: Suppression of carbamazepine-induced rash with prednisone. Neurology 41:144–145, 1991

Nightingale SL: From the Food and Drug Administration. JAMA 263:1896, 1990

Okuma T: Therapeutic and prophylactic effects of carbamazepine in bipolar disorders. Psychiatr Clin North Am 6:157–174, 1983

Okuma T: Effects of carbamazepine and lithium on affective disorders. Neuropsychobiology 27:138–145, 1993

Okuma T, Inanaga K, Otsuki S, et al: Comparison of the antimanic efficacy of carbamazepine and chlorpromazine: a double-blind controlled study. Psychopharmacology (Berlin) 66:211–217, 1979

Okuma T, Inanaga K, Otsuki S, et al: A preliminary double-blind study on the efficacy of carbamazepine in prophylaxis of manic-depressive illness. Psychopharmacology (Berlin) 73:95–96, 1981

Okuma T, Yamashita I, Takahashi R, et al: Double-blind controlled studies on the therapeutic efficacy of carbamazepine in affective and schizophrenic patients. (Abstract of paper presented at 16th Congress of CINP [Collegium Internationale Neuro-Psychopharmacologicum].) Psychopharmacology (Berlin), abstract TH18.05 (96–102), 1988

Okuma T, Yamashita I, Takahashi R, et al: Comparison of the antimanic efficacy of carbamazepine and lithium carbonate by double-blind controlled study. Pharmacopsychiatry 23:143–150, 1990

Pichard L, Gillet G, Fabre I, et al: Identification of the rabbit and human cytochromes P-450111A as the major enzymes involved in the N-demethylation of diltiazem. Drug Metab Dispos 18:711–719, 1990

Pisani F, Fazio A, Oteri G, et al: Differential interactions of valproic acid and valproamide with carbamazepine in humans, in Advances in Epileptology, Vol 16. Edited by Wolf P, Dam M, Janz F, et al. New York, Raven, 1987, pp 431–433

Pitterle ME, Collins DM: Carbamazepine-10-11-epoxide elevation associated with coadministration of loxapine or amoxapine (abstract). Epilepsia 39:654, 1988

Placidi GF, Lenzi A, Lazzerini F, et al: The comparative efficacy and safety of carbamazepine versus lithium: a randomized, double-blind 3-year trial in 83 patients. J Clin Psychiatry 47:490–494, 1986

Post RM: Time course of clinical effects of carbamazepine: implications for mechanisms of action. J Clin Psychiatry 49:35–48, 1988

Post RM: Carbamazepine treatment of bipolar affective disorder. Directions in Psychiatry 9 (lesson 19):1–12, 1989

Post RM, Uhde TW, Ballenger JC, et al: Carbamazepine and its -10-11-epoxide metabolite in plasma and CSF. Relationship to antidepressant response. Arch Gen Psychiatry 40:673–676, 1983a

Post RM, Uhde TW, Ballenger JC, et al: Prophylactic efficacy of carbamazepine in manic-depressive illness. Am J Psychiatry 140:1602–1604, 1983b

Post RM, Ballenger JC, Uhde TW, et al: Efficacy of carbamazepine in manic-depressive illness: implications for underlying mechanisms, in Neurobiology of Mood Disorders. Edited by Post RM, Ballenger J. Baltimore, MD, Williams & Wilkins, 1984a, pp 777–816

Post RM, Uhde TW, Wolff EA: Profile of clinical efficacy and side effects of carbamazepine in psychiatric illness: relationship to blood and CSF levels of carbamazepine and its -10-11-epoxide metabolite. Acta Psychiatr Scand Suppl 313:104–120, 1984b

Post RM, Berrettini W, Uhde TW, et al: Selective response to the anticonvulsant carbamazepine in manic-depressive illness: a case study. J Clin Psychopharmacol 4:178–185, 1984c

Post RM, Uhde TW, Roy-Byrne PP, et al: Antidepressant effects of carbamazepine. Am J Psychiatry 143:29–34, 1986

Post RM, Uhde TW, Roy-Byrne PP, et al: Correlates of antimanic response to carbamazepine. Psychiatry Res 21:71–83, 1987

Post RM, Leverich GS, Rosoff AS, et al: Carbamazepine prophylaxis in refractory affective disorders: a focus on long-term follow-up. J Clin Psychopharmacol 10:318–327, 1990

Post RM, Weiss SRB, Chuang DM, et al: Mechanisms of action of carbamazepine in seizure and affective disorders, in Anticonvulsants in Psychiatry. Edited by Joffe RT, Calabrese JR. New York, Marcel Dekker, 1994, pp 43–92

Price WA, DiMarzio LR: Verapamil-carbamazepine neurotoxicity [letter]. J Clin Psychiatry 49:80, 1988

Prien RF, Gelenberg AJ: Alternatives to lithium for preventive treatment of bipolar disorder. Am J Psychiatry 146:840–848, 1989

Raitasuo V, Lehtovaara R, Huttunen MO: Carbamazepine and plasma levels of clozapine (letter). Am J Psychiatry 150:169, 1993

Rapeport WG, McInnes GT, Thompson GG, et al: Hepatic enzyme induction and leucocyte delta-aminolaevulinic acid synthase activity: studies with carbamazepine. Br J Clin Pharmacol 16:133–137, 1983

Renaud JP, Cullin C, Pompon D, et al: Expression of human liver cyto-chrome P450 111A4 in yeast: a functional model for the hepatic en-zyme. Eur J Biochem 194:889–896, 1990

Rosa FW: Spina bifida in infants of women treated with carbamazepine dur-ing pregnancy. N Engl J Med 324:674–677, 1991

Sitland-Marken PA, Richman LA, Wells BG, et al: Pharmacologic manage-ment of acute mania in pregnancy. J Clin Psychopharmacol 9:78–87, 1989

Small JG, Klapper MH, Milstein V, et al: Carbamazepine compared with lithium in the treatment of mania. Arch Gen Psychiatry 48:915–921, 1991

Stoll KD, Bisson HE, Fischer E, et al: Carbamazepine versus haloperidol in manic syndromes: first report of a multicentric study in Germany, in Biological Psychiatry 1985. Edited by Shagass C. Amsterdam, Nether-lands, Elsevier, 1986, pp 332–334

Tartara A, Galimberti CA, Manni R, et al: Differential effect of valproic acid and enzyme-inducing anticonvulsants on nimodipine pharmacokinetics in epileptic patients. Br J Clin Pharmacol 32:335–340, 1991

Tohen M, Castillo J, Pope H Jr, et al: Concomitant use of valproate and carbamazepine in bipolar and schizoaffective disorders. J Clin Psycho-pharmacol 14:67–70, 1994

Tomson T: Interdosage fluctuations in plasma carbamazepine concentration determine intermittent side effects. Arch Neurol 41:830–834, 1984

Vick NA: Suppression of carbamazepine-induced skin rash with prednisone (letter). N Engl J Med 309:1193–1194, 1983

Vieweg V, Glick JL, Hering S, et al: Absence of carbamazepine-induced hyponatremia among patients also given lithium. Am J Psychiatry 144: 943–947, 1987

von Moltke LL, Greenblatt DJ, Harmatz JS, et al: Cytochromes in psycho-pharmacology (editorial). J Clin Psychopharmacol 14:1–4, 1994

Watkins SE, Callender K, Thomas DR, et al: The effect of carbamazepine and lithium on remission from affective illness. Br J Psychiatry 150:180–182, 1987

Wehr TA, Sack DA, Rosenthal NE, et al: Rapid cycling affective disorder: contributing factors and treatment responses in 51 patients. Am J Psy-chiatry 145:179–184, 1988

Yatham LN, Barry S, Mobayed M, et al: Is the carbamazepine-phenelzine combination safe? (letter). Am J Psychiatry 147:367, 1990

Zaccara G, Gangemi PF, Bendoni L, et al: Influence of single and repeated doses of oxcarbazepine on the pharmacokinetics profile of felodipine. Ther Drug Monit 15:39–42, 1993

CHAPTER 14

VALPROATE

Scott A. West, M.D.,
Paul E. Keck Jr., M.D., and
Susan L. McElroy, M.D.

V alproic acid was synthesized in the United States in 1882 and became commonly used as an organic solvent because of its simple, branched-chain fatty acid structure. Its use as a solvent led to the discovery in 1963 by Meunier in France that valproic acid had anticonvulsant properties, and it was subsequently approved for use in European countries in the 1960s in the treatment of epilepsy. Valproic acid later became available for use in the United States in the treatment of simple and complex absence seizures and in patients with multiple seizure types. Although it was not until the mid-1980s that its usefulness in the treatment of bipolar disorder began to be recognized in the United States, the first report of the effectiveness of valproic acid in the treatment of bipolar disorder appeared in France in 1966 (Lambert et al. 1966).

Over the past decade, numerous controlled and uncontrolled studies have demonstrated valproic acid to be an effective treatment for many patients with bipolar disorder. Subsequently, Abbott Laboratories, the manufacturer of valproic acid, has filed for an indication with the United States Food and Drug Administration (FDA) for the use of valproate in the treatment of bipolar disorder. Because several formulations of valproic acid are available, the term *valproate* is used to denote all these formulations. In this chapter, we review the research supporting the efficacy of valproate in the treatment of bipolar disorder and provide guidelines for its clinical use.

▶ Acute Mania

A substantial body of research has been done investigating the efficacy of valproate in the treatment of acute mania. At least 16 uncontrolled studies (for a review, see McElroy et al. 1992) and 6 controlled studies have evaluated the efficacy of valproate in the treatment of acute mania. Taken together, these studies have suggested that approximately two-thirds of patients, many of whom were previously refractory to lithium therapy, demonstrate a moderate to marked response to valproate. Five placebo-controlled studies (Bowden et al. 1994; Brennan et al. 1984; Emrich et al. 1985; Pope et al. 1991; Post et al. 1984) and two lithium-controlled studies (Bowden et al. 1994; Freeman et al. 1992) have demonstrated valproate to be more effective than placebo and as effective as lithium in the treatment of acute mania (see Table 14–1). In the first double-blind, placebo-controlled study of valproate in a large number ($N = 36$) of acutely manic and previously lithium-refractory or intolerant patients, Pope et al. (1991) found that 9 of 17 patients (53%) treated with valproate compared with 2 of 19 patients (11%) who received placebo demonstrated at least a 50% improvement in manic symptoms, as measured by decreases in Young Mania Scale scores. A median decrease of 54% on the scale occurred in patients who received valproate ($n = 17$) versus a 5% decrease in patients on placebo ($n = 19$), after 7–21 days of treatment. These differences in response between valproate and placebo were highly significant. Two additional patients in the valproate-treated group demonstrated a moderate response, with a reported improvement just below 50%, suggesting that 65% of patients may demonstrate moderate to marked improvement. Substantial antimanic effects were typically apparent 1–4 days after therapeutic blood concentrations were achieved, which were titrated to clinical response and tolerability and were maintained between 50 and 100 mg/L.

Table 14–1. Controlled studies of valproate in bipolar patients with acute mania

Investigators	N	Design	Outcome
Brennan et al. 1984	8	Double-blind, ABA, placebo-controlled	6/8 marked response, 2/8 no response
Post et al. 1984	1	Double-blind, crossover to placebo, carbamazepine, phenytoin, and valproate	No response to valproate, placebo, or phenytoin; marked response to carbamazepine
Emrich et al. 1985	5	Double-blind, ABA, placebo-controlled	4/5 marked response, 1/5 no response
Pope et al. 1991	36	Double-blind, placebo-controlled, parallel-group, 1- to 3-week trial	Valproate significantly superior to placebo; 9/17 valproate-treated patients, 2/19 placebo-treated patients responded
Freeman et al. 1992	27	Double-blind, lithium-controlled, parallel-group, 3-week trial	9/14 valproate-treated patients, 12/13 lithium-treated patients responded
Bowden et al. 1994	179	Double-blind, lithium- and placebo-controlled, parallel-group, 3-week trial	48% of valproate-treated patients, 49% of lithium-treated patients, 25% of placebo-treated patients responded; valproate and lithium significantly superior to placebo

In a large ($N = 179$), multicenter, double-blind, placebo-controlled study, Bowden et al. (1994) randomized acutely manic patients with bipolar disorder to treatment with valproate ($n = 69$), lithium ($n = 36$), or placebo ($n = 74$). Marked improvement, defined as at least a 50% reduction in the manic syndrome subscale score as measured by the Schedule for Affective Disorders and Schizophrenia, was observed in 48% of patients who received valproate and 49% of lithium-treated patients, compared with only 25% of patients who received placebo. Significant reductions in manic symptoms were evident by the fifth day of the study in patients treated with both valproate and lithium. Patients treated with valproate were more likely to complete all 21 days of the study; premature termination, largely due to lack of efficacy, occurred in 48% of patients in the valproate-treated group compared with 61% in the lithium-treated group and 64% in the in the placebo group. There have also been several reports on the use of valproate in children and adolescents with acute mania. Three uncontrolled, open trials including a total of 29 patients have been reported as of this writing (Kastner et al. 1990; Papatheodorou and Kutcher 1993; Papatheodorou et al. 1995; West et al. 1994).

Overall, 24 (83%) of patients demonstrated moderate to marked improvement based on reductions in mania rating scale scores. Side effects were minimal and well tolerated, with no serious adverse events reported in any of the studies. Although the safety and efficacy of valproate needs to be confirmed by controlled trials, these preliminary data suggest that valproate may be beneficial in children and adolescents.

These studies, taken together, suggest that approximately two-thirds of patients with acute mania demonstrate moderate to marked improvement with valproate, making it an excellent alternative to lithium, especially considering that the majority of patients studied to date have been refractory to or intolerant of lithium therapy.

▶ Acute Depression

Although there are no controlled studies of valproate in the treatment of either acute unipolar, bipolar, or schizoaffective depression, open studies have indicated that valproate is less effective in the treatment of acute depression than of acute mania. In four open studies (Calabrese et al. 1993a; Hayes 1989; Lambert 1984; McElroy et al. 1987) examining a total of 218 patients, 58 (27%) displayed a significant acute antidepressant response to valproate (for a review, see McElroy et al. 1992). In a cohort of 101 rapid-cycling bipolar patients followed by Calabrese and colleagues (Calabrese and Delucchi 1990; Calabrese et al. 1991, 1993a, 1993b), the acute antidepressant response rate to valproate was found to be 45% ($n = 58$ with 12 marked responders and 14 moderate responders), which may indicate that acute depressive episodes in patients with rapid cycling are more responsive to valproate compared with nonrapid cyclers. Additionally, patients with bipolar II disorder may demonstrate a better antidepressant response to valproate compared with bipolar I patients (Puzynski and Klosiewicz 1984).

▶ PROPHYLACTIC TREATMENT

Although there are no controlled studies evaluating the efficacy of valproate in the prevention of recurrent affective episodes in patients with bipolar or schizoaffective disorder, data from uncontrolled studies have suggested that valproate is an effective prophylactic treatment indeed, often reducing the frequency and/or intensity of recurrent affective episodes. Calabrese et al. (1993a), who followed patients for a mean period of 17.2 months, reported response rates of 72%–94% for the prevention of recurrent affective episodes, which included 68 of 94 patients (72%) who achieved effective prophylaxis for recurrent depressive episodes. These data suggest that valproate may be more effective in preventing affective episodes, especially recurrent depression, than in treating acute episodes. Numerous additional open studies (Emrich and Wolf 1992; Hayes 1989; McElroy et al. 1992; Puzynski and Klosiewicz 1984; Suppes et al. 1992) also suggest that valproate is effective in reducing or preventing recurrent depressive, manic, and mixed episodes and that concurrent treatment with other mood stabilizers, antipsychotics, and antidepressants may augment response to valproate.

In a 1995 study (Oral and Verimli 1995), 32 bipolar I patients, diagnosed according to DSM-III-R, participated in an open trial of valproate with lithium after lithium alone had failed. Failure was defined as having an episode despite therapeutic lithium concentration. Patients were placed on a combination of lithium (0.8–1.0 mEq/L) and valproate (45–110 µg/mL): half on sodium valproate and half on valproic acid. No patients met criteria for dysphoric mania or rapid cycling. Both groups showed acute response with reduction of mean mania scores from 39.2 to 22.9 after 10 days, as well as prophylactic response to valproate with continued remission of 68% in the first year, 57% in the second year, and 43% in the third year. Another recent naturalistic report contrasted patterns of recovery from bipolar disorder on lithium, carbamazepine, divalproex sodium, or combined regimens (Goldberg et al. 1996). In this review of 169 bipolar I patients, significant overall benefits were found for more than 40% of patients prescribed any of the treatment regimens. One-way analyses of variance (ANOVAs), based on the Clinical Global Impression (CGI) scale, showed that the combination of lithium and anticonvulsants did better than did single-agent therapies. "Mixed" bipolar patients were less likely than were "pure" manic patients to recover fully; among mixed bipolar patients, no significant differences were found in recovery between lithium and lithium plus anticonvulsants. Another study recently showed that divalproex given for an average of 286 days in a retrospective analysis adequately controlled symptoms in 85.1% of patients with a reduction in rehospitalization rates from 0.41 per patient to 0.03 per patient (Burks and Kulkarni 1996). Another study of continuation and maintenance treatment of bipolar I disorder reported results of a placebo-controlled trial of divalproex sodium (Solomon et al. 1997). Twelve patients, all of whom were also maintained on lithium at a serum level of 0.8–1.0 mmol/L, were less likely to relapse on divalproex ($P = 0.14$), but, perhaps as expected, were more likely to have at least one moderate or severe side effect ($P = .041$).

▶ PREDICTORS OF RESPONSE

A number of factors have been reported to be associated with a therapeutic response to valproate, although data are preliminary at this time. As reviewed by West et al. (1995), factors related to diagnosis, comorbidity, previous treatment, neurological conditions, and family history have all been reported to correlate with successful valproate therapy. Freeman et al. (1992), in a double-blind comparison of valproate and lithium in patients with acute mania, found that high depression scores correlated with a favorable response to valproate (Clothier et al. 1992). This finding was also reported by Calabrese et al. (1993a, 1993b), who found that 80%–89% of patients with mixed mania responded favorably to valproate, both acutely and prophylactically. The presence of rapid cycling (the occurrence of four or more affective episodes per year) has also been associated with a favorable response to valproate (Calabrese et al. 1991, 1993a, 1993b; McElroy et al. 1988a, 1988b), with rates of response ranging from 64% to 100%. However, in a controlled study by Pope et al. (1991), neither mixed mania nor rapid cycling were associated with a therapeutic response to valproate; it therefore remains unclear whether valproate is more effective in patients with these features. Possible predictors of response from the study by Bowden et al. (1994) have not as of this writing been reported. Bipolar patients with comorbid panic disorder have been reported to respond very well to treatment with valproate, with significant improvement of both affective and panic symptoms (Calabrese and Delucchi 1990; Keck et al. 1993b). Indeed, Calabrese and Delucchi reported that 21 of 22 patients (96%) with rapid-cycling bipolar disorder and comorbid panic attacks markedly improved on valproate therapy.

Additionally, numerous other factors have been associated with a favorable response to valproate, including comorbid mental retardation (Sovner 1989), nonparoxysmal electroencephalogram (EEG) abnormalities (McElroy et al. 1988a, 1992), a history of head trauma (Pope et al. 1988), a family history of mood disorders (Calabrese et al. 1993b), and rapid titration of valproate (McElroy et al. 1991; Pope et al. 1991). Patients who are lithium-naive have also been reported to have a favorable response to valproate (Calabrese et al. 1993a); however, in a controlled study by Bowden et al. (1994) that included a total of 179 patients, no association was found between previous lithium treatment and valproate response. Although some of these factors may indeed be legitimate predictors of response to treatment with valproate, in the absence of controlled data examining correlates of response, these issues remain unclear.

▶ FORMULATIONS, PHARMACOLOGY, AND PHARMACOKINETICS

Valproate is commercially available in several formulations: divalproex sodium (Depakote), an enteric-coated compound of equimolar portions of sodium valproate and valproic acid; valproic acid (Depakene); sodium valproate (Depakene syrup); and divalproex sodium sprinkle capsules (Depakote Sprinkle Capsules), which can be ingested intact or pulled apart and sprinkled on food.

Valproate facilitates the activity of gamma-aminobutyric acid (GABA), the primary inhibitory neurotransmitter in the central nervous system, by inhibiting its catabolism, increasing its synthesis and release, and increasing GABA-B receptor density (Emrich et al. 1981; Post et al. 1992; Rimmer and Richens 1985). These changes are thought to account, at least in part, for the mood-stabilizing effects of valproate. However, other pharmacologic effects of valproate include alterations of excitatory neurotransmitters, such as decreased dopamine turnover (Post et al. 1992), decreased aspartate release (Bernasconi et al. 1984), and decreased N-methyl-D-aspartate–mediated depolarization (Zeise et al. 1991), which may also play a role in the therapeutic activity of valproate.

The bioavailability of valproate is essentially complete with all of the formulations (Wilder 1992). The rate of absorption varies among the formulations, but peak serum concentrations typically occur 1–4 hours after ingestion. Valproate is highly bound (90%) to albumin and other plasma proteins, and the elimination half-life ranges from 6 to 16 hours.

Virtually all of the drug (97%) undergoes hepatic degradation via conjugation and mitochondrial beta-oxidation, resulting in numerous metabolites, most of which are inactive, but some of which have anticonvulsant activity. Metabolism is minimal in the P450 microsomal system, except when valproate is used concurrently with drugs that induce this pathway, such as carbamazepine, which may result in the accumulation of toxic metabolites and increased adverse effects (for review, see Keck et al. 1994). In contrast to carbamazepine, valproate also tends to increase serum concentrations of other anticonvulsants, including carbamazepine, phenobarbital, and phenytoin. Valproate does not induce its own metabolism or that of tricyclic antidepressants, antipsychotics, and oral contraceptives (Rimmer and Richens 1985).

❱ Guidelines for Clinical Use

Before initiating treatment with valproate, patients should be screened for hematologic and hepatic disease, because the most worrisome potential adverse effects include coagulopathy and hepatitis. If clinical circumstances permit, preliminary laboratory studies, including a complete blood count with platelets, bleeding time, and liver function studies, should be obtained before valproate administration; however, it is often more feasible to obtain these studies when patients are psychiatrically stable. There are no rigid guidelines available for monitoring these parameters, and in general it is not necessary to continue laboratory monitoring of hepatic and hematalogic function (Pellock and Willmore 1991). It is more important to monitor patients clinically and obtain laboratory studies only if they are clinically indicated. However, because the use of valproate in psychiatric patients is less extensive compared with that in neurological patients, periodic laboratory evaluations (every 6 months to 2 years) are generally recommended (Keck et al. 1994). It is also helpful to educate patients on bleeding abnormalities and the early signs and symptoms of hepatitis so that prompt recognition and intervention may occur. Clinically insignificant and transient elevations (two- to threefold increases from baseline) in hepatic transaminase levels often occur during the initial stages of treatment; these elevations typically resolve with continued treatment or dose reduction.

Treatment with valproate is typically initiated at 500–1,000 mg/day taken in two to four divided doses. This dosage can be titrated upward by 250–500 mg every 1–3 days based on clinical response and tolerability, and most patients will require 15–20 mg/kg per day. In patients who are acutely manic or agitated, an oral loading dose of 20 mg/kg may be given to achieve a more rapid clinical response; this dose is typically tolerated as well as gradual titration (Keck et al. 1993a; McElroy et al. 1993). After the initial loading dose, the same dose can be continued either in divided doses or as a single bedtime dose and should be further titrated based on clinical response and tolerability.

Serum concentrations of valproate are obtained 12 hours after the last dose (through levels) every 2–4 days and should be maintained between 50 and 125 µg/mL. Once an optimal dose has been achieved, the total daily dose may be given at bedtime to maximize compliance and convenience.

Valproate can be used concurrently with other psychotropic medications, and it is often used in conjunction with lithium, carbamazepine, antipsychotics (including clozapine and risperidone), tricyclic antidepressants, selective serotonin reuptake inhibitors (SSRIs), and benzodiazepines. Medications that have demonstrated some benefit are typically continued, and those that have been ineffective are tapered and eventually discontinued as valproate is titrated upward.

▶ Drug-Drug Interactions

Drug-drug interactions with valproate may occur with other drugs that are highly protein bound, including salicylates and warfarin. Salicylates have been reported to increase plasma valproate concentrations by protein displacement and metabolism inhibition (Abbott et al. 1986, Goulden et al. 1987). Valproate has been reported to displace warfarin from plasma proteins in vitro, resulting in increased unbound (active) warfarin concentrations (Urien et al. 1981), so caution is advisable when prescribing valproate to patients requiring warfarin, especially in light of the potential coagulopathies that may occur with valproate.

When valproate is administered with drugs that induce hepatic metabolism, such as carbamazepine, serum concentrations of valproic acid often decrease (Davis et al. 1994), necessitating increases in the dose of valproate. Conversely, drugs that inhibit hepatic metabolism have been reported to increase serum valproic acid concentrations; these drugs include fluoxetine (Sovner and Davis 1991), diazepam (Monfort 1993), chlorpromazine (but not haloperidol) (Ishizaki et al. 1984), and felbamate (Wagner et al. 1991). Because valproate tends to inhibit drug oxidation, serum concentrations of oxidatively metabolized drugs—namely, tricyclic antidepressants—can be increased (Keck et al. 1994). Minor elevations in serum concentrations of clozapine metabolites have also been reported to occur (Centorrino et al.

1994). Unlike carbamazepine, valproate does not increase the metabolism of oral contraceptives, so there is no increased risk of pregnancy in patients using this form of birth control (Crawford et al. 1986).

▶ ADVERSE EFFECTS

Valproate is typically well tolerated, and adverse effects are generally limited and most often responsive to dose reductions, changing the dosing schedule (e.g., giving a single bedtime dose), and/or administration of medications to alleviate adverse effects (e.g., H_2-blockers) (Beghi et al. 1986; Dreifuss et al. 1989; Smith and Bleck 1991).

The most common dose-related side effects are gastrointestinal (i.e., nausea, indigestion, flatulence, mild diarrhea, and, to a much lesser extent, vomiting). These effects often subside or resolve with continued treatment, but if persistent, they are usually responsive to dose reduction and/or the addition of H_2-blockers such as famotidine and ranitidine (Stoll et al. 1991). In our experience, divalproex sodium (Depakote) has caused the least amount of gastrointestinal distress. Other dose-related side effects include sedation, tremor, and mild elevations in hepatic transaminases; all are typically transient, but if persistent, they often respond to dose reduction.

Beta-blockers are useful in alleviating problematic tremors. To minimize sedation, it is often helpful to prescribe the total daily dose of valproate at bedtime, especially in patients with insomnia. In addition, weight gain and hair loss may occur; for weight gain, instituting a strict diet may be helpful, and for transient hair loss, the administration of zinc and selenium supplements may help minimize the problem (Hurd et al. 1984). Coagulopathies due to thrombocytopenia and impaired platelet function are infrequent and resolve with drug discontinuation.

There have been reports of rare, idiosyncratic reactions to valproate, including necrotizing hepatitis, hemorrhagic pancreatitis, and agranulocytosis, all of which are potentially fatal (Dreifuss et al. 1989; Pellock and Willmore 1991; Rimmer and Richens 1985; Smith and Bleck 1991). Irreversible, necrotizing hepatitis has been reported to occur in children younger than 10 years old with epilepsy, all of whom were neurologically and medically complicated and on multiple anticonvul-

Mania: Clinical and Research Perspectives

sant medications (Dreifuss et al. 1989). As of this writing, there have been no reports of fatal hepatitis occurring in adolescents or adults or in patients with primary psychiatric disorders requiring valproate monotherapy or polypharmacology with other mood stabilizers (e.g., carbamazepine) or psychotropic medications. Nevertheless, it is prudent to monitor patients for the development of early signs and symptoms of hepatitis, including fever, nausea, vomiting, abdominal pain, malaise, lethargy, and jaundice. It is noteworthy that there is no association between asymptomatic transient elevations in hepatic transaminase concentrations that commonly occur with valproate and the development of necrotizing hepatitis. In addition, pancreatitis and agranulocytosis are extremely rare, so there are no guidelines for routine laboratory monitoring. Patients should be monitored for new onset of abdominal pain or infection, and serum amylase concentrations and white blood cell counts should be evaluated as clinically indicated.

Valproate has been found to be teratogenic, with an increased risk of neural tube defects estimated to occur in 1 of 100 live births in patients with first trimester exposure (Rosa 1991). Although the co-administration of folate may reduce this risk (Delgado-Escueta and Janz 1992), careful consideration of the risks and benefits of valproate treatment should be taken in patients who are pregnant or desire to become so during treatment.

▌ Conclusion

Numerous studies have demonstrated valproate to be an effective and well-tolerated treatment in patients with bipolar disorder. Controlled studies have shown valproate to be as effective as lithium in the treatment of acute mania, and numerous open studies have consistently reported valproate to be effective prophylaxis for recurrent manic episodes, and, to a lesser extent, depressive episodes. Indeed, these studies have demonstrated that valproate reduces both the frequency and intensity of recurrent manic and depressive episodes over extended periods of time. Additionally, preliminary, uncontrolled trials suggest that valproate may be effective and well tolerated in children and adolescents with acute mania. Preliminary predictors of response include bipolar patients with rapid cycling, mixed affective states, and comorbid panic disorder. Valproate has a favorable side-effect profile and is well tolerated when used adjunctly with lithium, carbamazepine, antipsychotics, and antidepressants. In short, valproate is an excellent treatment option for patients with bipolar disorder and may be particularly helpful in patients who are intolerant of or refractory to lithium and/or carbamazepine.

▶ References

Abbott FS, Kassam J, Orr JM, et al: The effect of aspirin on valproic acid metabolism. Clinical Psychopharmacology and Therapeutics 40:94–100, 1986

Beghi E, DiMascio R, Sasanelli F, et al: Adverse reactions to antiepileptic drugs: a multicenter survey of clinical practice. Epilepsia 27:323–330, 1986

Bernasconi R, Hauser K, Martin P, et al: Biochemical aspects of the mechanism of action of valproate, in Anticonvulsants in Affective Disorders. Edited by Emrich HM, Okuma T, Müller AA. Amsterdam, Netherlands, Elsevier Science Publishers, 1984, pp 14–32

Bowden CL, Brugger AM, Swann AC, et al: Efficacy of divalproex vs lithium and placebo in the treatment of mania. JAMA 271:918–924, 1994

Brennan MJW, Sandyk R, Borsook D: Use of sodium valproate in the management of affective disorders: basic and clinical aspects, in Anticonvulsants in Affective Disorders. Edited by Emrich HM, Okuma T, Müller AA. Amsterdam, Netherlands, Excerpta Medica, 1984, pp 56–65

Burks S, Kulkarni S: The safety and efficacy of divalproex in bipolar disorder: a retrospective analysis of maintenance treatment. American Psychiatric Association 1996 Annual Meeting New Research Program and Abstracts (NR 332). Washington, DC, American Psychiatric Association, 1996, p 157

Calabrese JR, Delucchi GA: Spectrum of efficacy of valproate in 55 patients with rapid-cycling bipolar disorder. Am J Psychiatry 147:431–434, 1990

Calabrese J, Markovitz P, Wagner S: Predictors of valproate response in rapid-cycling bipolar disorder. Biol Psychiatry 29:166A–176A, 1991

Calabrese JR, Woyshville MJ, Kimmel SE, et al: Predictors of valproate response in bipolar rapid cycling. J Clin Psychopharmacol 13:280–283, 1993a

Calabrese JR, Rapport DJ, Kimmel SE, et al: Rapid cycling bipolar disorder and its treatment with valproate. Can J Psychiatry 38:S57–S61, 1993b

Centorrino F, Baldessarini RJ, Kando J, et al: Serum concentrations of clozapine and its major metabolites: effects of cotreatment with fluoxetine or valproate. Am J Psychiatry 151:123–125, 1994

Clothier JL, Swann AC, Freeman T: Dysphoric mania. J Clin Psychopharmacol 12:13S–16S, 1992

Crawford P, Chadwick D, Cleland P, et al: The lack of effect of sodium valproate on the pharmacokinetics of oral contraceptive steroids. Contraception 33:23–29, 1986

Davis R, Peters DH, McTavish D: Valproic acid: a reappraisal of its pharmacological properties and clinical efficacy in epilepsy. Drugs 47:332–372, 1994

Delgado-Escueta AV, Janz D: Consensus guidelines: preconception counseling management, and care of the pregnant woman with epilepsy. Neurology 42 (suppl 5):149–160, 1992

Dreifuss FE, Langer DH, Moline KA, et al: Valproic acid hepatic fatalities II: U.S. experience since 1984. Neurology 39:201–207, 1989

Emrich HM, Wolf R: Valproate treatment of mania. Prog Neuropsychopharmacol Biol Psychiatry 16:691–701, 1992

Emrich HM, von Zerssen D, Kissling W, et al: On a possible role of GABA in mania: therapeutic efficacy of valproate, in GABA and Benzodiazepine Receptors. Edited by Costa E, Dicharia G, Gessa GL. New York, Raven, 1981, pp 287–296

Emrich HM, Dose M, von Zerssen D: The use of sodium valproate, carbamazepine, and oxcarbazepine in patients with affective disorders. J Affect Disord 8:243–250, 1985

Freeman TW, Clothier JL, Pazzaglia P, et al: A double-blind comparison of valproate and lithium in the treatment of acute mania. Am J Psychiatry 149:108–111, 1992

Goldberg JF, Garno JL, Leon AC, et al: Single agent vs. multiple agent mood stabilizers in acute mania. Poster 59, annual meeting of NCDEU, Boca Raton, FL, May 1996

Goulden KJ, Dooley JM, Camfield PR, et al: Clinical valproate toxicity induced by acetylsalicylic acid. Neurology 37:1392–1394, 1987

Hayes SG: Long-term use of valproate in primary psychiatric disorders. J Clin Psychiatry 50 (suppl):35–39, 1989

Hurd RW, van Rinsvelt HA, Wilder BJ, et al: Selenium, zinc, and copper changes with valproic acid: possible relation to drug side effects. Neurology 34:1394–1395, 1984

Ishizaki T, Chibak, Saito M, et al: The effects of neuroleptics (haloperidol and chlorpromazine) on the pharmacokinetics of valproic acid in schizophrenic patients. J Clin Psychopharmacol 4:254–261, 1984

Kastner T, Friedman DL, Plummer AT, et al: Valproic acid for the treatment of children with mental retardation and mood symptomatology. Pediatrics 86:467–472, 1990

Keck PE, McElroy SL, Tugrul KC, et al: Valproate oral loading in the treatment of acute mania. J Clin Psychiatry 54:305–308, 1993a

Keck PE, Taylor VE, Tugrul KC, et al: Valproate treatment of panic disorder and lactate-induced panic attacks. Biol Psychiatry 33:542–546, 1993b

Keck PE, McElroy SL, Bennett JA: Pharmacology and pharmacokinetics of valproic acid, in Anticonvulsants in Psychiatry. Edited by Joffe RT, Calabrese JR. New York, Marcel Dekker, 1994, pp 27–42

Lambert P-A: Acute and prophylactic therapies of patients with affective disorders using valpromide (dipropylacetamide), in Anticonvulsants in Affective Disorders. Edited by Emrich HM, Okuma T, Müller AA. Amsterdam, Netherlands, Excerpta Medica, 1984, pp 33–44

Lambert P-A, Cavaz G, Borselli S, et al: Action neuropsychotrop d'un nouvel antiepileptique: le Depamide. Ann Med Psychol (Paris) 1:707–710, 1966

McElroy SL, Keck PE, Pope HG: Sodium valproate: its use in primary psychiatric disorders. J Clin Psychopharmacol 7:16–24, 1987

McElroy SL, Keck PE, Pope HG, et al: Valproate in primary psychiatric disorders: literature review and clinical experience in a private psychiatric hospital, in Use of Anticonvulsants in Psychiatry: Recent Advances. Edited by McElroy SL, Pope HG. Clifton, NJ, Oxford Health Care, 1988a, pp 25–41

McElroy SL, Keck PE, Pope HG, et al: Valproate in the treatment of rapid-cycling bipolar disorder. J Clin Psychopharmacol 8:275–279, 1988b

McElroy SL, Keck PE, Pope HG, et al: Correlates of antimanic response to valproate. Psychopharmacol Bull 27:127–133, 1991

McElroy SL, Keck PE, Pope HG, et al: Valproate in the treatment of bipolar disorder: literature review and clinical guidelines. J Clin Psychopharmacol 12:42S–52S, 1992

McElroy SL, Keck PE, Tugrul KC, et al: Valproate as a loading treatment in acute mania. Neuropsychobiology 27:146–149, 1993

Monfort J-C: Diazepam increases the serum level of free valproate. Paper presented at the annual meeting of the American Psychiatric Association, San Francisco, CA, May 27, 1993, Abstract 735, 1993

Oral T, Verimli A: Valproate-lithium combination in the prophylaxis of bipolar disorder: three years of open followup. Address presented at II International Congress on Advances in Affective Disorders, Jerusalem, Israel, September 1991

Papatheodorou G, Kutcher SP: Divalproex sodium treatment in late adolescent and young adult acute mania. Psychopharmacol Bull 29:213–219, 1993

Papatheodorou G, Kutcher SP, Katic M, et al: The efficacy and safety of divalproex sodium in the treatment of acute mania in adolescents and young adults: an open clinical trial. J Clin Psychopharmacol 15:110–116, 1995

Pellock JM, Willmore LJ: A rational guide to routine blood monitoring in patients receiving antiepileptic drugs. Neurology 41:961–964, 1991

Pope HG, McElroy SL, Satlin A: Head injury, bipolar disorder, and response to valproate. Compr Psychiatry 29:34–38, 1988

Pope HG, McElroy SL, Keck PE, et al: Valproate in the treatment of acute mania: a placebo-controlled study. Arch Gen Psychiatry 48:62–68, 1991

Post RM, Berettini W, Uhde TW, et al: Selective response to the anticonvulsant carbamazepine in manic-depressive illness: a case study. J Clin Psychopharmacol 4:178–185, 1984

Post RM, Weiss SRB, Chuang D-M: Mechanism of action of anticonvulsants in affective disorders: comparison with lithium. J Clin Psychopharmacol 12 (suppl):23–35, 1992

Puzynski S, Klosiewicz L: Valproic acid amide as a prophylactic agent in affective and schizoaffective disorders. Psychopharmacol Bull 20:151–159, 1984

Rimmer E, Richens A: An update on sodium valproate. Pharmacotherapy 5:171–184, 1985

Rosa FW: Spina bifida in infants of women treated with carbamazepine during pregnancy. N Engl J Med 324:674–677, 1991

Smith MC, Bleck TP: Convulsive disorders: toxicity of anticonvulsants. Clin Neuropharmacol 14:97–115, 1991

Solomon DA, Ryan LE, Keitner GJ, et al: A pilot study of lithium carbonate plus divalproex sodium for the continuation and maintenance treatment of patients with bipolar I disorder. J Clin Psychiatry 58:91–99, 1997

Sovner R: The use of valproate in the treatment of mentally retarded persons with typical and atypical bipolar disorders. J Clin Psychiatry 50 (suppl): 40S–43S, 1989

Sovner R, Davis JM: A potential drug interaction between fluoxetine and valproic acid. J Clin Psychopharmacol 11:389, 1991

Stoll AL, Vuckovic A, McElroy SL: Histamine 2-receptor antagonists for the treatment of valproate-induced gastrointestinal distress. Ann Clin Psychiatry 3:301–304, 1991

Suppes T, McElroy SL, Gilbert J, et al: Clozapine in the treatment of dysphoric mania. Biol Psychiatry 32:270–280, 1992

Urien S, Albengres B, Tillement JP: Serum protein binding of valproic acid in healthy subjects and in patients with liver disease. Int J Clin Pharmacol Ther Toxicol 19:319–325, 1981

Wagner ML, Graves NM, Leppik IE, et al: The effect of felbamate on valproate disposition (abstract). Epilepsia 32 (suppl 3):15, 1991

West SA, Keck PE, McElroy SL, et al: Open trial of valproate in the treatment of adolescent mania. Journal of Child and Adolescent Psychopharmacology 4:263–267, 1994

West SA, McElroy SL, Keck PE Jr: Valproate, in Predictors of Response in Mood Disorders. Edited by Goodnick PJ. Washington, DC, American Psychiatric Press, 1995, pp 133–146

Wilder BJ: Pharmacokinetics of valproate and carbamazepine. J Clin Psychopharmacol 12 (suppl):64–68, 1992

Zeise ML, Kasparow S, Zieglgansberger W: Valproate suppresses N-methyl-D-aspartate-evoked, transient depolarizations in the rat neocortex in vitro. Brain Res 544:345–348, 1991

CHAPTER 15

NOVEL ANTIPSYCHOTICS

Frances R. Frankenburg, M.D.,
Mary C. Zanarini, Ed.D., and
Paul J. Goodnick, M.D.

I n the past few years, clinicians and researchers have paid increasing attention to the treatment of bipolar affective disorder, or manic-depressive illness, with agents other than lithium salts. Although lithium is the cornerstone of treatment of bipolar disorders, there is a large number of people for whom lithium salts are inadequate treatment. Prien et al. (1984) noted in a double-blind, long-term, follow-up study of 117 bipolar patients that only one-third of lithium-treated patients remained euthymic when studied for up to 2 years. Various agents, such as the anticonvulsant agents, and calcium-channel blockers have been successfully used in the treatment of this disorder.

Neuroleptic agents are also often used for prophylaxis in the ongoing treatment of bipolar affective disorder. In an early study, Ahlfors et al. (1981) treated 93 patients who had not responded to lithium therapy with flupentixol decanoate (an antipsychotic agent not available in the United States) and found a significant decrease in mania-associated morbidity (although an increase in depressive illness) and concluded that flupentixol was "worth trying" in some patients with manic-depressive illness. Although there have been few other large studies examining the efficacy of maintenance neuroleptics, the use of neuroleptics in the prophylaxis of manic-depressive episodes is common clinical practice for patients who have not responded to lithium

(Sachs 1990; Sachs et al. 1994). For example, in a naturalistic study, Peselow et al. (1994) reviewed 305 patients with bipolar affective disorder who had been euthymic for 6 months while being treated with lithium alone and found that only 37% remained free of affective episodes by the fifth year of follow-up. Sixteen patients had had a manic episode and had then been treated with neuroleptic agents. Of these patients, 38% remained well.

Neuroleptic agents cause extrapyramidal side effects, which can be intolerable to patients and which often lead to noncompliance (Van Putten 1974). Patients with bipolar affective disorder may be particularly vulnerable to the development of tardive dyskinesia (Casey 1984). Therefore, there is much interest in the use of clozapine, a novel antipsychotic agent, because of its relative freedom from extrapyramidal side effects and tardive dyskinesia (Baldessarini and Frankenburg 1991), as well as other novel antipsychotic agents, such as risperidone and olanzapine.

▶ CLOZAPINE AS MAINTENANCE TREATMENT FOR BIPOLAR AFFECTIVE DISORDER

Individual Case Studies

Suppes et al. (1992) reported in detail on seven patients diagnosed with dysphoric mania refractory to standard treatments who were treated with clozapine. All patients had been very ill and had required multiple hospitalizations. Four of the seven patients had a neurological abnormality, and at least two patients had rapid-cycling disorder. The average dose of clozapine was 500 mg and usually replaced medication regimens that were previously very complicated. Clozapine was used as monotherapy in only three cases. Follow-up lasted 3–5 years and revealed substantial improvements. For example, the six patients who continued on clozapine (one patient developed agranulocytosis and was taken off the drug) required no further hospitalizations.

Calabrese et al. (1991) reported two cases of middle-aged women with rapid-cycling affective disorder who responded fairly well to clozapine or to the combination of clozapine and valproate. Interestingly, one of the women was not described as having any psychotic symptoms.

Frankenburg (1993) described a young man with severe bipolar disorder who responded well to 100 mg/day of clozapine and 2 mg/day of lorazepam. Since the publication of that case report, he has continued on clozapine therapy and has had no mood swings for 4 years.

Large Open Studies Including Patients With Schizophrenia and Bipolar Affective Disorders

Several large uncontrolled retrospective studies, mostly from Europe, have reported on the efficacy of clozapine in the treatment of patients with psychotic illnesses. Although most patients in these studies had schizophrenic illnesses, the studies included patients with schizoaffective and bipolar affective disorders who also had not responded well to previous neuroleptic treatments. These studies have been reviewed elsewhere (Frankenburg and Zanarini 1994). In this chapter, we review the findings that specifically concern the bipolar patients.

Battegay et al. (1977) reviewed the treatment of 93 patients treated with clozapine. Of these, 10 patients were diagnosed with "mixed psychoses"; 7 of these had manic-depressive psychoses. Of the 10 patients, 7 responded well and 2 fared badly. One patient discontinued treatment because of side effects.

Müller and Heipertz (1977) treated 52 manic patients with clozapine, in one-half of the cases with clozapine alone. Patients did well and were able to leave the hospital sooner than patients treated with other agents. The patients preferred clozapine because of the absence of extrapyramidal side effects. The average dose was 375 mg/day.

Leppig et al. (1989) reported on the effects of long-term clozapine therapy in 121 outpatients at the Psychiatric Hospital of the University of Munich. Mean length of treatment was 32 ± 43 months. Average dose was 131 mg/day. Ten patients were diagnosed with mania. The manic patients did less well than the schizophrenic patients. Of the manic patients, 23% showed no response to clozapine at all. Overall, only 5% of the patients showed no response, and all of the schizophrenic patients had some response to clozapine.

In another German study, Naber et al. (1992) reviewed the efficacy of clozapine in a large sample of patients, but gave few details other than noting that the response rate was between 55% and 72% in

25 patients with mania and 54 patients with psychotic depression.

McElroy et al. (1991) were one of the first groups to assess directly the question of whether diagnosis predicted response to clozapine. They surveyed treating clinicians and reviewed chart data of 25 patients with schizoaffective disorder, 14 patients with bipolar disorder, and 39 patients with schizophrenia. They concluded that the patients with affective disorders responded better to clozapine than did the patients with schizophrenia. Calabrese et al. (1996) carried out a prospective trial of clozapine monotherapy in 25 patients with either mania ($N = 10$) or schizoaffective disorder ($N = 15$) who had responded poorly or been unable to tolerate other agents. They concluded that clozapine is an effective agent for this population.

As can be seen from these studies, although most of the patients in the large open studies had schizophrenic illnesses, patients with bipolar disorder were often included and responded well except in the Leppig et al. (1989) study.

Mclean Study of Clozapine in Patients With Bipolar Affective Disorder

At McLean Hospital, Belmont, Massachusetts, our group (F.R.F. and M.C.Z.) is following more than 100 patients being treated with clozapine. A particular area of interest is the effect of diagnosis on response to clozapine. This study has been reported in detail elsewhere (Frankenburg and Zanarini 1994). We report here on the patients with bipolar affective disorder.

Patients were referred to the study by their treating psychiatrist. To be eligible, subjects had to meet DSM-III-R (American Psychiatric Association 1987) criteria for a psychotic illness and to have failed trials of at least three different antipsychotic medications. All bipolar patients had also failed trials of lithium and anticonvulsant agents. Each subject agreed to weekly blood tests and periodic examinations and interviews.

All patients gave written informed consent. The study was approved by the McLean Hospital Institutional Review Board. At entry into the study, one of the authors (Frankenburg) interviewed all patients, using the Structured Clinical Interview for DSM-III-R Axis I Disorders

(Spitzer et al. 1987). All patients were rated with the Brief Psychiatric Rating Scale (BPRS) (Overall and Gorham 1962), Clinical Global Impression (CGI) (Guy 1976), and Global Assessment Scale (GAS) (Endicott et al. 1976).

Sixteen patients had bipolar affective disorder. Their mean age was 35 ± 10 years; seven were female. The mean length of illness at the time that they started clozapine therapy was 12 ± 6.4 years. Eight patients had not responded to previous treatments, and eight patients had not responded and had also been unable to tolerate previous treatments. At the time of entry into the study, they were severely ill as reflected by their scores on the rating scales: BPRS, 52.8 ± 11.7; CGI, 5.0 ± 1.0; and GAS, 33.6 ± 9.5.

At the time of the first follow-up, the patients had been treated with clozapine for 6.3 ± 1.7 months with a mean dose of 284 ± 213 mg/day. Eight patients were also being treated with lithium; 5 were also being treated with divalproex sodium (Depakote); 2 were also being treated with an antidepressant agent. Side effects were very common. All patients complained of sedation, 14 of drooling, 7 of akathisia, and 8 of weight gain. There were no cases of leukopenia.

The patients showed clear clinical improvement on clozapine. Their scores on the rating scales improved: BPRS, 36.0 ± 13.8; CGI, 4.1 ± 1.4; and GAS, 45.8 ± 14.1 (all differences from baseline were significant at $P < .0001$). There were no cases of mania breaking through clozapine treatment. Two patients did become depressed, but they responded well to the addition of antidepressant agents.

In this large, prospective, open-label study, the earlier reports suggesting that clozapine may be an effective agent in the treatment of bipolar affective illnesses were strongly supported. These patients had chronic, severe illnesses that had not responded to conventional pharmacotherapy, and all had marked functional impairments due to their bipolar disorder. These patients in general improved on clozapine and, in several cases, have been able to avoid hospitalizations for up to 5 years after the initiation of clozapine, despite a history of lengthy and repeated hospitalizations prior to clozapine therapy.

Our study has two methodological limitations. First, patients were treated with clozapine in an open manner, and use of adjunctive medications was allowed. However, because all patients were entered into the trial because of their chronic treatment resistance, it is probable that at least some of their subsequent improvement was due to clozapine.

Second, bipolar illness is a cyclic illness, and thus, difficult in some aspects to rate. However, two of the rating measures (CGI and GAS), which were overall ratings, took this into account, and patients did show significant improvement on these measures.

In summary, these findings, taken together with the results from the earlier studies, suggest that patients with bipolar affective disorders who have not responded to or been able to tolerate conventional treatment may benefit from clozapine treatment. Side effects were common, but despite that, all patients were compliant with the drug.

▌ Treatment of the Acute Episode

Neuroleptic agents are useful for the treatment of the acute manic episode because of the lag time in response to lithium (Chou 1991; Goodwin and Jamison 1990). They may be indicated for the agitated, psychotic, and hyperactive patient (Vestergaard 1992). Disadvantages of neuroleptics include acute dystonias, the risk of tardive dyskinesia, extrapyramidal symptoms, and the risk of precipitating an episode on neuroleptic malignant syndrome (particularly if used rapidly and in high doses). Clozapine causes few extrapyramidal symptoms and is probably significantly freer of the risk of causing tardive dyskinesia (Baldessarini and Frankenburg 1991; Kane et al. 1993). Some limited evidence also suggests that clozapine may be particularly effective in reducing aggression and agitation (even when it does not diminish psychotic symptoms) (Ratey et al. 1993) and hence might be particularly useful in manic patients who are very agitated.

However, there is little in the literature describing the actual use of clozapine in acute cases of mania. In a review of the use of physostigmine to reverse clozapine-induced delirium, Schuster et al. (1977) described the use of clozapine to treat a manic episode in a 25-year-old woman. The patient had not responded to outpatient therapy with clopenthixol (a neuroleptic agent not available in the United States) and was treated vigorously with clozapine 100 mg three times a day. She developed a severe delirium, with visual and auditory hallucinations, and was unable to continue with clozapine therapy. As demonstrated by this case report, it is difficult to "load" patients with clozapine because of the possibility of the development of delirium. This is a problem particularly in geriatric patients who are very sensitive to the anticholinergic effects of clozapine (Frankenburg and Kalunian 1994).

Clozapine is not widely used in the short-term treatment of manic episodes, partly because it is widely perceived as an agent to be used for the long-term treatment of chronic refractory psychotic affective disorders. There is little in the literature to guide the clinician in the treatment of the acutely manic patient with clozapine, except for the report of Müller and Heipertz (1977) mentioned earlier (written in German and therefore not easily accessible to most English-speaking clinicians).

Clozapine and Depression

Will the use of clozapine in manic patients precipitate or induce depressive episodes? Kukopulos et al. (1980) showed that conventional neuroleptic agents may be "depressogenic" in the treatment of affective disorders in that they intensify and lengthen the postmanic depressions often seen in affective illnesses. Many authors have posited a role of neuroleptics in the genesis of depressive episodes in schizophrenic patients (Harrow et al. 1994). Many patients in our clinical experience who are treated with clozapine do become depressed, although in many cases it is difficult to distinguish between a medication-induced illness and depression as part of the natural course of the illness. In one study of patients being treated with clozapine at McLean Hospital, 18% were also being treated with fluoxetine (Centorrino et al. 1994).

Will the concurrent use of clozapine prevent the antidepressant-induced development of mania or rapid-cycling disorder in bipolar disorder (Kukopulos et al. 1980; Prien et al. 1973; Wehr and Goodwin 1979)? Although this question cannot be definitively answered yet, there have been few cases of manic episodes in patients receiving both clozapine and antidepressants.

Some anecdotal evidence also suggests that clozapine may have antidepressant properties. Privitera et al. (1993) described the treatment of a 44-year-old woman with bipolar II disorder with clozapine. She had suicidal ideation, mood-congruent delusions, anhedonia, and a Hamilton Rating Scale for Depression score of 29. The patient responded well to clozapine at 125 mg/day. Dassa et al. (1993) treated a 40-year-old woman with psychotic depression who had failed to respond to other drugs and electroconvulsive therapy (ECT). She responded to clozapine at doses of up to 500 mg/day. Ranjan and Meltzer (1996) described three additional patients with refractory psychotic depression who responded well to clozapine monotherapy.

In larger studies, evidence has also supported the role of clozapine as an antidepressant. Gross and Langner (1970) treated 15 schizoaffective patients and reported better success in the depressed than manic patients. Leppig et al. (1989) described clozapine at doses between 12.5 and 62.5 mg/day as having antidepressant properties in one-third of their patients with depressive features. They also described a surprisingly high rate of failure of their manic patients to respond to clozapine (see earlier). Because the average dose used in the Leppig et al. study was low (131 mg/day), perhaps lower doses are more effective antidepressants, whereas higher doses are better antimanic agents. On the other hand, in most case series, clozapine seems to have had, as described by Suppes et al. (1992), "bidirectional mood stabilization properties," in that the number of both depressions and manic episodes is decreased.

The synthesis of clozapine arose from a program in Switzerland involving tricyclic compounds. There is a structural similarity between an antidepressant that did arise from that program—dibenzepin—and clozapine, which may explain why clozapine possesses some antidepressant properties (Schmutz and Eichenberger 1982).

▶ Clozapine and Adjunctive Therapy

Because clozapine is used with treatment-resistant patients, it is perhaps not surprising that it is often used in conjunction with other agents, as noted earlier. Many patients with bipolar affective illness are treated with lithium and neuroleptics, anticonvulsants, or antidepressants. Peselow et al. (1994) concluded that lithium combined with another agent may be more effective treatment for patients who have already relapsed while being treated with lithium alone. However, the question of whether mood stabilizers and clozapine in particular offer any advantage over clozapine alone has yet to be answered. The combination of clozapine and valproic acid has been studied carefully by Kando et al. (1994) and found to be efficacious, safe, and free of increased side effects, with the exception of increased sedation and mild elevation in liver function tests.

Frankenburg et al. (1993) described the successful concurrent use of clozapine and ECT in 12 patients, of whom 1 had bipolar affective disorder and 1 had schizoaffective disorder. The manic patient (a 48-year-old male) also had mild mental retardation and a history of a severe head injury at the age of 12. He responded very well to the combined treatments. The schizoaffective patient (a 32-year-old male) had only minimal response.

Centorrino et al. (1994) showed that the simultaneous use of fluoxetine and clozapine led to a 76% increase in serum clozapine levels. Theoretically, this could lead to an increase in side effects, such as sedation or seizures, but in clinical practice the combination is well tolerated.

The efficacy of polypharmacy involving clozapine has not yet been studied in a controlled manner. Could patients on clozapine and either lithium or valproic acid have the second agent stopped? Suppes et al. (1991) showed that discontinuation of lithium in bipolar disorder may lead to an exacerbation of the illness. If lithium is to be discontinued because of patients' complaints of side effects (such as weight gain), it probably is safest to discontinue it over a period of at least 4 weeks (Suppes et al. 1993). Recent studies from Cleveland (Calabrese et al. 1996; Ranjan and Meltzer 1996) have suggested that clozapine monotherapy can be successful even in refractory patients.

Other Indications for Clozapine

Substance abuse is common in patients with affective disorder and may be associated with poor response to conventional therapy. Himmelhoch and Garfinkel (1986) noted that 12 of their 26 patients with dysphoric mania had histories of substance abuse. These patients tended to do poorly with lithium alone. Our group (M. Banov, C. A. Zarate, B. M. Cohen, F. R. Frankenburg, D. Scialabba, M. Kolbrener, J. D. Wines, P. Choras, and M. Tohen, April 1993, unpublished data) and Meltzer's group (Buckley et al. 1994) have noted that, in diagnostically heterogeneous groups, substance abuse does not predict poorer response to clozapine. Anecdotally, there have been several reports of patients with severe substance abuse problems doing well on clozapine and ending their substance abuse (Albanese et al. 1994). These reports are supported by animal work in which low doses of conventional neuroleptic agents increased the self-administration of psychomotor stimulants in rats; clozapine produced a dose-dependent decrease in cocaine self-administration (Roberts and Vickers 1984).

Finally, there is an intriguing association between neurological abnormalities and bipolar affective disorder. Neurological insults again may predict poor response to lithium. Himmelhoch and Garfinkel (1986) noted that most of their patients (the exact number cannot be obtained from their data) also had other neurological complications, such as seizures, migraine, or history of a severe head injury. Pope et al. (1988) reviewed the literature linking closed head injury to the development of cycling affective disorders and noted that their two patients with head injuries did poorly with lithium and well with valproate. Despite the fact that clozapine leads to abnormal electroencephalograms (EEGs) and increases the risk of seizures (Toth and Frankenburg 1994), clozapine has been used in neurologically abnormal patients with good effects, although, in one series of nine brain-injured patients, two patients did have seizures (Michals et al. 1993). Three case reports from Cleveland described the successful use of clozapine in patients with neurological illnesses and affective symptoms. Parsa et al. (1991) described the successful clozapine therapy of a 45-year-old woman with a manic-depression-like illness who presented with a psychotic depression and parkinsonian symptoms. She was treated with clozapine (dose not given) and remained fairly well for longer than 1 year. Sajatovic et al. (1991) treated a patient with Huntington's chorea and psychotic depression successfully with 175 mg/day of clozapine. Parsa et al. (1993) treated a 57-year-old woman with multiple system atrophy and a psychotic depression successfully with 100 mg/day of clozapine.

❱ Risperidone in Bipolar Disorder

Recently the new antipsychotic, risperidone—an agent that is a potent serotonin S_2 and dopamine D_2 receptor antagonist and that does not carry with it the risk of causing agranulocytosis—has been used in the treatment of psychotic affective disorders (Borison et al. 1992). Until now, there have been nine reports on the use of risperidone in mania and three on its use in depression.

Risperidone in Mania

Of nine reports on the use of risperidone in mania, four are case studies, one is a retrospective review, and four are open-label studies. The four case studies (Goodnick 1995; Kanagaratnam 1994; Madhusoodanan et al. 1995; Singh and Catalan 1994) all indicate successful results. Singh and Catalan indicated that four patients with mania and AIDS responded at a dose of 2–4 mg/day in 7–10 days with a decrease in the Young Mania Scale of 77%. Goodnick showed that two patients with psychotic mania who were previous nonresponders to lithium improved significantly within 7–10 days at a dose of 3–10 mg/day. Madhusoodanan et al. gave the medication to two geriatric patients with mixed bipolar disorder for 15 and 27 days; there were no side effects, and one of the two showed a significant response.

There have been one retrospective review (Keck et al. 1995) and four open studies (Ghaemi et al. 1995; Jacobsen 1995; Sajatovic 1995; Tohen et al. 1996). The retrospective review of risperidone by Keck et al. (1995), in a large series of patients, included 9 manic (7 pure and 2 "mixed") and 3 depressed patients. All 9 manic patients responded at a dose of 6–7 mg/day in a period of 8 weeks in conjunction with a mood stabilizer. Tohen et al. showed that a dose of 2–6 mg/day administered for at least 2 weeks led to a reduction of more than 50% in the Young Mania Scale in 10 of 13 patients. Side effects caused early dropout in only 1 patient (due to dizziness). Risperidone, as an adjunctive treatment to improve response, was used by Ghaemi et al. (1995) (2.8 mg/day, mean) and Jacobsen (1995) (1–6 mg/day). Their reported rates of improvement, respectively, were 9 of 14 (CGI > 2) and 6 of 6 (mean CGI level of severity of illness was reduced from 4.7

to 2.5, $P < .001$). The latter reported particular improvement in agitation, psychosis, sleep disturbance, and rapid cycling. In contrast, Sajatovic reported that none of the five patients placed on a dose of greater than 2 mg for an average of 5 weeks responded; two showed increased manic symptoms. This group had previously failed trials on lithium, anticonvulsants, and standard neuroleptics.

It is important further to note that in a trial of its use in schizoaffective disorder, four of six patients with bipolar schizoaffective disorder showed exacerbation of mania (Dwight et al. 1994). However, three of these four had significant mixed symptoms of both mania (Young Mania Scale > 18) and of depression (Hamilton Rating Scale for Depression > 15) at baseline. Perhaps in patients with mixed mania and depression, risperidone should be used only with extreme caution.

Risperidone in Depression

There have been only three published reports on the use of risperidone in psychotic depression (Hillert et al. 1992; Jacobsen 1995; Keck et al. 1995). Hillert et al. studied the use of risperidone in an open trial including seven patients with psychotic depression and three with schizoaffective depression at a dose of 4–10 mg/day for a period of 6 weeks. Patients were required to have baseline scores of at least 35 on the BPRS and of at least 20 on the Bech Rafaelsen Melancholia scale. There were improvements reported on both scales: the mean BPRS improved from 55.6 (baseline) to 42.7 (1 week) to 31.3 (final), and the mean Bech scale improved from 26.8 (baseline) to 18.8 (1 week) to 11.1 (final). In terms of individual patients, four of seven with psychotic depression showed significant improvement. Side effects reported included dizziness, sedation, mild tremor, and akathisia, each reported in 3 of the 10 patients. In terms of other open reports, Jacobsen showed that one patient with psychotic depression given 1.5 mg/day had a significant response, and Keck et al. indicated that a dose of 8 mg/day led to significant improvement when used as an adjunctive treatment for 8 weeks.

Thus, overall, in limited open trials of 55 patients with mania and 11 with depression, risperidone has produced significant improvement in more than 70% of patients. However, there are two important caveats: 1) none of these reports met the standard of research of being double-blind and placebo-controlled, and 2) there may be a significant risk of induction of mania in those patients with a mixed picture of both mania and depression.

▶ Olanzapine

Another recently released atypical antipsychotic is a relative of clozapine: olanzapine. This tranquilizer shows affinity at the D_1, D_4, 5-HT_2, 5-HT_3, 5-HT_6, muscarinic, and adrenergic (α_1) and histaminergic binding sites (Tollefson et al. 1997). In reports of a multicenter international trial, 1,996 patients were included that met criteria for schizophrenia, schizoaffective disorder, and schizophreniform disorder (DSM-III-R). Patients receiving a mean dose of 13.2 mg/day showed twice as good an improvement on the Montgomery-Asberg Depression Rating Scale (MADRS) as those receiving a mean haloperidol dose of 11.8 mg/day (6.0 versus 3.1, $P = .001$).

▶ Summary

Although currently indicated by the U.S. Food and Drug Administration (FDA) only for schizophrenic patients, clozapine has long been used successfully in the treatment of nonschizophrenic patients. In many large, open studies, clozapine has shown to be a useful agent in the treatment of bipolar affective disorder. Although it cannot be recommended as a first-line agent because of the risk of agranulocytosis (Alvir et al. 1993), patients with bipolar disorder who have not responded to lithium salts or anticonvulsant agents may be good candidates for clozapine therapy. In particular, clozapine may be indicated in the treatment of patients with dysphoric mania, rapid-cycling bipolar disorder, concurrent substance abuse, or history of neurological abnormality. More research is needed to delineate the role of clozapine in nonpsychotic bipolar illnesses, the correct dosing strategy, whether doses should differ according to the affective state of the patient, and whether there is a role for polypharmacotherapy in patients with treatment-resistant bipolar disorder. The role of risperidone, a new antipsychotic agent, in the treatment of psychotic affective disorder shows promise in the limited few case reports and open studies so far completed, but it needs further clarification in well-designed, controlled clinical trials. Olanzapine, similarly, needs more investigation.

▶ **REFERENCES**

Ahlfors UG, Baastrup PC, Dencker SJ, et al: Flupenthixol decanoate in recurrent manic-depressive illness: a comparison with lithium. Acta Psychiatr Scand 64:226–237, 1981

Albanese MJ, Khantzian EJ, Murphy SL, et al: Decreased substance abuse in chronically psychotic patients treated with clozapine. Am J Psychiatry 151:780–781, 1994

Alvir JMJ, Lieberman JA, Safferman AZ, et al: Clozapine-induced agranulocytosis: incidence and risk factors in the United States. N Engl J Med 329:162–167, 1993

American Psychiatric Association: Diagnostic and Statistical Manual of Mental Disorders, 3rd Edition, Revised. Washington, DC, American Psychiatric Association, 1987

Baldessarini RJ, Frankenburg FR: Clozapine: a novel antipsychotic agent. N Engl J Med 325:746–754, 1991

Battegay R, Cotar B, Fleischhauer J, et al: Results and side effects of treatment with clozapine (Leponex ®). Compr Psychiatry 18:423–428, 1977

Borison RL, Diamond BL, Pathiraja A: Clinical overview of risperidone, in Novel Antipsychotic Drugs. Edited by Meltzer HY. New York, Raven, 1992, pp 233–239

Buckley P, Thompson P, Way L, et al: Substance abuse among patients with treatment-resistant schizophrenia: characteristics and implications for clozapine therapy. Am J Psychiatry 151:385–389, 1994

Calabrese JR, Meltzer HY, Markovitz PJ: Clozapine prophylaxis in rapid cycling bipolar disorder. J Clin Psychopharmacol 11:396–397, 1991

Calabrese JR, Kimmel SE, Woyshville MJ: Clozapine for treatment refractory mania. Am J Psychiatry 153:759–764, 1996

Casey DE: Tardive dyskinesia and affective disorders, in Tardive Dyskinesia and Affective Disorders. Edited by Gardos G, Casey DE. Washington, DC, American Psychiatric Press, 1984, pp 2–19

Centorrino F, Baldessarini RJ, Kando JC, et al: Serum concentrations of clozapine and major metabolites: effects of cotreatment with valproate and fluoxetine. Am J Psychiatry 151:123–125, 1994

Chou JC-Y: Recent advances in treatment of acute mania. J Clin Psychopharmacol 11:3–21, 1991

Dassa D, Kaladjian A, Azorin JM, et al: Clozapine in the treatment of psychotic refractory depression. Br J Psychiatry 163:822–824, 1993

Dwight MM, Keck PE, Stanton SP, et al: Antidepressant activity and mania associated with risperidone treatment in schizoaffective disorder. Lancet 344:554–555, 1994

Endicott J, Spitzer RL, Fleiss JL, et al: The Global Assessment Scale (GAS). Arch Gen Psychiatry 33:766–771, 1976

Frankenburg FR: Clozapine and bipolar disorder. J Clin Psychopharmacol 13:289–290, 1993

Frankenburg FR, Kalunian D: Clozapine in the elderly. J Geriatr Psychiatry Neurol 7:131–134, 1994

Frankenburg FR, Zanarini MC: The uses of clozapine in nonschizophrenic patients. Harvard Review of Psychiatry 2:142–150, 1994

Frankenburg FR, Suppes T, McLean PE: Combined clozapine and electroconvulsive therapy. Convulsive Therapy 9:176–180, 1993

Ghaemi SN, Sachs GS, Baldassano CF, et al: Management of bipolar disorder with adjunctive risperidone: response to open treatment. American Psychiatric Association 1995 Annual Meeting New Research Program and Abstracts (NR 82). Washington, DC, American Psychiatric Association, 1995, p 77

Goodnick PJ: Risperidone treatment of refractory acute mania. J Clin Psychiatry 56:431–432, 1995

Goodwin FK, Jamison KR: Manic-Depressive Illness. New York, Oxford University Press, 1990

Gross H, Langner E: Das neuroleptikum 100-129/HF-1854 (Clozapin) in der Psychiatrie. International Pharmacopsychiatry 4:220–230, 1970

Guy N: ECDEU Assessment Manual for Psychopharmacology. Washington, DC, U.S. Department of Health, Education & Welfare, 1976

Hamilton M: A rating scale for depression. J Neurol Neurosurg Psychiatry 23:56–62, 1960

Harrow M, Yonan CA, Sands JR, et al: Depression in schizophrenia: are neuroleptics, akinesia, or anhedonia involved? Schizophr Bull 20:327–338, 1994

Hillert A, Maier W, Wetzel H, et al: Risperidone in the treatment of disorders with a combined psychotic and depressive syndrome: a functional approach. Pharmacopsychiatry 25:213–217, 1992

Himmelhoch JM, Garfinkel ME: Mixed mania: diagnosis and treatment. Psychopharmacol Bull 22:613–620, 1986

Jacobsen FM: Risperidone in the treatment of affective illness and obsessive-compulsive disorder. J Clin Psychiatry 56:423–429, 1995

Kanagaratnam G: Case report 3: Risperidone in bipolar affective disorder. JDD Case History Series No 1:11–12, 1994

Kando JC, Tohen M, Castillo J, et al: Concurrent use of clozapine and valproate in affective and psychotic disorders. J Clin Psychiatry 55:255–257, 1994

Kane JM, Woerner MG, Pollack S, et al: Does clozapine cause tardive dyskinesia? J Clin Psychiatry 54:327–330, 1993

Keck PE, Wilson DR, Strakowski SM, et al: Clinical predictors of acute risperidone response in schizophrenia, schizoaffective disorder, and psychotic mood disorders. J Clin Psychiatry 56:466–470, 1995

Kukopulos A, Reginaldi D, Laddomada P, et al: Course of the manic-depressive cycle and changes caused by treatments. Pharmakopsychiatria Neuropsychopharmakologia 13:156–167, 1980

Leppig M, Bosch B, Naber D, et al: Clozapine in the treatment of 121 out-patients. Psychopharmacology 99:S77–S79, 1989

Madhusoodanan A, Brenner R, Araujo L, et al: Efficacy of risperidone treatment for psychoses associated with schizophrenia, schizoaffective disorder, bipolar disorder, or senile dementia in 11 geriatric patients: a case series. J Clin Psychiatry 56:514–518, 1995

McElroy SL, Dessain EC, Pope HG, et al: Clozapine in the treatment of psychotic mood disorders, schizoaffective disorder, and schizophrenia. J Clin Psychiatry 52:411–414, 1991

Michals ML, Crismon ML, Roberts S, et al: Clozapine response and adverse effects in nine brain-injured patients. J Clin Psychopharmacol 13:198–203, 1993

Müller P, Heipertz R: Zur Behandlung manischer Psychosen mit Clozapin. Fortschr Neurol Psychiatr 45:420–424, 1977

Naber D, Holzbach R, Perro C, et al: Clinical management of clozapine patients in relation to efficacy and side-effects. Br J Psychiatry 160 (suppl 17):54–59, 1992

Overall JE, Gorham DR: The Brief Psychiatric Rating Scale. Psychol Rep 10:799–812, 1962

Parsa MA, Ramirez LF, Loula EC, et al: Effect of clozapine on psychotic depression and Parkinsonism. J Clin Psychopharmacol 11:330–331, 1991

Parsa MA, Simon M, Dubrow C, et al: Psychiatric manifestations of olivoponto-cerebellar atrophy and treatment with clozapine. Int J Psychiatry Med 23:149–156, 1993

Peselow ED, Fieve RR, Difiglia C, et al: Lithium prophylaxis of bipolar illness: the value of combination treatment. Br J Psychiatry 164:208–214, 1994

Pope HG, McElroy SL, Satlin A, et al: Head injury, bipolar disorder, and response to valproate. Compr Psychiatry 29:34–38, 1988

Prien RF, Klett CJ, Caffey EM Jr: Lithium carbonate and imipramine in prevention of affective episodes: a comparison in recurrent affective illness. Arch Gen Psychiatry 29:420–425, 1973

Prien RF, Kupfer DJ, Mansky PA, et al: Drug therapy in the prevention of recurrences in unipolar and bipolar affective disorder. Arch Gen Psychiatry 41:1096–1104, 1984

Privitera MR, Lamberti JS, Maharaj K: Clozapine in a bipolar depressed patient. Am J Psychiatry 150:986, 1993

Ranjan R, Meltzer HY: Acute and long-term effectiveness of clozapine in treatment-resistant psychotic depression. Biol Psychiatry 40:253–258, 1996

Ratey JJ, Leveroni C, Kilmer D, et al: The effects of clozapine on severely aggressive psychiatric inpatients in a state hospital. J Clin Psychiatry 54:219–223, 1993

Roberts DCS, Vickers G: Atypical neuroleptics increase self-administration of cocaine: an evaluation of a behavioral screen for antipsychotic activity. Psychopharmacology (Berlin) 82:135–138, 1984

Sachs GS: Use of clonazepam for bipolar affective disorder. J Clin Psychiatry 51 (suppl):31–34, 1990

Sachs GS, Lafer B, Truman CJ, et al: Lithium monotherapy: miracle, myth and misunderstanding. Psychiatric Annals 24:299–306, 1994

Sajatovic M: A pilot study evaluating the efficacy of risperidone in treatment refractory acute bipolar and schizoaffective mania (poster 19). NCDEU Annual Meeting, Orlando, FL, May 31–June 3, 1995, p 35

Sajatovic M, Verbanac P, Ramirez LF, et al: Clozapine treatment of psychiatric symptoms resistant to neuroleptic treatment in patients with Huntington's chorea. Neurology 41:156, 1991

Schmutz J, Eichenberger E: Clozapine, in Chronicles of Drug Discovery, Vol 1. Edited by Bindra JS, Lednicer D. New York, Wiley, 1982, pp 39–58

Schuster P, Gabriel E, Küfferle B, et al: Reversal by physostigmine of clozapine-induced delirium. Clinical Toxicology 10:437–441, 1977

Singh AN, Catalan J: Risperidone in HIV-related manic psychosis. Lancet 344:1029–1030, 1994

Spitzer RL, Williams JBW, Gibbon M: Structured Clinical Interview for DSM-III-R Axis I Disorders (SCID I). New York, New York State Psychiatric Institute, 1987

Suppes T, Baldessarini RJ, Faedda GL, et al: Risk of recurrence following discontinuation of lithium treatment in bipolar disorder. Arch Gen Psychiatry 48:1082–1088, 1991

Suppes T, McElroy SL, Gilbert J, et al: Clozapine in the treatment of dysphoric mania. Biol Psychiatry 32:270–280, 1992

Suppes T, Baldessarini RJ, Faedda GL, et al: Discontinuation of maintenance treatment in bipolar disorder: risks and implications. Harvard Review of Psychiatry 1:131–144, 1993

Tohen M, Zarate CA Jr, Centorrino F, et al: Risperidone in the treatment of mania (NR 286). J Clin Psychiatry 57:249–253, 1996

Tollefson GD, Beasley CM, Tran PV, et al: Olanzapine vs. haloperidol in the treatment of schizophrenia and schizoaffective and schizophreniform disorders: results of an international collaborative study. Am J Psychiatry 154:457–465, 1997

Toth P, Frankenburg FR: Clozapine and seizures: a review. Can J Psychiatry 151:123–124, 1994

Van Putten T: Why do schizophrenic patients refuse to take their drugs? Arch Gen Psychiatry 31:67–72, 1974

Vestergaard P: Treatment and prevention of mania: a Scandinavian perspective. Neuropsychopharmacology 7:249–255, 1992

Wehr TA, Goodwin FK: Rapid cycling in manic-depressives induced by tricyclic antidepressants. Arch Gen Psychiatry 36:555–559, 1979

CHAPTER 16

CALCIUM ANTAGONISTS AND NEWER ANTICONVULSANTS

M. Beatriz Currier, M.D., and
Paul J. Goodnick, M.D.

Bipolar disorder is a recurrent, disabling, and potentially life-threatening illness that demands an effective treatment. Lithium is an effective treatment for the majority of patients with bipolar disorder and is considered to be the standard treatment for acute and preventive pharmaco-management of mania (Prien et al. 1973). Preventive treatment studies, however, have revealed that approximately one-third of bipolar disorder patients fail to respond adequately to this treatment (Prien and Gelenberg 1989). Effective management of severe manic states frequently requires neuroleptics, which may produce intolerable extrapyramidal side effects. Bipolar patients with certain clinical features tend to respond poorly to lithium—specifically, patients with rapid cycles (Dunner et al. 1977), patients with episodes characterized by mixed states (manic and depressive features) (Himmelhoch and Garfinkel 1986), and patients who have comorbid personality disturbances (Chou 1991). Adverse side effects with chronic lithium management and the teratogenic effects associated with lithium frequently result in patient noncompliance. For lithium-refractory patients and lithium-intolerant patients, alternative effective treatments for mania are greatly needed (Chou 1991; Prien and Gelenberg 1989).

In 1982, Dubovsky et al. reported the first case of acute mania successfully treated with verapamil. Since that report, attention has focused on the use of calcium antagonists in acute and prophylactic treatment of mania. In this chapter, we review the role of calcium in the proposed pathophysiology of affective disturbance; the mechanism of action, pharmacology, and clinical indications of the calcium antagonists available in the United States; and the guidelines for administering these medications. A review of the studies addressing the efficacy of calcium antagonists in the treatment of mania is summarized with a focus on controlled, double-blind studies (see Table 16–1 and Table 16–2).

▶ IMPACT OF CALCIUM ION DYSREGULATION ON THE CENTRAL NERVOUS SYSTEM

Several lines of evidence have suggested an association between calcium concentration and neuropsychiatric abnormalities (Dubovsky 1986; Dubovsky and Franks 1983; Pollack et al. 1987). Disturbances of extracellular calcium concentration in the serum have been linked to alterations in mood, cognition, thought process, and level of arousal. Hypercalcemia produces depression, stupor, and coma, whereas hypocalcemia may present with delirium, psychosis, mood irritability, anxiety, and mania. Extracellular calcium concentration in the cerebrospinal fluid (CSF) of bipolar disorder patients in a manic state and in a depressed state has also been measured (Carmen and Wyatt 1979; Dubovsky and Franks 1983). Manic patients had low CSF calcium concentration, whereas depressed patients had elevated CSF calcium concentration. In addition, recovery from depression was associated with a lowering of the CSF calcium concentration.

Elevated intracellular calcium in peripheral cells of patients with mania and depression has also been reported. Dubovsky et al. (1992) reviewed four studies from their center on platelet intracellular calcium in bipolar disorder. In their initial study (Dubovsky et al. 1989), it was reported that mean baseline and agonist-stimulated levels (nM) were, respectively: highest in untreated manic patients (157 ± 65.1, 855 ± 247.7), untreated bipolar depressed (136 ± 44.8, 769 ± 280.2), untreated unipolar depressed (124 ± 24.9, 388 ± 100.3), and control subjects (98 ± 15, 427 ± 152). The next study (Dubovsky et al. 1991a) reconfirmed these results: untreated bipolar depressed (231 ± 30.7,

Table 16–1. Verapamil treatment of mania

Investigators	Dose (mg/day)	Duration (days)	Result (No. improved)
Case reports			
Dubovsky et al. 1982	160	21	1/1
Dubovsky and Franks 1983	160–480	21	2/2
Gitlin and Weiss 1984	240	Acute/prophylaxis	1/1
Kennedy et al. 1986	320	30	0/1
Solomon and Williamson 1986	320	4 months	2/2
Patterson 1987	320	10	1/1
Jacobsen et al. 1987	160	6 months	1/1
Mathis et al. 1988	320	?	2/4
Helmuth et al. 1989	360	7	7/7
Diecken 1990	320	24 months	1/1
Goodnick 1993	240	Acute/prophylaxis	3/3 (1/1 acute)
Open studies			
Hoschl et al. 1986	120–480	30	5/5
Brotman et al. 1986	240–320	10	6/6
Barton and Gitlin 1987	160–240	Maximum 21	0/8
Dinan et al. 1988	320–400	21	5/6
Goodnick 1996	360	14	12/12

(continued)

340 Mania: Clinical and Research Perspectives

Table 16–1. Verapamil treatment of mania *(continued)*

Investigators	Dose (mg/day)	Duration (days)	Result (No. improved)
Double-blind studies			
Giannini et al. 1984	320	30	Verapamil: −68%; lithium: −73% BPRS
Dose et al. 1986	320–480	7	7/8
Dubovsky et al. 1986	480	24	5/7 (verapamil: −53% BPRS; placebo: −22%)
Giannini et al. 1986	320	20	Verapamil > clonidine (day 10)
Hoschl and Kozeny 1989	120–480	35	Verapamil: −45% BPRS; lithium + neuroleptic: −27%; neuroleptic: −39%
Garza-Trevino et al. 1992	320	28	Verapamil: −44% Peterson Mania Scale; lithium: −39%
Janiciak et al. 1994	480	21	Verapamil: 3/5; placebo: 1/9

Note. BPRS = Brief Psychiatric Rating Scale.

Table 16–2. Summary of calcium antagonists in treatment of mania

Medication	Case report	Study type Open study	Double-blind	Dose (mg/day)	Success (%)
Verapamil					
Successes/total studies	10/11	4/5	7/7	160–480	92
Patients: improved/total	14/17	28/37	16/20 (3 studies)		79
Diltiazem					
Successes/total studies	0/0	1/1	0/0	120–360	100
Patients: improved/total	0/0	5/7	0/0		72
Nimodipine					
Successes/total studies	1/1	1/1	1/1	90–720	100
Patients: improved/total	2/2	6/6	5/9		76

454 ± 120.4), untreated unipolar depressed (158 ± 33.6, 362 ± 103.3), and control subjects (151 ± 10.2, 330 ± 36.8). Elevated intracellular calcium in bipolar depression over control subjects was also replicated (baseline: 221 ± 45.4 versus 150 ± 11.3, P < .02; agonist-stimulated: 424 ± 123 versus 304 ± 109.5, P < .004) (Dubovsky et al. 1991b). Finally, both platelet and lymphocyte intracellular calcium were studied in baseline studies in a combination of samples from manic plus bipolar depressed patients versus control subjects. For both platelet, as expected (121 ± 23.8 versus 79 ± 8.7, P < .001) and lymphocyte (129 ± 32.2 versus 83 ± 7.8, P < .001), measures of intracellular calcium elevations were significantly greater in bipolar subjects than in control subjects. Mean membrane concentrations (nM) of calmodulin-activated calcium ATPase, which establishes the normal level of intracellular calcium in most cells, has been described as significantly higher in samples from 35 bipolar I patients (11.8 ± 3.99, P < .005) and 21 bipolar II patients (11.3 ± 2.98, P < .02) than in 35 control subjects (9.42 ± 2.67) (Meltzer et al. 1988).

The role of intracellular calcium on biogenic amine synthesis, as well as on the sensitivity of postsynaptic adrenergic receptors, further links calcium alteration with affective states (Dubovsky and Franks 1983; Hoschl 1991). The synthesis and release of dopamine, norepinephrine, and serotonin from sympatosomes is mediated by intracellular calcium, which binds to calmodulin, an effector protein (Dubovsky and Franks 1983; Pollack et al. 1987). This calmodulin-calcium complex then activates tyrosine hydroxylase and tryptophan hydroxylase, the rate-limiting enzymes for the synthesis of the biogenic amines (Dubovsky and Franks 1983). The sensitivity of postsynaptic α_1- and α_2-adrenoreceptors is altered via a calcium-stimulated membrane phosphorylase enzyme that modifies the postsynaptic membrane configuration (Dubovsky and Franks 1983).

Several psychotropic medications including lithium and phenothiazines have calcium-channel–blocking properties (Dubovsky 1986; Dubovsky and Franks 1983; Himmelhoch and Garfinkel 1986; Johnson et al. 1993; Wood 1985). As a result, lithium has frequently been shown to lead to elevated plasma calcium levels (Carman and Wyatt 1979; Gerner et al. 1977; Linder et al. 1993); for example, Linder et al. (1993) showed an increase in plasma calcium of greater than 2.6 mmol/L in 25.5% of patients. Similarly, Dubovsky et al. (1992) showed that levels of platelet intracellular calcium (nM) were lower by 25%–29% in bipolar depressed patient treated with lithium but only 20%–23% in untreated control subjects. Although it remains unclear whether this calcium-blocking property provides the antimanic effect (Dubovsky and Franks 1983; Dubovsky et al. 1992; Pollack et al. 1987), this mechanism of action does suggest that calcium may play a role in mood regulation in controlling release of catecholamines. Of interest, beta-blockers and calcitonin, both of which lower free intracellular calcium, have been shown to be effective in controlling agitation in manic patients (Dubovsky 1986).

▌ Calcium Antagonists: Mechanism of Action and Clinical Uses

Cellular calcium concentration gradients influence the activity of smooth muscle cells and neurons. The intracellular calcium concentration is typically four times lower than the extracellular concentration (Dubovsky and Franks 1983). Neurons and smooth muscle cells maintain this gradient via the following mechanisms: 1) active transport of calcium out of the cell via the Na-Ca counterexchange system and the Ca-hydrogen antiport system; 2) movement of calcium into intracellular storage sites, such as the endoplasmic reticulum; 3) binding calcium to an intracellular binding protein, calmodulin; and 4) preventing the influx of calcium by blocking calcium channels (Dubovsky and Franks 1983; El-Mallakh and Jaziri 1990; Hoschl 1991). In addition to calcium-channel entry, calcium influx also occurs through membrane leakage and the Na-Ca antiport pathways (i.e., calcium ions follow the sodium ion influx during cellular depolarization) (El-Mallakh and Jaziri 1990). There are two types of calcium ion influx channels. The voltage-sensitive channels are voltage dependent (i.e., opened by propagation of the action potential), whereas the receptor-operated channels are opened by a neurotransmitter binding with the receptor (El-Mallakh and Jaziri 1990).

The principal mechanism of action of calcium antagonists is to inactivate the voltage-sensitive calcium channel, thus blocking calcium influx (Dubovsky 1986; Dubovsky and Franks 1983; Hoschl 1991;

Mehta 1994; Pollack et al. 1987). By doing so, these medications inhibit smooth muscle contraction, neurotransmitter synthesis and release, and neural signal transmission. In addition, by preventing the calcium influx associated with hypoxia, the calcium-channel blocker nimodipine also ameliorates neuronal damage typically associated with ischemia (El-Mallakh and Jaziri 1990; Hoschl 1991).

Calcium antagonists have a wide variety of clinical uses for nonpsychiatric conditions. Cardiovascular indications include supraventricular tachycardia, angina, hypertrophic cardiomyopathy, myocardial ischemia, hypertension, and the treatment of excessive platelet aggregation (Dubovsky 1986; Hoschl 1991; Pollack et al. 1987). Furthermore, successful management of achalasia, esophageal spasm, diarrhea, asthma, dysmenorrhea, premature labor, migraine headaches, Tourette's syndrome, and cerebral vasospasm following intracerebral hemorrhage has also been reported with the use of calcium antagonists.

In addition to mood disorders, calcium antagonists have been applied to a variety of other neuropsychiatric conditions. Agitation associated with phencyclidine intoxication and with dementia in geriatric patients has successfully been treated with verapamil (Dubovsky 1986; Hoschl 1991). Four of seven patients with "treatment-resistant" panic disorder showed improvement on the calcium-channel inhibitors verapamil (240 mg/day) or diltiazem (60 mg/day) (Goldstein 1985; Pollack et al. 1987). In contrast, several double-blind, placebo-controlled studies have found verapamil to be ineffective in the treatment of chronic schizophrenic patients (Grebb et al. 1986; Pickar et al. 1987).

▶ PHARMACOLOGICAL PROFILE OF CALCIUM ANTAGONISTS

Calcium antagonists as a group are chemically heterogenous. To date, the four compounds available in the United States are verapamil, nifedipine, diltiazem, and nimodipine (Mehta 1994; Pollack et al. 1987). We now briefly review the therapeutic effects, standard dose ranges, most common side effects, and several reports of drug-drug interactions associated with these agents.

Verapamil

A diphenylalkylamine compound, verapamil is approved for treatment of angina and parenteral treatment of tachyarrhythmias (Mehta 1994). Its typical dose range is 240–480 mg/day in divided doses. The therapeutic cardiovascular effects are achieved through dilation of main coronary arteries and prevention of coronary vasospasm. Cardiac conduction is slowed through the atrioventricular node (Pollack et al. 1987). For this reason, it is contraindicated in patients with atrioventricular block. Verapamil is highly lipophilic and readily crosses the blood-brain barrier (Doran et al. 1985; Hoschl 1991). The CSF concentration is approximately 7% of the serum concentration following oral or parenteral administration of verapamil (Doran et al. 1985). To date, this calcium antagonist has been most extensively studied in the treatment of mood disorders. It is generally well tolerated and safe. The most commonly reported side effects have included nausea, vertigo, headache, dry mouth, and constipation (Hoschl 1991). Isolated case reports of adverse drug interactions with verapamil have included reports of lithium toxicity, as well as decreased lithium levels (Hoschl 1991; Prien and Gelenberg 1989). Neurotoxicity has been associated with combined use of carbamazepine and verapamil, as well as the combination of carbamazepine and diltiazem (Chou 1991). Profound bradycardia has also been reported with concomitant use of verapamil and lithium (Dubovsky et al. 1987). Verapamil has not been reported to have hypnotic or sedative effects.

Diltiazem

Diltiazem, a benzothiazepine-class calcium antagonist, is used for the treatment of angina. The typical dose range is 120–240 mg/day in divided doses (Mehta 1994). Similar to verapamil, diltiazem slows cardiac conduction through the atrioventricular node. Diltiazem has been reported to increase digoxin serum levels (Pollack et al. 1987).

Nifedipine

Nifedipine, a dihydropyridine calcium antagonist, is also used for the treatment of angina (Mehta 1994). Its typical dose range is 30–120 mg/day in divided doses with a maximum dose of 180 mg/day. Cimetidine inhibits the metabolism of nifedipine, which leads to elevated nifedipine plasma levels (Pollack et al. 1987). As compared with verapamil, nifedipine has an increased likelihood of producing hypotension and reflex tachycardia.

Nimodipine

Nimodipine is a compound from the phenyldihydropyridine class of calcium antagonists. This agent is the most lipophilic and thus crosses the blood-brain barrier to provide more robust action on the central nervous system (Langley and Sorkin 1989). This compound prevents cerebral vasospasm following a subarachnoid hemorrhage (Pazzaglia et al. 1993). In addition, it has an anticonvulsant effect and decreases cocaine-induced hyperactivity (Pazzaglia et al. 1993). Typical dose range is 180–360 mg/day to a maximum dose of 720 mg/day. It is generally well tolerated even at high doses, with reports only of low blood pressure in some cases (Brunet et al. 1990). A unique property of nimodipine as compared with the other calcium antagonists is its lack of effect on the myocardium (Brunet et al. 1990). It is also unique among the calcium-channel inhibitors in having anticonvulsant properties (de Falco et al. 1992).

Calcium Antagonists Versus Lithium

In comparing the calcium-antagonistic medications with lithium, verapamil has similar effects on cardiac conduction and various endocrine systems. Both verapamil and lithium slow conduction throughout the atrioventricular node and decrease the spontaneous depolarization of the sinoatrial node (Antman et al. 1980; Dubovsky and Franks 1983). They both decrease insulin secretion, leading to glucose intolerance (Devis et al. 1975; Dubovsky and Franks 1983), and they both interfere with thyroid function (Dubovsky and Franks 1983; Eto et al. 1974). Lithium, verapamil, and nifedipine all interfere with the synthesis and release of antidiuretic hormone (Dubovsky and Franks 1983; Russell and Thorn 1974).

▶ Preliminary Studies of Calcium-Channel Inhibitors in the Treatment of Mania

In this section, progressing from case reports to open trials to double-blind studies, the current status of the application of calcium-channel inhibitors to bipolar disorder is reviewed (see Table 16–1 and Table 16–2). Despite the fact that the first successful use of verapamil occurred longer than 10 years ago (Dubovsky et al. 1982), the lack of availability of funds to pursue this research has impeded its advance in contrast to that of other potential psychotropic agents (Dubovsky 1994).

Case Reports

Most of the case studies have focused on the use of verapamil in the treatment of mania, both acute and prophylactic (see Table 16–1 and Table 16–2) (Dubovsky and Franks 1983; Dubovsky et al. 1982; Gitlin and Weiss 1984; Goodnick 1993; Helmuth et al. 1989; Jacobsen et al. 1987; Kennedy et al. 1986; Mathis et al. 1988; Patterson 1987; Solomon and Williamson 1986; Wehr et al. 1988). Dubovsky et al. (1982) reported the first case of successful treatment of an acute manic episode, diagnosed by DSM-III (American Psychiatric Association 1980) criteria, in a double-blind, crossover design. After 3 weeks on verapamil 80 mg tid, the patient experienced significant clinical improvement. The Manic State Rating Scale (MSRS) score decreased from 35 to 14. The patient relapsed (the MSRS increased to 34) 4 days after crossing over to placebo. Two additional double-blind case reports revealed dramatic improvement of acute mania with verapamil doses ranging from 160 to 480 mg/day over a 3-week treatment period (Dubovsky and Franks 1983). The two patients showed MSRS improvements when they were switched from placebo to verapamil, followed by relapse on reintroduction of placebo (patient 1: 80 to 45 to 90; patient 2: 35 to 15 to 30). In a manic patient with grandiose delusions treated with verapamil 320 mg/day, Patterson et al. (1987) reported a noticeable decrease in psychomotor agitation and rate of speech within 18 hours of starting verapamil. After 36 hours on this medication, the patient's sleep patterns stabilized. The grandiose delusions significantly decreased after 96 hours on verapamil, and the patient was discharged 10 days after beginning this treatment.

Goodnick (1993) reported on the safe and effective use of verapamil in the acute and prophylactic treatment of mania in three patients during pregnancy. An acutely manic patient with psychosis early in the course of her pregnancy experienced remission of manic symptoms and better control of psychotic symptoms after 2 weeks on verapamil slow-release 240 mg once a day. This dose was maintained throughout her pregnancy with no neonatal complications and no postpartum mood changes. Two other women who had experienced manic episodes in previous pregnancies when noncompliant with lithium had effective prophylaxis with verapamil slow-release 240 mg throughout their pregnancies without complications or postpartum mood changes.

Gitlin and Weiss (1984) published a case of a 32-year-old woman with a history of multiple antidepressant-induced manias despite lithium prophylaxis maintained at 1.2 mEq/L. Verapamil at a dose of 80 mg tid successfully treated hypomania and maintained mood stability for at least 1 year.

Dubovsky et al. (1985) reported on the successful prophylactic treatment of phenelzine-induced mania with verapamil 400 mg/day. A bipolar patient with previous episodes of phenelzine-induced hypomania underwent a double-blind, placebo-controlled "off-on-off-on" design. On reaching 2 weeks on verapamil 400 mg/day, phenelzine 45 mg/day was added to the regimen for 4 weeks with no emergence of mania. Within 3 weeks of crossing over to placebo combined with phenelzine, the patient relapsed into mania, which was again resolved when verapamil was restarted. The patient continued on verapamil for 8 months with no relapse.

Case reports on the treatment efficacy of other calcium antagonists in mania are scarce. Lindelius and Nilsson (1992) described a patient with an approximate 20-year history of bipolar disorder with annual cycles who received effective prophylaxis with flunarizine. Because the patient was intolerant to lithium side effects, a trial on flunarizine 10 mg/day was started with no further affective episodes for 3 years. He tolerated the calcium antagonist well with no adverse side effects. The patient developed depression after 3 years and received electroconvulsive therapy (ECT) while taking flunarizine, with good results and no complications. This calcium antagonist is not available in the United States.

Goodnick (1995) found in two patients that nimodipine was an effective treatment for rapid- and "ultra"–rapid-cycling bipolar patients. Patient 1 with an increasing rate of frequency of mania did not respond to lithium, valproate, thyroid elevation, or verapamil; this patient reached a severity of rapid mood shifts occurring up to every hour. This patient did improve dramatically, however, with nimodipine 60 mg tid. This improvement has persisted for a full year. Patient 2 also had increased frequency of manic-depressive episodes, developing rapid-cycling status by early 1992. Because of a previous lack of response, nimodipine at a dose of 60 mg tid was used to replace a combination of lithium plus carbamazepine, among others. The patient's cycling slowed within 10 days and stopped after 3 weeks; improvement persisted on nimodipine alone for 5 months.

Open Clinical Trials

Five open trials with verapamil have addressed acute treatment of mania (Barton and Gitlin 1987; Brotman et al. 1986; Dinan et al. 1988; Goodnick 1996; Hoschl et al. 1986) (see Table 16–1 and Table 16–2). Hoschl presented results on five manic patients placed on verapamil at a dose of 120–480 mg/day who all achieved remission within 1 month. Brotman et al. reported that all six acutely manic bipolar patients, who were either lithium nonresponders or lithium intolerant, showed a prompt reduction in manic symptoms as measured by the Young Mania Scale and the Brief Psychiatric Rating Scale (BPRS) within 3 weeks on verapamil at doses ranging from 240 to 320 mg/day. Four of these patients who were psychotic required concomitant use of neuroleptics early in their hospitalization. Three of the patients relapsed within 3 weeks of discontinuing verapamil. There were no reports of adverse side effects.

Barton and Gitlin (1987) presented negative results on the use of verapamil in previous nonresponders (12 nonresponders to carbamazepine and 11 to lithium). None of the eight manic patients treated with 160–240 mg/day of verapamil responded, as determined by the

Young Mania Scale. It is quite possible that this dosage was too low to produce therapeutic benefit; most of the more successful studies (see later, Dubovsky et al. 1986; Garza-Trevino et al. 1992; Giannini et al. 1984) used much higher doses. These patients may also have been overall refractory to all treatments. In contrast, two of the four patients given 240–320 mg/day of verapamil for 18 months showed mild improvement in prophylaxis.

Dinan et al. (1988) had more encouraging results with verapamil given at a higher dose of 320–400 mg/day for 21 days to six acutely manic patients according to DSM-III criteria. Five of the six patients (83%) showed significant improvement in manic symptoms as measured by the Peterson Rating Scale by the second week. Two of the patients were also receiving neuroleptics. One patient dropped out secondary to severe mania. There were no reports of adverse side effects.

Goodnick (1996) administered verapamil for 2 weeks at a dose of 360 mg/day to 12 patients meeting DSM-III-R (American Psychiatric Association 1987) criteria for mania. All patients showed some improvement on verapamil. Overall, the change on the Young Mania Scale was 60%. Furthermore, improvement on the Young Mania Scale correlated significantly with increase in plasma calcium ($r = -.61$, $P < .05$). The most recent single-blind comparison of verapamil (240–360 mg/day) versus lithium showed reductions in the Brief Psychiatric Rating Scale (BPRS) and the Mania Rating Scale (MRS) for both treatments. However, reductions in both cases were greater for lithium ($P = .002$ and $P = .018$, respectively (Walter et al. 1996).

Diltiazem has also been studied in an open design study for acute treatment of mania. Caillard (1985) reported significant clinical improvement in five of seven patients treated for acute mania. Diltiazem was administered for 14 days at doses of 120–360 mg/day. The two patients who failed to respond had a secondary mania by Feighner's criteria (Feighner et al. 1972) (i.e., organic mood disorder by DSM-III-R criteria). Side effects were few but included headache, transient edema of the extremities, and vertigo without orthostasis. No sedative effect was noted.

In a 7-day controlled, open-trial design, the efficacy of nimodipine in the acute treatment of mild mania was tested. Brunet et al. (1990)

reported significant clinical improvement on day 7 in all six patients treated with nimodipine 360 mg/day. Mood and "speech activity" were most improved, whereas sleep was least improved. Two patients in the sample required prn droperidol. No adverse side effects occurred; no changes in blood pressure, heart rate, electrocardiogram, or electroencephalography were noted; and no sedative effects were noted. All patients did have increased serum calcium levels that remained within the normal range. In one study on the use of nimodipine in prophylaxis of bipolar disorder, Manna (1991) found that in nine rapid-cycling bipolar patients randomized in sequential 6-month periods to either nimodipine alone, lithium alone, or nimodipine plus lithium, the combination was more effective than either agent alone in reducing the number and duration of relapses into either mania or depression.

Double-Blind Controlled Studies

A variety of double-blind studies have been conducted on the calcium-channel inhibitors (see Table 16–1 and Table 16–2). With verapamil, three studies have been conducted against placebo (Dose et al. 1986; Dubovsky et al. 1986; Janiciak et al. 1994), two against lithium (Garza-Trevino et al. 1992; Giannini et al. 1984), and two against other agents (Giannini et al. 1985; Hoschl and Kozeny 1989). There has also been one lithium-controlled study of prophylaxis on verapamil (Giannini et al. 1987). With regard to other agents, there has been one placebo-controlled trial "off-on-off" paradigm for nimodipine against placebo (Pazzaglia et al. 1993) and one placebo-controlled, parallel-design protocol for D-600 (4-methoxy-verapamil) (Aldenhoff et al. 1986).

Regarding the verapamil studies, Dose et al. (1986) reported significant improvement among seven of eight patients with either mania or schizoaffective mania treated with a short 7-day trial of verapamil 320–480 mg/day in an A-B-A design preceded and followed by 1 week of placebo. On the Inpatient Multidimensional Psychiatric Scale, the mean percentage of maximum score for mania dropped from 18 (placebo 1) to 12 (verapamil) to 17 (placebo 2). The clinical improvement was noted within 3 days in some patients. Several patients had neuroleptic and lithium included in the treatment regimens. Minor changes in blood pressure and heart rate were noted. The short time trial, small sample, unknown diagnostic criteria, and use of concomitant psychotropics are limitations of this study.

In a longer trial of 24 days, Dubovsky et al. (1986) evaluated verapamil's efficacy in the acute treatment of moderate to severe mania (DSM-III criteria) among seven patients, including two with comorbid dementia, one due to past history of alcoholism, and one due to lithium-induced neurotoxicity. In a double-blind design, verapamil doses up to 480 mg were administered for 24 days, followed by placebo for another 24 days. Using the MSRS and the BPRS, five of the seven patients significantly improved on verapamil within 1–2 weeks. Overall, both the mean MSRS and the BPRS scores improved from baseline to verapamil and worsened on placebo (MSRS: 57.3 to 22.4 to 44.5; BPRS: 33.7 to 15.7 to 26.4). No adverse effects were noted.

The most recent report is preliminary, with the extension still in progress (Janiciak et al. 1994). This 3-week, double-blind, parallel-group, random-assignment, placebo-controlled trial of verapamil in DSM-III-R bipolar disorder, manic/mixed type employed the MRS and BPRS mania subscale (items 4, 6, 8, 10, 15, 17) for determination of response with at least 50% improvement in MRS for determination of response. To this point, blinds have been broken on 21 patients (11 females, 10 males) with a mean age of 35.8 years. Because of the small sample size, analysis of covariance based on change in the MRS and BPRS has not yet proved significant. However, of patients remaining at least 1 week in the double-blind phase, response has been seen in 3/5 (60%) of the verapamil versus only 1/9 (11%) of the placebo patients.

Giannini et al. (1984) compared the efficacy of lithium and verapamil in the acute treatment of mania among 12 patients with mild to moderate mania according to DSM-III criteria. Using a crossover design, patients were treated for 30 days with verapamil 320 mg, then crossed over to lithium after a 10-day washout with placebo. Lithium dosing ranged from 900 to 1,800 mg/day for the 30-day trial. Serum lithium levels ranged from 0.84 to 1.26 mmol/L. The investigators found that verapamil (−68%) and lithium (−73%) caused equivalent reduction in pathology as measured by the BPRS. All patients relapsed when verapamil was discontinued during the placebo washout, and no major side effects were reported.

Similarly, Garza-Trevino et al. (1992) found no significant difference in efficacy between lithium and verapamil for acute treatment of mania in a double-blind, controlled, and randomized trial. Twenty patients with acute mania (DSM-III-R criteria) were randomized to 4-week trials on either verapamil 320 mg/day ($n = 12$) or lithium at doses to achieve serum levels of 0.75–1.5 mEq/L ($n = 8$). The patients that were randomized to lithium were dropped: one voluntarily, one because of cardiotoxicity, and one because of assaultive behavior. Neuroleptic and clonazepam were administered as needed. Both treatment groups improved significantly with no significant difference between the two groups as measured by the Peterson Mania Scale, the Clinical Global Impression (CGI) scale, and the BPRS. For example, mean Peterson Mania Scale scores dropped from 23.92 to 13.29 (−44.5%) on verapamil and from 20.38 to 12.39 (−39.2%) on lithium.

Several studies have compared the efficacy of verapamil with other antimanic treatments. Giannini et al. (1985) compared the efficacy of verapamil to clonidine for acute treatment of mania in a double-blind, crossover study. Twenty lithium nonresponders with acute mania (DSM-III criteria) were randomly divided into treatment with either verapamil 320 mg/day or clonidine 17 μg/kg daily for 20 days, then were crossed over to the other medication following a 5-day washout on placebo. It was found that verapamil was significantly more effective than clonidine as measured by the BPRS. Using the nonparametric statistic, the Mann Whitney U Test, overall scores showed that verapamil was superior at day 10 ($U = 25$, $P < .05$) and at day 20 ($U = 8$, $P < .001$). During the trial, 60% of the patients reported subjective preference to verapamil, and there were no major side effects.

In a double-blind study, Hoschl and Kozeny (1989) compared the efficacy of verapamil ($n = 12$) versus neuroleptic ($n = 24$) and versus neuroleptic combined with lithium ($n = 11$) in the treatment of acute mania (DSM-III criteria). Verapamil dosage ranged from 120 to 480 mg/day; neuroleptic doses were equivalent to 375 ± 271 mg, and lithium serum levels were 0.75 ± 0.22 mEq/dL. Following a 35-day treatment period, Hoschl and Kozeny found that verapamil was equally effective as neuroleptic alone or neuroleptic in combination with lithium. The mean reduction in BPRS was from 40 to 22 (−45%) for verapamil; from 31 to 19 (−39%) for neuroleptic alone; and from

34 to 25 (−26.5%) for lithium plus neuroleptic. Low doses used in the lithium- and neuroleptic-treated groups may have affected the outcome. No major side effects were reported with verapamil.

One study contrasted the efficacy of verapamil versus lithium in the prophylactic treatment of mania (Giannini et al. 1987). In a double-blind, crossover design, 20 patients with bipolar disorder according to DSM-III criteria underwent a 1-year study with 6-month trials each on either verapamil 320 mg or lithium (a dose to generate a serum level of 0.8–1.0 mEq/L). For all patients, the most recent manic episode had been in the previous 21 months. According to monthly assessment of the BPRS, patients receiving verapamil showed overall improvement at day 60 ($P < .05$) and at day 180 ($P < .05$); for the lithium group, this improvement did not occur until the evaluation at day 180 ($P < .01$).

Two double-blind, controlled studies have evaluated calcium antagonists other than verapamil in the acute treatment of mania. Aldenhoff et al. (1986) tested D-600 in a double-blind, placebo-controlled, parallel design, randomized trial among 10 patients with acute mania (DSM-III criteria). The patients had been off other medications for 5 weeks prior to starting 75 mg of D-600 or placebo for a 15-day trial. Four of five patients improved marginally on D-600 within 8 days. The nonresponder had to be started on neuroleptic. The main therapeutic effect noted between the active drug group versus placebo group was decreased psychomotor activity. There were no sedative effects noted, and no effects on heart rate and blood pressure.

Pazzaglia et al. (1993) completed a double-blind, placebo-controlled study of nimodipine in the acute and prophylactic treatment of patients with lithium- and carbamazepine-refractory mania and in one case of depression. Eleven patients diagnosed with bipolar disorder (Research Diagnostic Criteria [Spitzer et al. 1978] and DSM-III-R criteria) who were lithium and carbamazepine refractory, and one unipolar depressed patient (DSM-III-R criteria) underwent an "off-on-off" design with off-drug phases lasting approximately 7.6 ± 1.6 weeks with active-drug phases of approximately 11.6 ± 6.5 weeks. Patients were not taking any other medications. Nimodipine dose ranged from 90 to 720 mg/day. Of the nine patients who completed the trial, five showed significant clinical improvement. All three of the patients with ultra-ultra–rapid-cycling bipolar disorders (cycle duration less than 24 hours) had significant improvement on nimodipine. On a Mood Analogue Scale, the scores of these three patients changed from an initial placebo rating of 1.09, 2.55, and 2.34, to 0.12, 1.74, and 1.63, respectively. The one patient with unipolar depression (ultra rapid = cycle less than 1 week) had complete prophylaxis of recurrent depression. Side effects noted with nimodipine included peripheral flushing, mild orthostasis, and gastrointestinal symptoms that were dose related. In an attempt at replication, more recent "off-on-off-on" single-case analysis by the same group (McDermut et al. 1994) indicated that a 42-year-old rapid-cycling bipolar II woman refractory to previous treatments underwent double-blind treatment with placebo (B), nimodipine (A), and verapamil (C) in a B-A-B-A-C-A design. The maximum daily doses used were 630 mg of nimodipine and 320 mg of verapamil. The results indicated in terms of "percentage of days euthymic" are as follows (numbers are approximate because they are based on reading graphs): nimodipine (88%, 97%, 95%) was better than placebo (42%, 30%) and better than verapamil (30%). In contrast, mean ratings for mania (Young Mania Scale) and for depression (Hamilton Rating Scale for Depression [Hamilton 1960]), respectively, showed nimodipine (2, 18; 4, 15; 3, 13) was better than verapamil (3, 15) and better than placebo (5, 28; 10, 28). The investigators suggest that cyclic rapidity may be a marker for nimodipine treatment.

▶ Calcium-Channel Blockers: Summary

The preliminary studies on the use of calcium-channel inhibitors in the acute and prophylactic treatment of mania have been promising. These studies reveal that calcium antagonists are generally well tolerated and provide several advantages over lithium. Blood drawing to monitor serum levels is not necessary with calcium-channel inhibitors, and these agents may be safe during pregnancy and free of the teratogenic effects associated with other antimanic therapies. However, further investigation with larger samples of manic patients in well-designed and controlled studies is needed to clarify and establish the efficacy of these agents in the treatment of mania. The utilization of these agents among the lithium- and carbamazepine-refractory sub-groups of bipolar disorder is particularly important. With the current state of knowledge regarding the study of calcium-channel inhibitors in the treatment of mania, it is reasonable to reserve calcium antago-nists for patients who are lithium or anticonvulsant refractory or intolerant.

▶ NEW ANTICONVULSANTS: LAMOTRIGINE AND GABAPENTIN

In recent years, two more anticonvulsants have been introduced, with early results indicating a possible role in the treatment and prophylaxis of bipolar disorder: lamotrigine and gabapentin. As recently reviewed (Cloyd and Leppik 1996), lamotrigine (similar to valproate) is used for localization-related and generalized epilepsies, and gabapentin (like carbamazepine) is predominantly used for only localization-related epilepsies. The mechanism of action for lamotrigine is sodium-channel, and for gabapentin, enhanced GABA inhibition. Lamotrigine's most important side effect is a 6% rate of skin rash, with a risk of Stevens-Johnson syndrome; at the time of writing, no specific side effects are known for gabapentin. Key features in kinetics are protein binding (lamotrigine 55%, gabapentin < 10%), plasma half-life (lamotrigine 18–30 hours, gabapentin 5–7 hours), and route of elimi-nation (lamotrigine, hepatic glucuronidation; gabapentin, renal). These parameters show less interaction risk with decreased protein binding than either carbamazepine or valproate, which have interac-tion risks of 85%–95%); gabapentin, with renal elimination, may be particularly beneficial in patients with compromised liver function.

There have been two reports on lamotrigine for bipolar disorder (Ascher et al. 1996; Calabrese et al. 1996). An initial case report (Calabrese et al. 1996) indicated that lamotrigine was successful as monotherapy for treatment of rapid-cycling bipolar disorder. The pa-tient, a 49-year-old male, had had a history of rapid cycling since age 14, with progressive worsening. He had a history of failure with both lithium (3 years) and carbamazepine (3 weeks, discontinued because of nausea). In the year before he took lamotrigine, he had experienced eight episodes, four each of mania and of depression. Over a period of 7 weeks, his maximal dose of lamotrigine reached 200 mg, which was maintained thereafter. In that time, his score on the Hamilton Rating Scale for Depression (HRSD) fell from 46 to 9, and his score on the Global Assessment Scale (GAS) increased from 32 to 69. He maintained euthymia without further cycling for the next 11 months of follow-up. Ascher et al. (1996) reported results of a multicenter trial from an open 6-month prospective trial, in which 75 patients (83% bipolar I) received lamotrigine at mean doses of 287 mg/day (monotherapy), 175 mg/day (with carbamazepine) and 105 mg/day (with valproate). As might be expected, mania ratings on the Schedule for Affective Disorders and Schizophrenia—Change (SADS-C) improved significantly in the subset of 31 with mania, hypomania, or mixed states within the first 4 weeks, from a mean of 21.1 to a mean of 8.0 ($P < .0001$).

Perhaps more impressive is the finding that of the 54.7% of patients who presented in the depressed phase of bipolar disorder, 28 (68%) had a moderate (7) or marked (21) response in reduction of their HRSD. In that same 4-week period, the mean fall in HRSD was from 31.5 to 18.0 ($P = .0001$).

There are also two reports concerning gabapentin: one case report (Stanton et al. 1997) and one study (Schaffer and Schaffer 1997). The case report concerned a 40-year-old male with bipolar disorder and alcohol dependence, complicated by a bilateral frontal lobe injury after a motor vehicle accident 2 years before gabapentin treatment. This patient refused lithium, and the physicians did not use carbamazepine or valproate because of the patient's impaired liver function. Gabapentin was initiated at a dose of 900 mg/day and increased over 4 days to 3,600 mg/day. According to the Young Mania Scale, the patient's mania score fell from 34 at baseline to 17 after 10 days of treatment. The Schaffer and Schaffer study included 28 patients with bipolar disorder (10 bipolar I, 10 bipolar II, 7 cyclothymia, and 1 not otherwise specified). None had responded well to lithium, carbamazepine, or valproate. With an average dose of 539 mg/day (range: 333–2,700), 18 of the 28 had a positive response. Of the responders, 83% have continued prophylactically for at least 6 months successfully. Of the 10 patients in which it was discontinued, 8 were discontinued because of side effects, either oversedation or overactivation.

▶ REFERENCES

Aldenhoff JB, Schlegel S, Hauser I, et al: Antimanic effects of the calcium-antagonist D-600: a double-blind placebo controlled study. Clin Neuro-pharmacol 9:553–555, 1986

American Psychiatric Association: Diagnostic and Statistical Manual of Mental Disorders, 3rd Edition. Washington, DC, American Psychiatric Association, 1980

American Psychiatric Association: Diagnostic and Statistical Manual of Mental Disorders, 3rd Edition, Revised. Washington, DC, American Psychiatric Association, 1987

Antman EM, Stone PH, Muller JE, et al: Calcium blocking agents in the treatment of cardiovascular disorders. Ann Intern Med 93:873–885, 1980

Barton BM, Gitlin MJ: Verapamil in treatment-resistant mania: an open trial. J Clin Psychopharmacol 7:101–103, 1987

Brotman AW, Farhadi AM, Gelenberg AJ: Verapamil treatment of acute mania. J Clin Psychiatry 47:136–138, 1986

Brunet G, Cerlich B, Robert P, et al: Open trial of a calcium antagonist, nimodipine, in acute mania. Clin Neuropharmacol 13:224–228, 1990

Caillard V: Treatment of mania using a calcium antagonist: preliminary trial. Neuropsychology 14:23–26, 1985

Calabrese JR, Fatemi SH, Woyshville MJ: Antidepressant effects of lamotrigine in rapid cycling bipolar disorder. Am J Psychiatry 153:1236, 1996

Carman JS, Wyatt RJ: Calcium: bivalent cation in the bivalent psychoses. Biol Psychiatry 14:295–336, 1979

Chou JC: Recent advances in treatment of acute mania. J Clin Psychophar-macol 11:3–21, 1991

Cloyd J, Leppik IE: Systematic approach to medical treatment of epilepsy, in Contemporary Epilepsy Evaluation and Treatment, Vol 2: The Ther-apy. Amsterdam, Netherlands, Elsevier Science Publishers, Excerpta Medica, 1996, pp 11–18

Corn T, Ascher J, Calabrese J, et al: Lamictal in the treatment of bipolar disorder. Poster presented at annual meeting of the American College of Neuropsychopharmacology, San Juan, PR, December 1996

de Falco FA, Bartiromo U, Majello L, et al: Calcium antagonist nimodipine in intractable epilepsy. Epilepsia 33:343–345, 1992

Deicken RF: Verapamil treatment of bipolar depression. J Clin Psychophar-macol 10:148–149, 1990

Devis G, Somers G, van Obberghen E, et al: Calcium antagonists and islet function. Diabetes 24:547–551, 1975

Dinan TG, Silverstone T, Cookson JC: Cortisol, prolactin, and growth hormone levels with clinical ratings in manic patients treated with verapamil. Int Clin Psychopharmacol 3:151–156, 1988

Doran AR, Norang PK, Meigs CY, et al: Verapamil concentrations in the cerebrospinal fluid after oral administration. N Engl J Med 312:1261–1262, 1985

Dose M, Emrich HM, Cording-Tommel C, et al: Use of calcium antagonists in mania. Psychoneuroendocrinology 11:241–243, 1986

Dubovsky SL: Calcium antagonists: a new class of psychiatric drugs? Psychiatric Annals 16:724–728, 1986

Dubovsky SL: Why don't we hear more about the calcium antagonists? Biol Psychiatry 35:149–150, 1994

Dubovsky SL, Franks RD: Intracellular calcium ions in affective disorders: a review and an hypothesis. Biol Psychiatry 18:781–797, 1983

Dubovsky SL, Franks RD, Lifschitz M, et al: Effectiveness of verapamil in the treatment of a manic patient. Am J Psychiatry 139:502–504, 1982

Dubovsky SL, Franks RD, Schrier D: Phenelzine-induced hypomania: effects of verapamil. Biol Psychiatry 20:1009–1014, 1985

Dubovsky SL, Franks RD, Allen S, et al: Calcium antagonists in mania: a double-blind study of verapamil. Psychiatry Res 18:309–320, 1986

Dubovsky SL, Franks RD, Allen S: Verapamil: a new antimanic drug with potential interactions with lithium. J Clin Psychiatry 48:371–372, 1987

Dubovsky SL, Christiano J, Daniell LC, et al: Increased platelet intracellular calcium ion concentration in patients with affective disorders. Arch Gen Psychiatry 46:632–638, 1989

Dubovsky SL, Lee C, Christiano J, et al: Elevated platelet intracellular calcium concentration in bipolar depression. Biol Psychiatry 29:441–450, 1991a

Dubovsky SL, Lee C, Christiano J, et al: Lithium decreases platelet intracellular calcium ion concentrations in bipolar patients. Lithium 2:167–174, 1991b

Dubovsky SL, Murphy DL, Christiano J, et al: The calcium second messenger system in bipolar disorders: data supporting new research directions. Journal of Neuropsychiatry 4:3–14, 1992

Dunner DL, Patrick V, Fieve RR: Rapid cycling manic-depressive patients. Compr Psychiatry 18:561–566, 1977

El-Mallakh RS, Jaziri WA: Calcium channel blockers in affective illness: role of sodium-calcium exchange. J Clin Psychopharmacol 10:203–206, 1990

Eto S, Wood JM, Hutchins M, et al: Pituitary Ca^{+2} uptake and release of ACTH, GH and BH: effect of verapamil. Am J Physiol 226:1315–1319, 1974

Feighner JP, Robins E, Guze SB, et al: Diagnostic criteria for use in psychiatric research. Arch Gen Psychiatry 26:57–63, 1972

Garza-Trevino ES, Overall JE, Hollister LE: Verapamil versus lithium in acute mania. Am J Psychiatry 149:121–122, 1992

Gerner RH, Post RM, Spiegel AM, et al: Effects of parathormone and lithium treatment on calcium and mood in depressed patients. Biol Psychiatry 12:145–151, 1977

Giannini AJ, Houser WL, Loiselle RH, et al: Antimanic effects of verapamil. Am J Psychiatry 141:1602–1603, 1984

Giannini AJ, Loiselle RH, Price WA, et al: Comparison of antimanic efficacy of clonidine and verapamil. J Clin Pharmacol 25:307–308, 1985

Giannini AJ, Tarasz R, Loiselle RH, et al: Verapamil and lithium in the maintenance therapy of manic patients. J Clin Pharmacol 27:980–982, 1987

Gitlin MJ, Weiss J: Verapamil as maintenance treatment in bipolar illness: a case report. J Clin Psychopharmacol 4:341–343, 1984

Goldstein JA: Calcium channel blockers in the treatment of panic disorder. J Clin Psychiatry 46:546, 1985

Goodnick PJ: Verapamil prophylaxis in pregnant women with bipolar disorder. Am J Psychiatry 150:1560, 1993

Goodnick PJ: Nimodipine treatment of rapid cycling bipolar disorder. J Clin Psychiatry 56:330, 1995

Goodnick PJ: Verapamil response in mania and changes in plasma calcium and magnesium. South Med J 89:225–226, 1996

Grebb JA, Shellon RC, Tayer ER, et al: A negative, double-blind, placebo controlled, clinical trial of verapamil in chronic schizophrenia. Biol Psychiatry 21:691–694, 1986

Hamilton M: A rating scale for depression. J Neurol Neurosurg Psychiatry 23:56–62, 1960

Helmuth D, Ljaljevic Z, Ramirez L, et al: Choreoathetosis induced by verapamil and lithium treatment. J Clin Psychopharmacol 9:454–455, 1989

Himmelhoch JM, Garfinkel ME: Sources of lithium resistance in mixed mania. Psychopharmacol Bull 22:613–620, 1986

Hoschl C: Do calcium antagonists have a place in the treatment of mood disorders? Drugs 42:721–729, 1991

Hoschl C, Kozeny J: Verapamil in affective disorders: a controlled, double-blind study. Biol Psychiatry 25:128–140, 1989

Hoschl C, Blahos J, Kabes J: The use of calcium channel blockers in psychiatry, in Biological Psychiatry 1985. Edited by Shagass CE, Josiassen RC, Bridger WH, et al. New York, Elsevier, 1986, pp 330–332

Jacobsen FM, Sack DA, James SP: Delirium-induced hypomania: effect of verapamil. Biol Psychiatry 20:1009–1014, 1987

Janiciak PG, Pandey GN, Sharma RP, et al: Verapamil for acute mania: preliminary results from a double-blind placebo-controlled study. Biol Psychiatry 35:679, 1994

Johnson FN, Birch NJ, Carstens M, et al: Mechanisms of lithium action. Review of Contemporary Pharmacotherapy 4:287–318, 1993

Kennedy S, Ozersky S, Robillard M: Refractory bipolar illness may not respond to verapamil. J Clin Psychopharmacol 6:316–317, 1986

Langley MS, Sorkin EM: Nimodipine: a review of its pharmacodynamic and pharmacokinetic properties, and therapeutic potential in cerebrovascular disease. Drugs 37:669–699, 1989

Lindelius R, Nilsson CG: Flunarizine as maintenance treatment of a patient with bipolar disorder. Am J Psychiatry 149:139, 1992

Linder J, Levin K, Saaf J, et al: Influence of lithium treatment on calcium and magnesium in plasma and erythrocytes. Lithium 4:115–123, 1993

Manna V: Disturbi affecttivi bipolari e ruolo del calcio interneuronale: effetti terapeutici del trattamento con sali di litio e/o calcio antogonista in pazienti con rapida inversione di polarita. Minerva Med 82:757–763, 1991

Mathis P, Schmitt L, Moron P: Efficacite du verapamil dans les acces maniaques. Encephale XIV:127–132, 1988

McDermut W, Pazzaglia P, Huggins T, et al: Use of single case analyses in off-on-off-on trials in affective illness: a demonstration of the efficacy of nimodipine. Depression 2:259–271, 1994

Mehta M: Physicians' Desk Reference, 48th Edition. Montvale, NJ, Medical Economics, 1994

Meltzer HE, Caesar S, Goodnick PJ, et al: Calmodulin-activated calcium ATPase in bipolar illness. Neuropsychobiology 20:169–173, 1988

Patterson JF: Treatment of acute mania with verapamil. J Clin Psychopharmacol 7:206–207, 1987

Pazzaglia PJ, Post RM, Keller TA, et al: Preliminary controlled trial of nimodipine in ultra-rapid cycling affective dysregulation. Psychiatry Res 49:257–272, 1993

Pickar D, Wolkowitz OM, Doran AR, et al: Clinical and biochemical effects of verapamil administration in schizophrenic patients. Arch Gen Psychiatry 44:113–118, 1987

Pollack MH, Rosenbaum JF, Hyman SE: Calcium channel blockers in psychiatry. Psychosomatics 28:356–369, 1987

Prien RF, Gelenberg AJ: Alternatives to lithium for preventative treatment of bipolar disorder. Am J Psychiatry 146:840–848, 1989

Prien RF, Caffey EM Jr, Klett CJ: Prophylactic efficacy of lithium carbonate in manic depressive illness. Arch Gen Psychiatry 28:337–341, 1973

Russell JT, Thorn NA: Calcium and stimulation-secretion coupling in the neurohypothesis. Acta Endocrinol (Copenh) 76:471–487, 1974

Schaffer CB, Schaffer LC: Gabapentin in the treatment of bipolar disorder. Am J Psychiatry 154:291–292, 1997

Solomon L, Williamson P: Verapamil in bipolar illness. Can J Psychiatry 31:442–444, 1986

Spitzer RL, Endicott J, Robins E: Research Diagnostic Criteria: rationale and reliability. Arch Gen Psychiatry 35:773–782, 1978

Stanton SP, Keck PE Jr, McElroy SL: Treatment of acute mania with gabapentin. Am J Psychiatry 154:287, 1997

Walter A, Burk M, Brook S: Superiority of lithium over verapamil in mania: a randomized, controlled single-blind trial. J Clin Psychiatry 57:543–546, 1996

Wehr TA, Sack BA, Rosenthal NE, et al: Rapid cycling affective disorder: contributing factors and treatment responses in 51 patients. Am J Psychiatry 145:179–184, 1988

Wood K: The neurochemistry of mania: the effect of lithium on catecholamines, indoleamines, and calcium mobilization. J Affect Disord 8:215–223, 1985

CHAPTER 17

PSYCHOTHERAPY

Charlene A. McAlpin, R.N.,
and Paul J. Goodnick, M.D.

Psychotherapy helps me to deal with my illness. . . . it is a
safe place where I can talk about my troubles and rebuild
my self-esteem.

The words of a manic patient in remission

The advances in medical sciences, including the discovery of
the biological origins and manifestations of bipolar illness,
have resulted in improved precision and efficacy of medical
treatment. Pharmacotherapy is essential and without dispute the
central treatment in bipolar illness. Yet as one observes in clinical
practice, there are limits of success for even the most beneficial medications. One cannot ignore that the manifestations of bipolar illness,
although biological in etiology, are behavioral and psychological in
expression, with significant personal, interpersonal, and social consequences. Psychotherapy can be of significant value to the individual
dealing with intense issues related to having bipolar disorder and has
been found to be an important adjunctive intervention in the treatment of this illness.

Psychological interventions are effective in improving an individ-

The authors thank Enrique F. Casero, Ph.D., for his contributions in the writing of
this chapter.

ual's coping and response to psychosocial stressors in his or her life. Research indicates that psychosocial stress may precipitate an affective episode and influence relapse and outcome (Post 1992). Psychotherapy is an important intervention that may diminish the occurrence and severity of exacerbations through improved coping of life stressors. This chapter, while making reference to bipolar illness, is dedicated to discussion of the psychotherapeutic management of manic patients.

▶ PRECIPITATION OF EPISODES BY STRESS

As humans we experience psychosocial stress in our lives related to the dynamic interplay of our personalities and intrapsychic conflicts with the external world. Individuals, such as the manic patient, who have problematic behavior that interferes with their personal, interpersonal, and social functioning, may experience relatively frequent stress. Add to their major affective disorder comorbidity with personality and addictive disorders, as sometimes occurs, and the effect of stress is multiplied (Kahn 1993).

Recent research has attempted to identify the role of stress in precipitating affective episodes in genetically vulnerable individuals. Biological and clinical data suggest that psychosocial factors may indeed play a role in precipitating acute episodes of bipolar illness (Post 1992; Post et al. 1984, 1986; Silverstone and Romas-Clarkson 1989). Post suggested that major life events and other psychosocial stressors may be the stimuli that set off a limbic system excitatory mechanism, especially early in the course of the illness, thereby triggering the occurrence of an affective episode. His research suggests that psychotherapeutic interventions are particularly important early in the course of illness before an autonomous pattern has set in (Post 1992; Post et al. 1984, 1986).

Other studies further support the role of psychosocial variables in the presentation of affective illness. A naturalistic study (Aronson and Shukla 1987) of bipolar patients in a lithium clinic immediately after a hurricane showed an overall increased relapse rate, and recently unstable patients were found to be at highest risk. A prospective study a few years later further supported the role of stress in precipitating acute affective episodes. It was found that bipolar patients experiencing severely stressful events over a 2-year period had a higher relapse rate than bipolar patients experiencing mildly stressful events or no stress (Ellicott et al. 1990).

▶ PERSONALITY AS A PRECURSOR TO ILLNESS AND AS ALTERED BY IT

The complex interaction of psychology and biology is paramount in the study of personality and bipolar illness. Although personality may play a role in predisposing an individual to an affective disorder (Akiskal 1988), personality may also be an expression and result of having bipolar illness. (This includes the distinct and unique traits that make up an individual and govern his or her behavior.) A major feature of personality is one's social behavior. *Character* is often used interchangeably with *personality* and is used accordingly in this chapter. *Temperament,* on the other hand, is often viewed as having a more biological and genetic basis of origin (Goodwin and Jamison 1990).

Personality as a Precursor to Illness

In his study, Akiskal (1988) described personality styles in relation to mania and bipolar illness in general. He suggested that personality may predispose one to an affective disorder. His work outlines the relationship of "affective temperaments," or personality styles, to various affective disorders. Four temperaments were described, which as one progresses along a continuum of severity may become a subaffective disorder. The "hyperthymic" temperament correlates to hypomania. Similar to the other personality styles, Akiskal believes that a significant proportion of this temperament is biological and represents a potential precursor for hypomania, contending that the hyperthymic temperament, along with the others, may respond to medication. The remaining proportion is described as "character spectrum" disorders generally unresponsive to psychopharmacological interventions. These disorders result from social and nonaffective constitutional factors (Akiskal 1988). Although the affective temperament model of character does not provide a comprehensive explanation, it does describe a strong influence on personality functioning for bipolar illness and supports the role of psychotherapy as a treatment modality in combination with pharmacotherapy. However, additional research to substantiate this premise is warranted.

Personality as Altered by Illness

In addition to the role that personality may play in predisposing one to an affective disorder, personality may also be an expression and result of having bipolar illness. The narcissism, egocentricity, need for approval, perfectionism, rigidity, and grandiosity that are often seen in manic patients, like the characteristic denial of their maladaptive behavior, are suggestive of defensive postures to psychic pain caused by the intense and frequent mood swings. Studies by Davenport et al. (1979, 1984) described patterns of maladaptive behaviors occurring over multigenerations in families with bipolar illness. The researchers described the affective instability of the illness as the root of the defensive behaviors and that, over time, these behaviors shaped one's personality. The patterns of these behaviors observed over generations included avoidance and denial of intense emotions of anxiety and anger, unrealistic standards of conformity and self-expectations, lack of intimate relationships outside of the family constellation, parental low self-esteem displaced onto the children, and fears related to issues of the heritable aspects of the illness. They noted a resistance to change and lack of awareness, expression, and resolution of needs.

Earlier psychoanalytic studies of bipolar patients showed interesting behavioral parallels, and several of their conclusions overlap with those of Davenport (M. B. Cohen et al. 1954; Fromm-Reichmann 1959). These studies tended to focus on the role of rigid conformity within the family system. The psychoanalysts concluded that manic-depressive families avoided affect and used denial to manage hostility and anxiety. They observed that the families had difficulty simultaneously tolerating hostility or competitiveness and intimacy. Like Fromm-Reichmann, Cohen et al. described the hypomanic as carrying out a relatively stereotyped social performance that is lacking of any close-relatedness or genuine interest in others. The psychoanalysts suggest that the concept of reciprocity is missing in manic individuals and such individuals use others as interchangeable objects, often utilizing morality and conventionality as tools for bargaining (M. B. Cohen et al. 1954; Fromm-Reichmann 1959). They explain that these behavior patterns mobilize narcissistic defenses to the point of mania in genetically vulnerable individuals.

Goodwin and Jamison (1990) described developmental tasks as being interrupted by the illness. The onset of the illness coincides with late adolescence and early adulthood, when developmental tasks such as separating from parents, solidifying a sense of identity, forming intimate relationships, and career development are impaired or blocked. These maturational issues later become concerns for the patient in remission.

▌ PSYCHOLOGICAL ISSUES

The experience of having bipolar illness and the pain of recalling one's behavior during a manic episode in particular is traumatic. When patients are coming down from mania, they often disclose terror and shame over their actions while high. One has the challenge of learning to trust and accept oneself despite the uncontrollable mood swings. Often patients disclose being guarded against experiencing extremes of pleasure or spontaneity because they fear it will herald hypomania. The fear of wondering when the next episode will occur is overwhelming and constant for many.

Denial

An account of hospital admissions for a manic patient often follows an episode of violence or a behavior so disruptive to the patient's family that they are forced to initiate involuntary inpatient care. In the acute stage of illness, the manic person often lacks the insight and judgment to recognize the inappropriateness of his or her behavior. Denial as a defense is a common characteristic used by manic patients to cope with their illness.

Denial, although clearly pronounced in the manic phase of illness, is often employed as a coping strategy beyond the acute episode. Along with the passage of time, exploring the meaning of the illness, the thoughts and feelings related to having the illness, and gentle interpretations in the context of a therapeutic relationship can help the individual decrease the use of this defensive mechanism.

Anger

In the process leading from denial to the recognition of the reality of a lifelong illness, with all its disruptions and losses, anger is aroused in many patients. A natural reaction to loss, anger can be adaptive and part of the process of acceptance. It may motivate patients to learn more about the illness and pursue quality care or urge them to resist and fight with vengeance their treatment regimen and caretakers.

Fears of losing control and the need to feel protected and safe from potentially destructive impulses usually directed at others may be of concern to the patient. A caring yet firm approach by competent caretakers and the use of external controls during agitated episodes are helpful in calming the patient and helping him or her feel secure.

Shame and Guilt

Shame, humiliation, and self-disgust are painfully experienced by many. Patients say they feel devastated as they see their world, which they fought so hard to rebuild during remission, crumble around them once again. Hopelessness and despair set in, and sometimes ambivalence, as the patient tries to assimilate the biological origins and treatment of the disorder with the psychological and interpersonal manifestations of it.

However, despite the common recurrent themes of shame and guilt, a study of bipolar patients (Pardoen et al. 1993) who were tested for self-esteem using the Rosenberg Self-Esteem Scale showed that these patients did not score significantly differently from the control group. The research suggests that although bipolar patients may experience multiple psychological traumas as a result of their illness, these traumas do not have a permanent impact on self-esteem.

Real and Imagined Losses

The bipolar patient may experience real and imagined losses due to the illness itself and sometimes related to treatment. Having a chronic mental illness requiring adherence to a structured medical regimen and compliance with medication for life creates feelings of defectiveness and disturbances in self-concept. The illness may be blamed for unrelated failures in life and opportunities gone adrift. Other treatments may also become the scapegoat for personal inadequacies. Real losses may also occur as a result of treatment. A study of manic-depressive patients in remission revealed that many patients believe their illness makes a positive contribution to their lives (Jamison et al. 1980).

Avoidance of Strong Emotions

Problems learning to discriminate normal from abnormal moods are frequent issues for the manic-depressive individual (M. B. Cohen et al. 1954; Fromm-Reichmann 1959). Whether a sign of illness or a normal emotion of everyday life, moods may confuse or frighten many bipolar patients. They often fear that intense emotions may provoke an affective episode. To compensate for their fears, some individuals maintain a self-imposed constriction of emotionally charged life experiences. Robbed of their feelings, their lives becomes gray and flat, but in their minds, safe. Psychotherapy and education can help recapture their feelings and separate the emotions of everyday living—joy, enthusiasm, excitability, lethargy, irritability, sadness—from hypomania and depression.

Fears of Recurrence

Along with an understanding of the chronic nature of bipolar illness and the limits of medical interventions come the fear and uncertainty of when the next episode will occur. Many patients maintain a grave pessimism about being at the mercy of their moods. An overwhelming sense of powerlessness and despair is experienced by many as they watch their moods fluctuate despite any action on their part. For rapid cyclers, the anxiety is even more pronounced.

Concerns About Genetics

In addition to the insecurities brought on by fears of recurrence, many patients express anxiety and guilt related to the heritability of their illness. Having the traumatic experience of growing up in a family affected by this illness, many patients verbalize fears about ending up like an affected parent and repeating the cycle with their own children.

▌ INTERPERSONAL BEHAVIORS

Mood changes associated with mania affect not only manic patients but those around them as well. The interpersonal problems are often severe, leaving the patient frustrated and often rejected by others. Individuals in an acute manic episode often alienate themselves from others as a result of their actions, which place others in embarrassing situations and positions of lowered self-esteem and self-doubt. Those in contact with the manic patient frequently find themselves on the defensive, trying to justify their actions and motivations. The reactions from family and friends often include anger, frustration, rejection, and withdrawal because they are not able to make sense of their loved one's emotional lability, devastating financial transactions, sexual acting out, and otherwise inappropriate and damaging behavior. For some, there is an underlying feeling that the manic patient can control his or her actions.

From an analytical perspective, manic patients' style of interacting is explained as representing a compromise in the issue of achieving true intimacy. As described by Janowsky et al. (1970, 1974), their relationships tend to be characterized by lack of reciprocity and maturity with interpersonal maneuvers that are simultaneously "cementing and distancing." On the basis of clinical observations, Janowsky and colleagues found that manic patients demonstrated particular interpersonal characteristics and behaviors while in the acute stage of the illness. These behaviors included shifting responsibility for their actions to others, exploiting other's weaknesses, testing limits, manipulating the self-esteem of others, provoking anger, and dividing staff (Janowsky et al. 1974). The study indicated that these interpersonal characteristics are predictable and correlate in intensity with the severity of the manic state as defined by the severity of symptoms such as flight of ideas, pressured speech, grandiosity, and hyperactivity. It was observed by the researchers that when the manic episode remitted, the interpersonal characteristics disappeared. In other words, the changes in the acutely manic patient's style of interpersonal interactions fluctuated with the phases and acuity of the illness. The researchers contended that conceptualization of the manic patient's interpersonal activity provides a valuable framework for interpreting and intervening in their style of relating (Janowsky et al. 1970).

▶ Psychotherapeutic Interventions

Psychological support may take many forms when working with a manic patient—ranging from brief interventions during medication management sessions to formal individual or group psychotherapy on an ongoing basis. The primary clinician is in a unique position to assess the general psychological state of the patient and the emotional issues the patient may be facing. Formal psychotherapy is extremely beneficial to some patients and of less critical value to others. In the acute stage of illness, manic patients generally require inpatient hospitalization for stabilization and treatment. The therapeutic milieu plays an essential role in the treatment of manic patients.

Individual Psychotherapy

Psychotherapy can be extremely beneficial to manic patients by helping them deal with issues arising as a result of the illness, in addition to more deeply rooted intrapsychic conflicts. Research indicates that clinicians sometimes de-emphasize the role of psychotherapy in the treatment regimen of bipolar patients. Patients, on the other hand, generally place a greater value on psychotherapy and often find it an important adjunct to medication (Vasile et al. 1987). Empirical research is lacking on the efficacy of psychotherapy as independent of medication; however, it is believed that psychotherapy may have an additive and independent impact on the course of illness (Kahn 1990). Specific research on combined pharmacological treatment and psychotherapy is described in the literature, yet methodological limitations make the outcomes difficult to interpret. Research is also inconclusive as to the indications and effectiveness of individual therapy over group or family therapy. Few of the studies used pre- or poststudy measurements or control groups for the analysis of treatment outcomes. Of the better controlled studies, Cochran (1984) supports the treatment plan of individual psychotherapy in combination with lithium as resulting in an improved clinical outcome and lithium compliance. In this study, patients who participated in six sessions of cognitive-behavioral therapy had improved medication compliance and fewer hospitalizations than patients who were treated with only standard clinic care.

Beyond Cochran's (1984) work, little is known about the efficacy of one theoretical orientation over another for treatment of manic patients. Post (1992) suggested that affective episodes precipitated by psychosocial stressors in which behavioral sensitization and electrophysiological kindling play a significant role may best respond to cognitive and behavioral therapies. This approach can target the "automaticity" or habit mechanisms associated with the repetitions of episodes. The goal of the initial phases of this therapy includes the detection and analysis of a central theme, followed by an interpretation and working through of the manic defenses to help reshape behavior to a more adaptive level (Mester 1986).

In working with a manic patient, the therapist is confronted with the task of determining to what degree one's character is a result of having the affective illness, as opposed to the role of developmental factors or ego defenses. A difficult challenge of the therapist is to judge what behavior is an unconsciously motivated defense as opposed to a biologically driven action. For instance, is grandiosity a defensive compensation for low self-esteem, or an uncontrollable manifestation of mania? Perhaps a better relatedness may occur through action, as when the clinician or another significant figure in the patient's life strongly disapproves of a behavior. This disapproval provokes rage in the patient and may make the patient more receptive to gaining insight into his or her conflicting wishes to control and to be loved. Kahn (1990) suggested that the greatest "psychotherapeutic leverage" for helping the patient consciously control manic behavior occurs when there is a shift from "manipulation or rejection to open dependency" in the therapeutic relationship. Once the patient has been stabilized on medication, residual dysphoria or maladaptive behaviors should be explored in therapy with the premise that at this point they are most likely the result of intrapsychic conflicts. Kahn (1993) stated that denial, the avoidance of responsibility for actions, irritability, manipulation of others, attention-seeking behavior, and unhappiness are but a few of the behaviors that may have deeper psychological origins not overtly evident until the manic cycle is under control pharmacologically.

It is essential for the therapist to maximize the patient's sense of control over his or her behavior and treatment. This process empowers the patient and may result in increased self-esteem and improved compliance. The meaning and symbolic value of medication as an introject and transitional object for the patient may be an important issue to be explored in psychotherapy. As a result of the internalization of the transitional object, the patient may experience medication as an introject possessing powerful properties for good or evil (Hyland 1991). In this manner, medication assumes an intrapsychic function in addition to its pharmacologic one, and the effect should be evaluated in terms of the unconscious mental conditioning as well as its biochemical properties (Haussner 1986).

Countertransference Problems

The therapist needs to be aware of his or her feelings and responses toward the patient on an ongoing basis, but especially in situations in which the patient decompensates. These situations may give rise to feelings of anger and inadequacy in the therapist. Anger is also commonly experienced by the therapist when the patient is manic and keenly senses and attacks the therapist's personal vulnerabilities (Janowsky et al. 1970). Kahn (1990) related the main countertransference problems as excessive fear as well as profound anger. Urges to punish and punitive wishes may be manifest by overmedication and prematurely "firing" the patient, or the desire to see the patient get into trouble. Fear may be acted out more covertly by inappropriate termination or failure to hospitalize or involve family and police when needed. Mania may be seductive and appealing to the therapist because of his or her own narcissistic issues. Countertransference envy and identification may occur. Special attention should be given to increase the therapists' awareness of their feelings and responses to decrease any possibility of acting out through their patients.

Group Therapy

Studies suggest that group psychotherapy can ameliorate the course of illness in bipolar illness (Graves 1993; Shakir et al. 1979; Shaw 1986; Volkmar et al. 1981). Although strictly controlled studies are lacking, decreased hospitalization and improved social function have been noted (Shakir et al. 1979; Volkmar et al. 1981). Observations by Wulsin et al. (1988) support the efficacy of group therapy because of the patient's need for education and support about the illness, the need to reinforce medication management, and the interpersonal issues that present during the course of illness. A retrospective clinical study of outpatient group psychotherapy by Graves (1993) found that many individuals in the group felt "ostracized" by their families and subsequently perceived the group as a surrogate family offering support from both family and social criticism.

Research on inpatient groups for patients with bipolar disorder is limited. In a study of inpatients participating in short-term group psychotherapy sessions, Pollack (1993) utilized content analysis procedures to identify the emergence of five core categories: understanding the illness, relating with others, managing daily life, relating with self, and living in society. The group process events that the participants described as personally important to them were guidance, universality, and self-understanding. Applying the results of these data, Pollack (1995a) later developed the Self-Management of Bipolar Disorder Group Model as a model to provide therapy and education to this patient population. In the self-management group, the topic is preplanned by the therapist, as compared with the interactional group, in which the identification of the session topic is the result of the immediate needs of the participants. The new model directly addresses areas of concern identified by inpatients and is a response to the patients' evaluations of the interactional therapy group. Preliminary results of the new model have been positive, although research controls are lacking to date (Pollack 1995b).

Couples and Family Therapy

A study of couples group therapy as an adjunct to lithium maintenance of manic patients found that patients who participated in couples psychotherapy had better social functioning and family interactions with fewer life disruptions than patients on standard maintenance treatment in a lithium outpatient clinic (Davenport et al. 1977).

Fitzgerald (1972) described family therapy in acute mania as a beneficial modality to deal with a manic patient's behavior as "an attempt to communicate both his distress and his needs in his interpersonal situation and as a cry for help" (p. 550). He described family therapy in combination with lithium as "enhancing" the treatment outcome. Studies by Glick et al. (1985) also support family psychotherapy as a treatment modality in the care of manic patients. The results indicated that patients who were treated with inpatient family intervention experienced fewer hospitalizations at the 6-month follow-up evaluation and better work and social role functioning as compared with those who participated in a standard inpatient treatment program.

Acutely manic individuals often act out and create conflicts with family members, who in turn may react with behavior that further escalates the manic patient's outbursts. Family therapy may help members to disengage and remain calm in response to outbursts while maintaining a protective stance that may help patients be in better control (Kahn 1990). Likewise, studies by Haas and Spencer and colleagues (Haas et al. 1988; Spencer et al. 1988) regarding the effectiveness of inpatient family intervention of a psychoeducational nature found improved hospital treatment outcome for the family intervention group as compared with those who did not have this treatment.

Milieu Therapy

The rules and structure of the milieu play a significant role in providing a stable environment within which a decompensated patient can regain self-regulatory capacities and have a reparative emotional experience. Therapeutic responses from the clinical team are central healing factors in the milieu. Anticipating disruption of the milieu when a manic patient is hospitalized is important in order to plan cogent interventions and reduce anger and dissension among the health care team members. The team members need to process their interactions continuously to decrease manipulation and to maintain staff cohesion. The rules and structure of the therapeutic community, as well as clearly delineated staff roles, must be maintained. Exploring a manic patient's ability to create defensive responses in the therapist and successfully manipulate the therapist is a point of self-growth for the therapist.

An interesting study of the hospitalization effect in acute mania suggests that manic patients show greater improvement in a highly structured and nonstimulating environment (S. Cohen et al. 1988). The researchers compared the treatment outcomes of manic patients on an open ward and psychiatric intensive care unit. Other variables controlled, significantly greater improvement and shorter length of stay occurred in the patients hospitalized in the psychiatric intensive care unit in comparison with the open ward. The findings suggest that the hospitalization effect is of major significance in the early management of acutely manic patients.

Patient and Family Education

Patients frequently ask many questions and request information about bipolar illness and its treatment. Clinicians have a professional responsibility and legal duty under their professional practice act to provide education and informed consent to their patients. Patient education materials are routinely available in the acute care environment as well as in some practitioners' offices. Patients should be encouraged to participate actively in the education process and ask questions about their treatment regimen. Reliance on pamphlets and other written materials is insufficient. Patients should be provided with opportunities to interact with the clinician on an ongoing basis to clarify information and to obtain needed support. An unhurried, receptive, and collaborative approach is essential for encouraging the patient to ask questions and become involved in the education process.

Education programs should include information about the natural course of bipolar illness, including its characteristic chronic and highly recurrent nature. Theories of etiology, biological aspects, and behavioral manifestations should be presented according to each patient's interest and cognitive ability. The patient needs to understand the heritability of the illness and to be informed about genetic counseling. All patients need to know the signs and symptoms of an impending episode and the roles that medication noncompliance and psychosocial stress may play in precipitating an episode. The clinician should counsel patients about the benefits of practicing stress management in their lives. Because sleep deprivation may precede mania, patients need to be taught the importance of a stable sleep routine and to avoid situations that may cause disruptions in the normal pattern. Wehr et al. (1987) indicated that a single night of unexplained sleeplessness in bipolar patients should be seen as a possible early warning sign of an impending manic episode.

Family and significant others should be actively involved in the education about the illness and treatment to enable them to give support to the patient. In turn, educating the family is supportive to them and reduces their distress. Conceptualizing bipolar illness as a biological disorder with psychological and behavioral symptomatology can be beneficial, because it may decrease anger and dispel false perceptions that mood changes and behavior are the result of personal weakness. By gaining a better understanding of the illness, the family may be more accepting of the mood and behavior changes and better able to provide support. For example, when a patient is in a manic phase, the family may assist the patient to "slow down," steer the patient away from social situations, and institute financial controls. Education may also help to minimize the social stigma attached to the illness.

Community Resources

A number of community-based resources that provide self-help, support, education, and referrals are available for patients and families. National and local mental health associations, such as the National Depressive and Manic-Depressive Association, National Alliance for the Mentally Ill, National Mental Health Association, and Community Advocates for the Mentally Ill, sponsor support groups and formal education programs. These associations can be beneficial to the patient and family in providing services in times of crisis as well as on an ongoing basis.

▶ SUMMARY

Medications are essential for treating the biological aspects of bipolar illness. Psychotherapy in combination with lithium or other medications can be extremely beneficial in helping patients deal with issues and traumas in how they perceive themselves, are perceived by others, and interact with the outside world. Psychological support and therapy may also improve the individual's coping abilities and response to psychosocial stress in his or her life. Life stressors may play a role in precipitating affective episodes and may affect the outcome of illness. The optimum treatment regimen includes psychopharmacological intervention and psychotherapy.

The experience of mania is emotionally traumatic for the individual and creates many psychotherapeutic issues. Common issues that are frequently the focus of psychotherapy sessions include denial, anger, shame and guilt, real and imagined loss, avoidance of strong emotions, fears of recurrence, and concerns about the genetic aspects of the illness.

Individuals in an acute manic episode generally create interpersonal conflicts and alienate themselves from others. This behavior is usually the result of their actions, which place others in embarrassing situations and positions of lowered self-esteem and self-doubt. Those in contact with manic patients frequently find themselves on the defensive, trying to justify their actions and motivations. Reactions from family, friends, and sometimes staff include anger, frustration, rejection, and withdrawal. Family and significant others may find themselves without the necessary coping skills to deal with the unpredictability of mood and behavior, the damage to relationships, and the economic losses that occur as a result of mania. Janowsky et al. (1974) observed that manic patients demonstrated particular interpersonal characteristics and behaviors while in the acute stage of the illness, including shifting responsibility for their actions to others, exploiting other's weaknesses, testing limits, manipulating the self-esteem of others, provoking anger, and dividing staff. These interpersonal characteristics are thought to be predictable and correlate in intensity with the severity of the manic state.

Psychological support and psychotherapeutic interventions may take many forms when working with manic patients, ranging from brief interventions to formal individual or group psychotherapy on a long-term basis. No single theoretical model has proven more effective over another for treatment of a particular problem. To date, research is inconclusive regarding the effectiveness of individual therapy as compared with group or family therapy. Studies support the efficacy of group therapy in combination with individual and family psychotherapy and lithium treatment as resulting in an improved clinical outcome (Cochran 1984; Glick et al. 1985; Wulsin et al. 1988).

Therapists need to be aware of countertransference issues that commonly occur when working with manic patients. Anger is a frequent reaction to patients' manipulative efforts. Manic patients may be difficult to manage, especially during an acute episode. In the hospital setting, the acting out is often targeted at undermining and sabotaging the milieu. Consistent interventions from the health care team can be a therapeutic experience for manic patients as they learn that their behaviors are controllable and that the team is caring and powerful enough to protect them from self-destructive activities. Medication compliance is a common concern for patients. Educating patients and families regarding the illness and treatment regimen can help empower them and provide a sense of control and participation in care, which in turn encourages compliance and collaboration with the primary care provider for early intervention in an impending episode. Trends in health care emphasize community-based care and brief hospitalization. A number of community-based resources that provide self-help, support, education, and referrals are available for manic patients and their families.

▶ REFERENCES

Akiskal HS: Cyclothymic and related disorders, in Depression and Mania. Edited by Georgotas A, Cancro R. New York, Elsevier, 1988, pp 86–97

Aronson TA, Shukla S: Life events and relapse in bipolar disorder: the impact of a catastrophic event. Acta Psychiatr Scand 75:571–576, 1987

Cochran SD: Preventing medical noncompliance in the outpatient treatment of bipolar affective disorders. J Consult Clin Psychol 52:873–878, 1984

Cohen MB, Baker G, Cohen RA, et al: An intensive study of twelve cases of manic-depressive illness. Psychiatry 17:103–137, 1954

Cohen S, Khan A, Clark A, et al: Hospitalization effect in acute mania. Gen Hosp Psychiatry 10:138–141, 1988

Davenport YB, Ebert MH, Adland ML, et al: Couples group therapy as an adjunct to lithium maintenance of the manic patient. Am J Orthopsychiatry 47:495–502, 1977

Davenport YB, Adland ML, Gold PW, et al: Manic-depressive illness: psychodynamics features of multigenerational families. Am J Orthopsychiatry 49:24–35, 1979

Davenport YB, Zahn-Waxler C, Adland ML, et al: Early child rearing practices in families with a manic-depressive parent. Am J Psychiatry 141:230–235, 1984

Ellicott A, Hammen C, Gitlin M, et al: Life events and the course of bipolar disorder. Am J Psychiatry 147:1194–1198, 1990

Fitzgerald RG: Mania as message: treatment with family therapy and lithium carbonate. Am J Psychiatry 26:547–555, 1972

Fromm-Reichmann F: Intensive psychotherapy of manic-depressives, in Psychoanalysis and Psychotherapy: Selected Papers. Edited by Bullard DM, Weigert EV. Chicago, IL, University of Chicago Press, 1959, pp 221–227

Glick ID, Clarkin JF, Spencer JH, et al: A controlled evaluation of inpatient family intervention: preliminary results of the six-month follow-up. Arch Gen Psychiatry 42:882–886, 1985

Goodwin FK, Jamison KR: Clinical description and diagnosis, in Manic-Depressive Illness. Edited by Goodwin FK, Jamison KR. New York, Oxford University Press, 1990, pp 13–55

Graves JS: Living with mania: a study of outpatient group psychotherapy for bipolar patients. Am J Psychother 47:113–126, 1993

Haas GL, Glick ID, Clarkin JF, et al: Inpatient family intervention: a randomized clinical trial: II—results at hospital discharge. Arch Gen Psychiatry 45:217–224, 1988

Haussner RS: Medication and transitional phenomena. International Journal of Psychoanalysis and Psychotherapy 11:375–398, 1986

Hyland J: Integrating psychotherapy and pharmacotherapy. Bull Menninger Clin 55:205–215, 1991

Jamison KR, Gerner RH, Hammen C, et al: Clouds and silver linings: positive experiences associated with primary affective disorders. Am J Psychiatry 137:198–202, 1980

Janowsky D, Leff M, Epstein R: Playing the manic game: interpersonal maneuvers of the acutely manic patient. Arch Gen Psychiatry 22:252–261, 1970

Janowsky D, Khaled El-Yousef M, Davis J: Interpersonal maneuvers of manic patients. Am J Psychiatry 131:250–255, 1974

Kahn D: The psychotherapy of mania. Psychiatr Clin North Am 13:229–240, 1990

Kahn D: The use of psychodynamic psychotherapy in manic-depressive illness. J Am Acad Psychoanal 21:441–455, 1993

Mester R: The psychotherapy of mania. Br J Med Psychol 59:13–19, 1986

Pardoen D, Bauwens F, Tracy A, et al: Self-esteem in recovered bipolar and unipolar outpatients. Br J Psychiatry 163:755–762, 1993

Pollack LE: Content analysis of groups for inpatients with bipolar disorder. Applied Nursing Research 6:19–27, 1993

Pollack LE: How do inpatients with bipolar disorder evaluate diagnostically homogeneous groups? J Psychosoc Nurs Ment Health Serv 31:26–32, 1995a

Pollack LE: Treatment of inpatients with bipolar disorders: a role for self-management groups. J Psychosoc Nurs Ment Health Serv 33:11–16, 1995b

Post RM: Transduction of psychosocial stress into the neurobiology of recurrent affective disorder. Am J Psychiatry 149:999–1010, 1992

Post RM, Rubinow DR, Ballenger JC: Conditioning, sensitization, and kindling: implications for the course of affective illness, in Neurobiology of Mood Disorders. Edited by Post RM, Ballenger JC. Baltimore, MD, Williams & Wilkins, 1984, pp 432–466

Post RM, Rubinow DR, Ballenger JC: Conditioning and sensitization in the longitudinal course of affective illness. Br J Psychiatry 149:191–201, 1986

Shakir SA, Volkmar FR, Bacon S, et al: Group psychotherapy as an adjunct to lithium maintenance. Am J Psychiatry 136:455–456, 1979

Shaw E: Lithium noncompliance. Psychiatric Annals 10:583–587, 1986

Silverstone T, Romas-Clarkson S: Bipolar affective disorder: causes and prevention of relapse. Br J Psychiatry 154:321–335, 1989

Spencer JH, Glick ID, Haas GL, et al: A randomized clinical trial of inpatient family intervention, III: effects at 6-month and 18-month follow-ups. Am J Psychiatry 145:1115–1121, 1988

Vasile RG, Samson JA, Bemporad J, et al: A biopsychosocial approach to treating patients with affective disorders. Am J Psychiatry 144:341–344, 1987

Volkmar FR, Shakir SA, Bacon S, et al: Group therapy in the management of manic-depressive illness. Am J Psychother 35:226–234, 1981

Wehr TA, Sack DA, Rosenthal NE: Sleep reductions as a final common pathway in the genesis of mania. Am J Psychiatry 144:201–204, 1987

Wulsin L, Bachop M, Hoffman D: Group therapy in manic depressive illness. Am J Psychother 42:263–271, 1988

CHAPTER 18

SUMMARY

Alan G. Mallinger, M.D., and
Samuel Gershon, M.D.

T he diagnostic concepts with regard to affective disorders and bipolar disorder have undergone considerable evolution and development over the past 100 years.

▌ HISTORICAL PERSPECTIVE AND BACKGROUND

Before the major binational diagnostic study (Cooper et al. 1970), there was a major difference in the apparent higher diagnosis of affective disorders in the United Kingdom as compared with the United States. Many more of these cases were categorized as schizophrenia in the United States. Over the intervening years, there seems to have been a progressive shift in both countries toward assigning an affective disorder diagnosis more frequently. In the 1950s, in initial editions of the textbook *Clinical Psychiatry* by Mayer-Gross, Slater, and Roth (Mayer-Gross et al. 1969), there was a demand for a higher level of purity of diagnosis for bipolar disorder than is currently the case in DSM-III-R (American Psychiatric Association 1987) and DSM-IV (American Psychiatric Association 1994) classifications. In the *Clinical Psychiatry* textbook, there was a demand that affect- and content-congruent delusions and hallucinations be accepted only as part of a primary diagnosis of affective disorder. This matter requires serious deliberation about where the distinctions are placed and where the cutoffs in diagnostic criteria apply, significantly affecting treatment outcome and prognosis. For example, in describing the delusions that might appear in mania, Mayer-Gross et al. stated, "there is no sharp boundary between the natural conceit of the manic and grandiose ideas which may become delusional; but fixed delusions are very uncommon, and what is seen is, instead, a playful fabrication, readiness to accept any grandiose suggestion offered" (p. 213). They went on to say that manic excitement in its most severe form leads to confusion, in which the typical symptoms of mania are obscured. Consciousness, which is clear in the least severe states, becomes clouded; illusions and hallucinations may be observed; and the condition may resemble a delirium. Therefore, it is clear that, at this end of the diagnostic continuum, a strict criterion was established with regard to concomitant delusions and hallucinations in bipolar disorder.

As mentioned, the diagnostic criteria may significantly affect prognosis and treatment outcome. It is also clear that lithium, the most widely used treatment for mania, does not result in response in all cases. In fact, it is calculated that perhaps only 60% or 70% of cases may be lithium responders. To what extent is it possible to determine the prognostic features that determine such outcome? Many studies have addressed this issue. The most common significant features that affect outcome and have been reported to predict an unfavorable outcome include poor occupational status prior to the index episode, history of alcoholism, psychotic features and symptoms of depression during the index manic episode, and interepisode affective symptoms at 6-month follow-up (Tohen et al. 1990). To highlight the unfavorable outcome contributed by psychotic features, the authors stated that the "use of neuroleptic drugs was associated with poor occupational status at 48 months and poor residential status at 6 and 48 months" (p. 1110). Because the presence of psychotic features was also associated with poor outcome, this association suggests that more severely ill patients were treated with neuroleptic drugs, probably in response to more severe dysfunction in this group. Another critical feature is the stability of the clinical condition in the interepisode. The Tohen et al. study and others have suggested that those cases that can be restored to optimal interepisode status also carry the likelihood of a more favorable treatment outcome. The effect of mixed states in contributing to unfavorable outcome to lithium and other related therapies was reported in a study by Calabrese et al. (1993) and also in a report by Himmelhoch and Garfinkel (1986), who observed lithium resistance in mixed states and noted increased substance abuse and organic factors. In a study by Prien et al. (1988), only 36% of the 69 patients with mixed states were sufficiently stabilized on open treatment to be entered into a maintenance phase for follow-up. Furthermore, patients with mixed features at the index episode responded least well to acute treatment and were more likely to suffer recurrences during the maintenance phase.

Thus, diagnostic issues play an important role in the evaluation of patients and in studies of treatment response. Again, in this context, child and adolescent diagnosis of mania and affective disorders historically is an area of ongoing change and development, and the ability to make this diagnosis in this population has become an issue of serious discussion. These concerns are highlighted by the fact that in most controlled studies of depression in children and adolescents, the agents found to be effective for these conditions in adults have essentially been shown not to be effective with children and adolescents. This finding raises a series of issues that may relate to developmental neurobiology or other concerns in trying to understand the unique features in this population.

▶ DIRECTIONS FOR FUTURE RESEARCH

Implications of the Lithium Mode of Action

It has been almost four decades since the beginning of the "modern era" of lithium treatment, yet despite the widely recognized efficacy of this agent, a clear understanding of its mode of action remains elusive. Psychopharmacologists have classically focused on studies of neurotransmitter and receptor function, but it seems clear that this approach is insufficient to explain the therapeutic actions of lithium. Rather, lithium appears to exert substantial effects on second-messenger systems, which, through the process of signal transduction, link receptor activation to cellular metabolic events. For example, the inositol phospholipid second-messenger system involves the cascade of activation diagramed in Figure 18–1. As this figure illustrates, for-

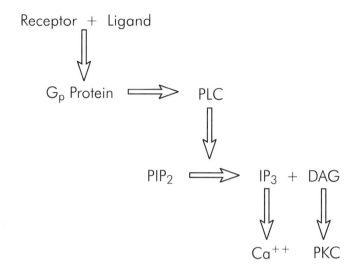

Figure 18–1.   Signal transduction cascade. PLC = phospholipase C; PIP$_2$ = phosphatidylinositol-4,5-bisphosphate; IP$_3$ = inositol-1,4,5-triphosphate; DAG = diacylglycerol; PKC = protein kinase C.

mation of a receptor-ligand complex leads to activation of G$_p$ protein, which in turn activates the enzyme phospholipase C. This enzyme then catalyzes the hydrolysis of membrane phosphatidylinositol-4,5-bisphosphate (PIP$_2$) to the second messengers inositol-1,4,5-triphosphate (IP$_3$) and diacylglycerol. IP$_3$ subsequently acts to elevate free intracellular calcium (Ca^{++}) by releasing this ion from storage sites, and diacylglycerol modulates protein kinase C activity. An analogous cascade of events links receptors (through G protein) to the enzyme adenylate cyclase, which then catalyzes formation of the second messenger cyclic adenosine monophosphate (cAMP); this then modulates the activity of protein kinase A.

Lithium affects these second-messenger systems in several important ways. For example, lithium has long been known to dampen the activity of the adenylate cyclase second-messenger system, an effect that likely is mediated through inhibition of G$_s$ proteins that ordinarily stimulate adenylate cyclase, and possibly by activation of phosphodiesterase (the enzyme that breaks down cAMP) as well. Indeed, this mechanism is widely recognized as responsible for common lithium side effects such as polyuria and hypothyroidism.

More recently, it has been recognized that lithium dampens receptor-mediated responses of the inositol phospholipid second-messenger system. The exact mechanism for this effect has yet to be elucidated. However, it is known that lithium reduces the activity of the G protein that mediates activation of phospholipase C in response to receptor occupancy (Avissar et al. 1988; Drummond 1988). Furthermore, lithium strongly inhibits the enzyme myo-inositol-1-phosphatase, and by so doing may interfere with the synthesis of PIP_2. IP_3 (produced from PIP_2 hydrolysis) is converted by sequential enzymatic removal of phosphate groups to inositol 1-phosphate and then myo-inositol. However, the enzyme that converts inositol 1-phosphate to myo-inositol (myo-inositol-1-phosphatase) is inhibited by lithium. This inhibition is specific and occurs at therapeutically appropriate drug concentrations, with a K_i of approximately 0.8 Mm (Hallcher and Sherman 1980). As a result, lithium can decrease tissue myo-inositol content and concomitantly increase the amount of inositol 1-phosphate (Sherman et al. 1981). With less myo-inositol available, the resynthesis of membrane PIP_2 could be diminished, providing less substrate for phospholipase C. In this way, cellular responses to receptor activation could potentially be attenuated (Berridge et al. 1982; Michell 1982; Sherman et al. 1981). Indeed, it has been found in experiments that lithium dampens the response to stimulation of several phosphoinositide-linked muscarinic and adrenergic receptor systems (Casebolt and Jope 1987; Kendall and Nahorski 1987; Menkes et al. 1986; Worley et al. 1988). Kofman and Belmaker (1993) suggested that myo-inositol-1-phosphatase inhibition is a key mechanism of action for lithium and that new inositol monophosphate inhibitors might be designed and synthesized as novel antimanic agents.

An examination of this area must take into account the considerable cross-talk that occurs between second-messenger systems. For example, protein kinase C produced in the inositol phospholipid cascade phosphorylates and thus deactivates G_i, a G protein that ordinarily inhibits adenylate cyclase. Therefore, protein kinase C produced by the inositol phospholipid second-messenger system can ultimately affect the adenylate cyclase second-messenger system by releasing adenylate cyclase from inhibition and increasing intracellular cAMP and subsequently protein kinase A.

The complexity of the second-messenger systems described precludes any simple extrapolation from drug action to the pathophysiology of bipolar disorder itself. Nevertheless, a number of studies have pursued aspects of second-messenger functioning in bipolar disorder, utilizing peripheral cells from untreated patients. These studies, discussed next, provide a conceptual link between the pharmacodynamics of lithium and pathological second-messenger functioning in bipolar disorder.

Evidence From Studies of Peripheral Cells in Bipolar Disorder

The abnormalities of second-messenger functioning that have been reported to occur in peripheral blood components of untreated bipolar patients include 1) hyperfunctional G proteins in white blood cells from manic or depressed patients, 2) increased PIP_2 in platelets from manic patients, and 3) increased intracellular free Ca^{++} in platelets and white blood cells from patients in both the manic and depressed phases of the disorder.

Schreiber et al. (1991) investigated binding of the nonhydrolyzable guanosine triphosphate analog Gpp(NH)p to membrane preparations from mononuclear leukocytes. In untreated manic patients, isoproterenol- and carbamylcholine-stimulated Gpp(NH)p binding was elevated as compared with healthy volunteers. Thus, G protein responses to muscarinic and β-adrenergic agonists were higher in drug-free manic patients as compared with control subjects, although lithium-treated euthymic bipolar patients showed G protein responses that were similar to those of the healthy volunteer control subjects. In a study by Young et al. (1994), G protein α subunit levels were measured in mononuclear leukocytes and was found to be higher in bipolar depressed patients than in control subjects. Unipolar patients with major depressive disorder did not differ from control subjects, however.

A preliminary study at our center (Brown et al. 1993) indicated that platelet membrane PIP_2 was significantly elevated in seven drug-free, bipolar manic patients as compared with seven healthy control subjects. Such an increase in the level of substrate for phospholipase C could ultimately contribute to an exaggerated response to receptor stimulation, such as elevated free intracellular calcium.

A series of reports by Dubovsky and associates lent support to the link between bipolar disorder and abnormal intracellular calcium. Dubovsky et al. (1989) found higher baseline intracellular calcium concentrations in blood platelets from manic patients as compared with control subjects. In addition, intracellular calcium concentration after stimulation with platelet-activating factor and thrombin was higher in manic and depressed bipolar patients than in treated euthymic bipolar patients, unipolar depressed patients, or control subjects. Subsequently, Dubovsky et al. (1991) replicated their finding for depressed bipolar patients and also reported that intracellular calcium in lymphocytes as well as platelets were higher in bipolar patients than in control subjects (Dubovsky et al. 1992). On the basis of these latter data, the investigators suggested that bipolar disorder may be associated with a generalized abnormality of the cell membrane, a G protein, or some other mechanism of intracellular calcium homeostasis.

Bowden et al. (1988) previously suggested that bipolar patients may have pathophysiological disturbances in calcium metabolism as compared with unipolar patients. These investigators subsequently reported that both the basal and the thrombin-stimulated increase of ionic intracellular calcium were higher in euthymic, lithium-treated bipolar patients as compared with healthy control subjects (Tan et al. 1990).

Implications of the Use of Calcium-Channel Blockers as Antimanic Agents

Between 20% and 40% of acutely manic patients fail to respond to lithium treatment (Chou 1991; Kramlinger and Post 1989), and the management of such cases is often a difficult clinical problem. Neuroleptics are frequently used alone or adjunctly with lithium, especially to help control hyperactivity and to provide sedation (Chou 1991), but studies indicate that these agents are less effective than lithium on the affective and ideational dimensions of mania, as compared with behavioral manifestations (Menza et al. 1988). Anticonvulsants, particularly carbamazepine and valproic acid, are widely used as second-choice treatments (Prien and Potter 1990). The data from previous double-blind, controlled studies indicate that carbamazepine is more effective than placebo, comparable in effect with lithium, and at least as effective as neuroleptics (Chou 1991). Nevertheless, clinical improvement has generally been observed in less than two-thirds of patients (Gerner and Stanton 1992; Kramlinger and Post 1989; Okuma et al. 1990; Small 1990; Small et al. 1991). Response rates for other anticonvulsant agents, such as valproic acid or benzodiazepines (e.g., clonazepam), are probably similar, although somewhat less well documented. Calcium-channel blockers such as verapamil potentially represent a class of therapeutic agents with a novel mechanism of action.

A number of controlled studies have supported the use of calcium-channel blockers in acute mania, although the number of patients studied to date is limited. Most of these investigations were performed with verapamil. In one case reported by Dubovsky et al. (1982), the patient's manic symptoms improved during verapamil administration, but subsequently returned after double-blind placebo substitution. This observation was later replicated with two additional patients (Dubovsky and Franks 1983). Giannini et al. (1984) studied 12 patients who were sequentially treated with verapamil-placebo-lithium for 30 days under double-blind conditions. Both active drugs produced significant improvement, and there was no difference between verapamil and lithium for symptom ratings measured at any point of the study. Giannini et al. (1985) subsequently compared verapamil with clonidine in 20 manic patients who were previously unresponsive to lithium, using a double-blind, crossover design. They found that verapamil was significantly more effective than clonidine. Dubovsky et al. (1986) compared verapamil with placebo in a double-blind, crossover study and reported that five of seven patients showed symptomatic improvement on verapamil but not placebo. Dose et al. (1986) compared verapamil with placebo, using a double-blind, placebo-drug-placebo design. In five of eight patients, manic symptoms improved on verapamil and worsened on placebo. Two additional patients improved on verapamil but did not relapse on placebo. Hoschl and Kozeny (1989) treated 12 manic patients with verapamil, 24 patients with neuroleptic, and 11 patients with neuroleptic plus lithium. Verapamil was comparable in efficacy to the other treatments. More recently, Garza-Trevino et al. (1992) treated 20 acutely manic patients with verapamil or lithium in a double-blind, randomized trial. Both treatment groups improved significantly, and there was no difference between treatments. A number of open studies have also supported the potential utility of calcium-channel blockers in the treatment of mania, but are not detailed here (e.g., see Barton and Gitlin 1987; Brotman et al. 1986; Brunet et al. 1990; Caillard 1985; Dubovsky et al. 1985; Patterson 1987; Slagle 1989).

New Hypothesis and Suggested Directions for Future Studies

As presented, the evidence from controlled and open studies support-ing the effectiveness of calcium-channel blockers in the treatment of acute mania is at least strongly suggestive. Furthermore, there is a compelling theoretical rationale for further study of the antimanic ac-tions of these agents. Although the exact pathophysiological mecha-nisms underlying manic episodes remain unknown, the clinical phenomenology of this disorder (e.g., racing thoughts, motor hyper-activity) is consistent with exaggerated neuronal activity. In this regard, it is noteworthy that intracellular calcium plays an important role in both the phasic and tonic release of neurotransmitters (Zucker and Lando 1986). When an action potential arrives at the presynaptic nerve terminal, calcium channels are opened, and influx of this ion leads to a rise of intracellular calcium that triggers phasic neurotransmitter release. Residual calcium also contributes to tonic release of neuro-transmitters, in which quanta of transmitters are released in the absence of action potentials.

Calcium also plays an important role in postsynaptic events. As detailed earlier, regulation of intracellular free calcium is linked to sig-nal transduction processes mediated by inositol-phospholipids. Thus, activation of α_1-adrenergic, muscarinic cholinergic, and several other types of receptors leads to production of IP_3, which in turn increases intracellular calcium ion concentrations by mobilizing calcium from intracellular stores. IP_3 can also be phosphorylated to form inositol-1,3,4,5-tetrakisphosphate (IP_4), which stimulates entry of extracellular calcium into the cell (Hill et al. 1988). The therapeutic action of lith-ium could be related to its ability to attenuate this receptor-mediated increase of intracellular calcium that arises from the inositol phospholipid signal transduction mechanism.

From this perspective, calcium-channel blockers such as verapamil are of substantial interest because of their potential to achieve a similar effect on intracellular free calcium through a separate mechanism. Indeed, as Meldolesi and Westhead (1989) noted, regarding the regulation of cellular functions in neurons, the effect of an intracellular calcium rise due to second-messenger systems is difficult to distinguish from the same effect due to activation of voltage-gated calcium channels. Thus, in the hypothetical case where lithium fails to act effectively on the inositol phospholipid signal transduction mechanism, calcium-channel blockers could nevertheless produce the desired effect on intracellular calcium because of their different cellular site of action. For this reason, agents such as verapamil constitute a particularly interesting therapeutic alternative for lithium-resistant mania.

To summarize, the treatment of acute mania remains problematic. Although lithium with or without a neuroleptic is well established as the treatment of first choice for this condition, and most clinicians now use anticonvulsants when indicated, there remains a subset of patients who either do not benefit from or cannot tolerate these therapies. For such individuals, alternative treatments are needed. Existing data from clinical investigations suggest that calcium-channel blockers such as verapamil may be effective as antimanic agents. Moreover, it could be argued that lithium, the prototypical antimanic drug, exerts its therapeutic action by attenuation of a receptor-mediated rise of intracellular calcium. Indeed, it has been reported in the literature that intraplatelet calcium is elevated in manic patients. However, the existing literature in this area is unsubstantial, especially with respect to controlled therapeutic studies. In particular, the therapeutic efficacy of calcium-channel blockers has not been subjected to definitive study with adequate numbers of subjects. This area remains vitally important for future research.

Implications of Purity of Diagnosis

It may well be that increased treatment specificity will be developed from a clearer understanding of these mechanisms of action in regard to diagnostic subtypes. For example, it has been proposed that carbamazepine is superior to lithium in rapid-cycling bipolar subjects. Also, new inositol monophosphate inhibitors may exhibit different therapeutic actions, and further work on calcium-channel blockers may further contribute to this goal.

▶ REFERENCES

American Psychiatric Association: Diagnostic and Statistical Manual of Mental Disorders, 3rd Edition, Revised. Washington, DC, American Psychiatric Association, 1987

American Psychiatric Association: Diagnostic and Statistical Manual of Mental Disorders, 4th Edition. Washington, DC, American Psychiatric Association, 1994

Avissar S, Schreiber G, Danon A, et al: Lithium inhibits adrenergic and cholinergic increases in GTP binding in rat cortex. Nature 331:440–442, 1988

Barton BM, Gitlin MJ: Verapamil in treatment-resistant mania: an open trial. J Clin Psychopharmacol 7:101–103, 1987

Berridge MJ, Downes CP, Hanley MR: Lithium amplifies agonist-dependent phosphatidyl-inositol responses in brain and salivary glands. Biochem J 206:587–595, 1982

Bowden CL, Huang LG, Javors MA, et al: Calcium function in affective disorders and healthy controls. Biol Psychiatry 23:367–376, 1988

Brotman AW, Farhadi AM, Gelenberg AJ: Verapamil treatment of acute mania. J Clin Psychiatry 47:136–138, 1986

Brown AS, Mallinger AG, Renbaum LC: Elevated platelet membrane phosphatidylinositol 4,5-bisphosphate in bipolar mania. Am J Psychiatry 150:1252–1254, 1993

Brunet G, Cerlich B, Robert P, et al: Open trial of a calcium antagonist, nimodipine, in acute mania. Clin Neuropharmacol 13:224–228, 1990

Caillard V: Treatment of mania using a calcium antagonist: preliminary trial. Neuropsychobiology 14:23–26, 1985

Calabrese JR, Woyshville MJ, Kimmel SE, et al: Mixed states and bipolar rapid cycling and their treatment with divalproex sodium. Psychiatric Annals 23:70–77, 1993

Casebolt TL, Jope RS: Chronic lithium treatment reduces norepinephrine-stimulated inositol phospholipid hydrolysis in rat cortex. Eur J Pharmacol 140:245–246, 1987

Chou JC: Recent advances in treatment of acute mania. J Clin Psychopharmacol 11:3–21, 1991

Cooper JE, Kendell RE, Gurland BJ, et al: Psychiatric Diagnosis in New York and London: A Comparative Study of Mental Health Admissions (Maudsley Monograph No 20). London, England, Oxford University Press, 1970

Dose M, Emrich HM, Cording-Tommel C, et al: Use of calcium antagonists in mania. Psychoneuroendocrinology 11:241–243, 1986

Drummond AH: Lithium affects G-protein receptor coupling. Nature 331:388, 1988

Dubovsky SL, Franks RD: Intracellular calcium ions in affective disorders: A review and an hypothesis. Biol Psychiatry 18:781–797, 1983

Dubovsky SL, Franks RD, Lifschitz M, et al: Effectiveness of verapamil in the treatment of a manic patient. Am J Psychiatry 139:502–504, 1982

Dubovsky SL, Franks RD, Schrier D: Phenelzine-induced hypomania: effect of verapamil. Biol Psychiatry 20:1009–1014, 1985

Dubovsky SL, Franks RD, Allen S, et al: Calcium antagonists in mania: a double-blind study of verapamil. Psychiatry Res 18:309–320, 1986

Dubovsky SL, Christiano J, Daniell LC, et al: Increased platelet intracellular calcium ion concentration in patients with bipolar affective disorders. Arch Gen Psychiatry 46:632–638, 1989

Dubovsky SL, Lee C, Christiano J, et al: Elevated platelet intracellular calcium concentration in bipolar depression. Biol Psychiatry 29:441–450, 1991

Dubovsky SL, Murphy J, Thomas M, et al: Abnormal intracellular calcium ion concentration in platelets and lymphocytes of bipolar patients. Am J Psychiatry 149:118–120, 1992

Garza-Trevino ES, Overall JE, Hollister LE: Verapamil versus lithium in acute mania. Am J Psychiatry 149:121–122, 1992

Gerner RH, Stanton A: Algorithm for patient management of acute manic states: lithium, valproate, or carbamazepine? J Clin Psychopharmacol 12:57s–63s, 1992

Giannini AJ, Houser WL Jr, Loiselle RH, et al: Antimanic effects of verapamil. Am J Psychiatry 141:1602–1603, 1984

Giannini AJ, Loiselle RH, Price WA, et al: Comparison of antimanic efficacy of clonidine and verapamil. J Clin Pharmacol 25:307–308, 1985

Hallcher LM, Sherman WR: The effects of lithium ion and other agents on the activity of myo-inositol-1-phosphatase from bovine brain. J Biol Chem 255:10896–10901, 1980

Hill TD, Dean NM, Boynton AL: Inositol 1,3,4,5-tetrakis-phosphate induces Ca^{2+} sequestration in rat liver cells. Science 242:1176–1178, 1988

Himmelhoch JM, Garfinkel ME: Mixed mania: diagnosis and treatment. Psychopharmacol Bull 22:613–620, 1986

Hoschl C, Kozeny J: Verapamil in affective disorders: a controlled, double-blind study. Biol Psychiatry 25:128–140, 1989

Kendall DA, Nahorski SR: Acute and chronic lithium treatments influence agonist and depolarization-stimulated inositol phospholipid hydrolysis in rat cerebral cortex. J Pharmacol Exp Ther 241:1023–1027, 1987

Kofman O, Belmaker RH: Biochemical, behavioral, and clinical studies of the role of inositol in lithium treatment and depression. Biol Psychiatry 34:839–852, 1993

Kramlinger KG, Post RM: Adding lithium carbonate to carbamazepine: antimanic efficacy in treatment-resistant mania. Acta Psychiatr Scand 79:378–385, 1989

Mayer-Gross W, Slater E, Roth M: Clinical Psychiatry, 3rd Edition. London, England, Bailliere, Tindall & Cassell, Ltd, 1969

Meldolesi J, Westhead EW: The nervous system, nerve cells and their models, in Inositol Lipids in Cell Signalling. Edited by Michell RH, Drummond AH, Downes CP. London, England, Academic Press, 1989, pp 311–335

Menkes HA, Baraban JM, Freed AN, et al: Lithium dampens neurotransmitter response in smooth muscle: relevance to action in affective illness. Proc Natl Acad Sci U S A 83:5727–5730, 1986

Menza MA, Easton J, Flaum MA, et al: Approaches to the treatment of lithium-resistant mania. Psychiatr Med 6:73–87, 1988

Michell R: A link between lithium, lipids and receptors? Trends Biochem Sci:387–388, 1982

Okuma T, Yamashita I, Takahashi R, et al: Comparison of the antimanic efficacy of carbamazepine and lithium carbonate by double-blind controlled study. Pharmacopsychiatry 23:143–150, 1990

Patterson JF: Treatment of acute mania with verapamil. J Clin Psychopharmacol 7:206–207, 1987

Prien RF, Potter WZ: NIMH workshop report on treatment of bipolar disorder. Psychopharmacol Bull 26:409–427, 1990

Prien RF, Himmelhoch JM, Kupfer DJ, et al: Treatment of mixed mania. J Affect Disord 15:9–15, 1988

Schreiber G, Avissar S, Danon A, et al: Hyperfunctional G proteins in mononuclear leukocytes of patients with mania. Biol Psychiatry 29:273–280, 1991

Sherman WR, Leavitt AL, Honchar MP, et al: Evidence that lithium alters phosphoinositide metabolism: chronic administration elevates primarily D-myo-inositol-1-phosphate in cerebral cortex of the rat. J Neurochem 36:1947–1951, 1981

Slagle DA: The acute withdrawal of diltiazem and atenolol: a possible challenge to affective stability. J Clin Psychopharmacol 9:381–382, 1989

Small JG: Anticonvulsants in affective disorders. Psychopharmacol Bull 26:25–36, 1990

Small JG, Klapper MH, Milstein V: Carbamazepine compared with lithium in the treatment of mania. Arch Gen Psychiatry 48:915–921, 1991

Tan CH, Javors MA, Seleshi E, et al: Effects of lithium on platelet ionic intracellular calcium concentration in patients with bipolar (manic-depressive) disorder and healthy controls. Life Sci 46:1175–1180, 1990

Tohen M, Waternaux CM, Tsuang MT: Outcome in mania: a 4-year prospective follow-up of 75 patients utilizing survival analysis. Arch Gen Psychiatry 47:1106–1111, 1990

Worley PF, Heller WA, Snyder SH, et al: Lithium blocks a phosphoinositide-mediated cholinergic response to hippocampal slices. Science 239: 1428–1429, 1988

Young LT, Li PP, Kamble A, et al: Mononuclear leukocyte levels of G proteins in depressed patients with bipolar disorder or major depressive disorder. Am J Psychiatry 151:594–596, 1994

Zucker RS, Lando L: Mechanism of transmitter release: voltage hypothesis and calcium hypothesis. Science 231:574–578, 1986

INDEX

Page numbers printed in **boldface** type refer to tables or figures.

Psychotherapy *(continued)*
personality and
as precipitator of illness, 365–366
real and imagined losses and, 368–369
shame and guilt and, 368
stress as precipitator of episodes and, 364–365
Pyridine-3-carboxylic acid (Lithonit), for alcoholism and bipolar disorder, 72

Rapid cycling bipolar disorder, 4, 7–8
valproate response and, 307
Recurrence, fears of, 369
Red blood cells, choline activity in, in bipolar disorder, 149–150
Relapse, following lithium discontinuation, 247
Renal function, lithium effects on, 250–251
Reserpine, depression and, 157
Restriction fragment length polymorphisms (RFLPs), 83
Risperidone, 329–331
for depression, 330–331
for mania, 329–330
Rubidium, cAMP effects of, 257–258

Salicylates, valproate interaction with, 310
Schizophrenia
acetylcholine precursor effects in, 146–147
blunted activation in, 214
mania differentiated from, 56
physostigmine effects in, 146
Secondary mania, brain regions involved in, 206–208, **207**
Sedation, valproate-induced, 311
Segregation analysis, 86–87
Self-help groups, for alcoholism and bipolar disorder, 75
Sensory event-related potentials, 178–180
Sequence-tagged sites (STS), 83
Serotonin (5-HT; 5-hydroxytryptamine), 103–113
brain stem location of, 119
buspirone-induced prolactin release and, 108
in cerebrospinal fluid, 104, **105**
cortisol response to 5-hydroxytryptophan and, 108, **109**
fenfluramine-induced changes in plasma cortisol and prolactin and, 108
plasma, 104
platelet studies of, 105–107
adenosine-phosphate-augmented 5-HT-induced platelet aggregation response, 106–107
calcium mobilization and, 107
content, 105
^{3}H-imipramine binding, 106, **107**
uptake, 106
postmortem studies of, 108, 110
treatment of bipolar disorder and, 110–113
lithium in, **112,** 112–113
tryptophan in, 110–112, **111**
urinary, 104
Shame, 368

Sibling pair analyses, 85
Simulation studies, computerized, 85
Single photon emission computed tomography (SPECT), 194, 196
in bipolar disorder at "rest," 216
following electroconvulsive therapy, 226
in unipolar depression, 208, **209**, 213
Sleep deprivation, brain changes in response to, 225–226
Sodium valproate (Depakene syrup). *See* Valproate
Spin-labeling and inversion recovery technique, 217, 220, **221–222**
Stress, precipitation of episodes by, 364–365
Strong emotions, avoidance of, 369
Structural scans. *See* Brain imaging
Substance abuse. *See also* Alcohol use and bipolar disorders
clozapine for patients with, 327–328
mania differentiated from, 57

Tardive dyskinesia, vulnerability to, 320
Temporal lobe, magnetic resonance imaging of, **200**
Teratogenicity
of carbamazepine, 282
of lithium, 242–244
of valproate, 312
Thermodynamic paradigm, open-systems, creativity and, 29–30

Thiothixene, carbamazepine interaction with, 288
Thyroid hormones, carbamazepine interactions with, 289–290
Thyrotropin-releasing hormone, carbamazepine interaction with, 289–290
Tranylcypromine, carbamazepine interaction with, 287
Tricyclic antidepressants. *See also specific drugs*
antidepressant effect of, 148
valproate interaction with, 310
Truncated episodes, 7–8
Tryptophan, for bipolar disorder, serotonin deficiency and, 110–112, **111**
Tuberoinfundibular tract, 119–120

Urine
dopamine in, **125**
lithium effects on, 127
epinephrine in, **125**
homovanillic acid in, **125**
5-hydroxyindoleacetic acid in, 104
lithium-induced polyuria and, 252–253
metanephrine in, **125**
3-methoxy-4-hydroxyphenylglycol in, 120–121, **122**
lithium effects on, 126–127
norepinephrine in, 121, **125**
lithium effects on, 127
normetanephrine in, **125**
serotonin in, 104

Valproate, 159–161, 301–313, 389
for acute depression, 304–305
for acute mania, 302, **303**, 304